# DOG BITES

# DOG BITES

## A Multidisciplinary Perspective

*Edited by Daniel S. Mills and*
*Carri Westgarth*

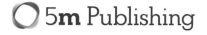

5m Publishing

First published 2017

Published by
5M Publishing Ltd,
Benchmark House,
8 Smithy Wood Drive,
Sheffield, S35 1QN, UK
Tel: +44 (0) 1234 81 81 80
www.5mpublishing.com

A Catalogue record for this book is available from the British Library

ISBN 978-1-910455-61-6

Book layout by Servis Filmsetting Ltd, Stockport, Cheshire
Printed by Replika Press Ltd, Pvt India
Photos as indicated in the text

**Warning to readers about pictures**
Due to the nature of the content some of the images and text may be distressing to some readers. Chapters containing images that the editors have identified as potentially upsetting will contain a warning at the beginning.

# CONTENTS

This book is dedicated to the many people around the world who lend their expertise and time to the efforts of dog bite prevention. We hope that this book helps you in your work.

# ACKNOWLEDGEMENTS

This book is the result of a collaborative effort. The editors wish to thank deeply all the authors for their time and expertise in writing their respective chapters. Many of these authors attended a meeting at the University of Lincoln in 2013 to discuss the topic of dog bite prevention, from which the need for such a book emerged. We thank all the attendees for their contribution and opinions. We further extend our thanks to 5M Publishing and Sarah Hulbert for believing in the value of this text to society and patiently guiding us through to publication. The editors are also extremely grateful to Barbara Burgess for her hard work and dedication in co-ordinating such a large project to completion. We could not have done it without your expert chasing of people (including ourselves!) and co-ordination. Carri Westgarth would also like to thank the UK Medical Research Council for the personal fellowship 'Understanding dog ownership and walking for better human health', which contributed to the research contained in this book and funded her academic position during the time of writing.

As researchers we extend our deepest thanks to all our research participants, for their time given towards furthering knowledge on the topic of dog bite prevention. Science cannot happen without subjects to study! We also appreciate the input of so many colleagues (too many to mention) who have given generously of their time to discuss ideas and make us the academics we are now.

Finally, thanks to our families (human and animal) for their patience and support and providing continual inspiration.

# CONTRIBUTORS

**Annamaria Passantino** obtained her DVM and PhD degrees at Messina University (Italy). From 1996 to 2001, she was appointed researcher in clinical veterinary medicine. In 2001, she became associate professor at the University of Messina. She has been co-ordinator of a university course (2008–12) and of a research doctorate on EU countries' norms concerning animal welfare and protection in the University of Messina. Currently, she is vice dean at the Department of Veterinary Sciences and president of the Animal-Welfare Body in the Messina University. Fields of interest: forensic veterinary medicine, veterinary legislation, animal protection and medical ethics. She has written or co-authored more than 250 publications.

**Barbara Schöning** is a board-certified veterinarian specialising in animal behaviour, animal welfare, and animal behaviour counselling. She completed her MSc at the University of Southampton on behavioural development of Rhodesian Ridgeback dogs and her PhD at the University of Bristol on aggressive behaviour in dogs with special emphasis on temperament testing and risk assessment. She runs a veterinary behavioural clinic in Hamburg, Germany, and works regularly as an expert in risk assessment cases in dogs, and welfare cases of dogs, horses and cats. In the last fifteen years she has assessed around 1,200 dogs, about half of them after they had bitten another dog or a human, and half because they belonged to a certain 'dangerous dog' breed listed in a German state's Dangerous Dogs Legislation (DDA) without a history of a previous biting incident.

**Carri Westgarth** is a research fellow at the University of Liverpool with a passion for understanding the relationships we have with our pets. With a background in animal behaviour and dog training, she has spent the past twelve years training and researching in veterinary epidemiology and human public health. Her research interests focus on the implications of dog ownership for human health and well-being, but also how owner management of their dogs can impact dog welfare. She recently completed a prestigious Medical Research Council-funded fellowship titled 'Understanding dog ownership and walking for better human health'. Both quantitative and qualitative research methods are used to tackle her primary research questions of how to improve population health through the promotion of dog walking, and how to prevent dog bites. She is a board member of the International Society for Anthrozoology and founder of the Merseyside Dog Safety Partnership. Her expertise on understanding and changing the behaviour of dog owners is sought by many organisations wishing to prevent dog bites and promote 'responsible' dog owner behaviour. She is also a full member of the Association of Pet Behaviour Counsellors, teaches dog training classes, and was previously a professional assistance dog instructor. Her practical experience in many areas relating to dogs, combined with a multi-disciplinary perspective, gives unique strength and relevance to her academic outputs.

**Christopher Mannion** qualified in dentistry from the University of Birmingham in 1995 and then in medicine from Guy's, King's and St Thomas' Medical school in 2001, and undertook his junior surgical training in London in a wide variety of surgical disciplines. His maxillofacial training, which he completed in 2011, was in the Yorkshire region. He received a European scholarship and spent a period of time in Madrid, Spain, where he worked with European facial surgeons, gaining experience.

Christopher works at Leeds Teaching Hospitals NHS Trust and has a varied practice. He has subspecialty interests in trauma and facial reconstruction, and is a qualified instructor in Advanced Trauma Life Support. He is a fellow of the Royal College of Surgeons of England. He is actively involved in the teaching and training of both undergraduate and postgraduate doctors and dentists. He is a senior lecturer at the University of Leeds Medical School, and is the training programme director in Oral and Maxillofacial Surgery for Yorkshire and Humber Deanery. He has authored more than twenty-five scientific publications.

**Daniel Mills** is an RCVS-, European- and ASAB-recognised specialist in clinical animal behaviour, who has been developing and exploring new interventions for behaviour problems at the University of Lincoln, where he is professor of veterinary behavioural medicine, for more than twenty years. He was recently awarded his Fellowship of Veterinarian Surgeons from the Royal College of Veterinary Surgeons in recognition of his contributions to veterinary behavioural medicine. He is the author of more than 100 full scientific papers and forty books and chapters. He has a strong research interest in the comparative psychology underpinning behaviour and behavioural interventions, with a particular interest in what makes an individual different and how this arises from his or her interaction with the environment. This links both his applied and fundamental research, for example by examining how we and non-human animals recognise and respond to the emotional state of another.

More recently, he has had opportunities to scientifically explore his interests in the potential value of our relationships with animals. His research in this area focuses on the benefits from pet keeping using a multidisciplinary approach, for example through collaborations with biologists, health care professionals, psychologists, lawyers and economists.

**Dingeman Rijken** is a forensic physician based at the Department of Forensic Medicine at the University Hospitals of Leuven and the Public Health Service of Amsterdam. He received his medical doctorate from the University of Utrecht and was senior house officer at Brighton and Sussex University Hospitals. He has previously worked in Africa with local governments, the Red Cross and UN.

**Esther Schalke** is a doctor in veterinary medicine who graduated from the University of Hanover, Germany, in 1996. She got her PhD in 2000, is a board-certified specialist in animal behaviour and a diplomate of the ECVBM-CA. She worked as a post-doctoral research fellow at the Institute of Animal Welfare and Behaviour, University of Veterinary Medicine, Hanover, from 1997 to 2012. Her research subject was aggressive behaviour in dogs and learning behaviour. In 2009 she founded the Lupologic GmbH: Centre of Applied Ethology and Veterinary Behaviour Medicine. She has published numerous publications about aggressive behaviour in dogs.

**Fernanda Fadel** was awarded a degree in biological sciences from the Universidade Federal do Paraná in Brazil, and then completed an MSc in evolution, ecology and systematics at Ludwig-Maximilians-Universität in Germany. She is currently carrying out her PhD studies at the University of Lincoln, UK, exploring the genetics of impulsivity and aggression in dogs through genome-wide association studies.

**Fiona Cooke** has a PhD in the implementation and enforcement of animal welfare and protection law in local government. She is a professional animal behaviourist specialising in dog and cat behaviour, and a qualified assistance dog trainer. Fiona lectures in law, advises various charities on animal law matters, and contributes to a number of initiatives in the field of animal welfare law.

**Francine Watkins** is a senior lecturer in public health at the University of Liverpool based in the Department of Public Health and Policy. She has more than fifteen years' experience teaching qualitative methods to public health postgraduate students. Her PhD was an ethnographic study of rural communities exploring the health implications of stigma and social exclusion. Her research interests are in qualitative research exploring access to health services by different groups and the use of health intelligence by public health stakeholders. More recently she has been exploring dog aggression towards humans in order to develop strategies for dog bite prevention.

**Graham Turton** has worked hands-on in the animal care sector for more than eighteen years, sixteen of which in kennels. He was kennel supervisor for ten years in one of the UK's busiest stray kennels, dealing with thousands of dogs every year, from the very friendly to the outright aggressive, and including classed 'dangerous dog' types. He currently cares for abused and case animals for one of the biggest UK animal charities.

**Heath Keogh** joined the Metropolitan Police Service in 2003 and is a Met-trained dog legislation officer. He gives presentations on the LEAD Initiative to local authorities and other police forces, and attends round table discussions with partner agencies, national dog organisations and government departments with regards to 'dangerous dogs'. He also owns and has shown Staffordshire Bull Terriers at international level, and is a qualified judge for the UK Kennel Club. Heath has appeared on national TV with Battersea Dogs Home promoting the rehoming of rescue dogs and Staffordshire Bull Terriers.

**Helen Zulch** is a veterinarian and European specialist in veterinary behavioural medicine. She is a senior lecturer in clinical animal behaviour in the School of Life Sciences, University of Lincoln and an honorary assistant professor at the University of Nottingham School of Veterinary Medicine and Science. Helen has worked in companion animal behaviour for many years and currently lectures on undergraduate and postgraduate programmes at the University of Lincoln. She consults in the University of Lincoln's Animal Behaviour Referral Clinic. Her research interests include problem prevention in pets, olfaction in dogs and the sciences explaining learning, including their practical application.

Retired Lieutenant (Inspector) **James W. Crosby** BS, CBCC-KA (Jacksonville Sheriff's Office, Jacksonville, Florida, USA) has extensive canine behavioural training and expertise and is an internationally recognised authority and court-accepted expert on canine attacks and aggression. James's specialty is investigating dog bite-related fatalities, especially evidentiary and behavioural factors involved in these deaths. His investigation of more than twenty fatalities and post-attack evaluation of more than forty subject dogs has been essential in numerous successful prosecutions. Holding a BS with concentration in psychology, James is completing his master's degree in veterinary forensics at the Veterinary College at the University of Florida.

**James Oxley** currently carries out independent research investigating human–animal interactions and animal welfare mainly focusing on perceptions and knowledge of dangerous dogs, dog bites and rabbit owner management practices. In March 2011, James acquired a masters by research in applied biology at Writtle College, the University of Essex, in the UK. This research looked not only into dog owners' perceptions of three dog-related laws in the UK, but also looked into the occurrence and types of dog identification, dog walking and public knowledge of parasitic transmission.

**Jenny Newman** began her career in human medicine, graduating from Liverpool University in 2002. In 2008 she rejoined the university, changing her focus to veterinary epidemiology, and in 2012 she completed an MPhil exploring the evidence for risk factors for dog aggression. Jenny's primary interests are now at the intersection of veterinary epidemiology and informatics, developing and utilising classifiers of free text in veterinary clinical records in order to facilitate novel approaches to surveillance via routinely recorded narrative information.

**Katharina Woytalewicz** is a board-certified veterinarian and worked for twenty-three years as a veterinarian for the Hamburg Society for the Prevention of Cruelty to Animals (Hamburger Tierschutzverein e.V.), before she became general welfare manager of the society's animal shelter in 2008. Her range of duties includes all necessary measures to ensure the well-being of the animals in the shelter.

**Kendal Shepherd** qualified from Bristol University in 1978. With extensive experience in small animal practice, she was the first veterinary surgeon to be accredited by ASAB as a certificated clinical animal behaviourist in 2005. She is currently heavily involved in the behavioural assessment of dogs for the courts under both sections 1 and 3 of the Dangerous Dogs Act 1991. Her present particular interests are: promoting the need for vet/medic co-operation in thorough and expert investigation of all dog bite incidents, including fatalities, to inform prevention; the routine education of children regarding dog bite prevention; and the encouragement of all veterinary surgeons and nurses to routinely safeguard the behaviour of their patients in all cases that they treat.

**Kenton Morgan** is an innovator. The first Professor of Epidemiology appointed to a UK Veterinary School, he experienced dog aggression aged ten, at a sprint, on a village milk round. At seventeen he learnt to drive on regardless of the sudden appearance of car-chasing farm dogs. His first dog bite was as a veterinary student in Cambridge in 1973. He has a passionate interest in the application of epidemiological design and analysis to solve real world problems and in training and promoting young veterinary researchers. His research portfolio includes terrestrial and aquatic animal diseases, human joint replacement, tooth decay and gun crime.

**Kerstin Meints** is a professor in developmental psychology at the University of Lincoln. She completed her PhD at Hamburg University. She then worked in experimental psychology, University of Oxford, and is member of Wolfson College, Oxford. Professor Meints is the director of the well-established Lincoln Infant and Child Development Lab. Alongside research on children's development of language, categorisation and trust, she focuses on comparative and applied research in human–animal interaction, especially dog bite prevention and assessing interventions. She carried out the first assessment of the dog bite prevention programme 'Blue Dog'.

**Kevin McPeake** qualified as a veterinary surgeon from the University of Glasgow University in 2005 and completed a postgraduate diploma in companion animal behaviour counselling from the University of Southampton in 2011. Kevin has worked both in first opinion small animal practice and has run his own behaviour referral practice. Kevin joined the Animal Behaviour Clinic team at the University of Lincoln in 2014 to research a prospective new canine anti-anxiety medication, and also regularly sees canine and feline behaviour referrals at the clinic. Kevin has been a committee member of the British Veterinary Behaviour Association since 2012.

**Lorraine McElhinney** graduated with a BSc (Hons) in microbiology from Leeds University in 1991. She then completed an MSc in animal parasitology at the University of North Wales, Bangor and a PhD in molecular virology at the University of Manchester. In April 1996, she joined the Rabies Team at VLA Weybridge as a post-doctoral researcher. She is currently the deputy of the UK, OIE and WHO reference laboratory for rabies, at APHA Weybridge (formerly VLA). She leads research and surveillance projects in emerging and zoonotic viruses (particularly lyssaviruses and hantaviruses). She lectures in rabies at Liverpool and Manchester Universities.

**Lorna Lancaster** has been working in the field of microbiology and biochemistry for fifteen years. Starting at the University of York, UK, Lorna studied mechanisms used by bacteria to eliminate competition in its surrounding environment. This work was continued at the Universitaet Witten/Herdecke, Germany researching the activity of toxins and antibiotics on bacterial cellular function. Lorna was then involved in the development of vaccines to prevent healthcare associated infections at the National Institute of Biological Standards and Control. At the University of Lincoln, UK, Lorna is currently researching the competition of bacteria within biofilms, focusing on healthcare-associated infections.

**Lynn Hewison** MSc is the behaviour clinic technician at the referral only Animal Behaviour Clinic within the School of Life Sciences at the University of Lincoln, UK. Prior to this, she completed her MSc in clinical animal behaviour, with her thesis focusing on whether a test for impulsivity could be developed for use within rescue centres. She has a strong interest in clinical animal behaviour in both research and its application, especially in the area of welfare assessment and development of treatment plans.

**Malgorzata Pilot** is a senior lecturer in the School of Life Sciences, University of Lincoln, UK. She specialises in mammalian evolutionary genetics, with a particular focus on wild and domestic canids. In her recent research projects, she has investigated the evolutionary history of grey wolves based on genome-wide data.

**Marcello Ruta** is senior lecturer at the University of Lincoln's School of Life Sciences. He received his PhD from University of London's Birkbeck College (Biology Department) and the London Natural History Museum (Palaeontology Department). He conducted research at University College London (Department of Biology), University of Chicago (Department of Organismal Biology and Anatomy), the Field Museum of Natural History in Chicago (Geology Department), and University of Bristol (School of Earth Sciences). His interests include the origin and diversification of major groups (especially limbed vertebrates), patterns and processes from the fossil record, and tempo and mode of macroevolutionary changes.

**Matt Burgess** is a medical physician and an officer in the United States Navy. He is currently a diagnostic radiology resident at Naval Medical Center San Diego in San Diego, California. Dr Burgess graduated from the University of South Florida College of Medicine in Tampa, Florida, and completed a paediatric internship at Naval Medical Center Portsmouth in Portsmouth, Virginia. He subsequently served three years as a flight surgeon with the United States Marine Corps in Iwakuni, Japan. He has served in places such as Okinawa, Guam, Thailand, Singapore, and Australia. He lives with his wife, Kathryn, and three children, Everett, Brody, and Emily, in San Diego.

**Maya Braem Dubé** is a behaviour veterinarian based in Switzerland. After finishing her veterinary studies at the University of Berne, her veterinary doctoral dissertation focused on evaluating aggression in dogs. After specialising in veterinary behaviour medicine in Switzerland, continued to work and study with Prof Daniel Mills at the University of Lincoln (UK). Since her return to Switzerland, she has been seeing behaviour cases at her own practice and at the veterinary hospital in Zürich. In 2012 she joined the animal welfare group at the University of Berne. Her research focuses on animal personality and its links to communication and behaviour problems.

**Melissa Starling** is an Australian post-doctoral fellow working in the field of animal welfare and behaviour. She completed a bachelor of science at the Australian National University. Her honours project was on brood parasitism in the Pallid cuckoo. She spent approximately four years in the workforce as an environmental consultant building skills in animal identification, habitat assessment, and survey techniques, and then embarked upon her PhD on cognitive bias as a measure of welfare and personality in the domestic dog at the University of Sydney in 2010. Her current research interests are the human–animal bond, cognitive bias, and applied animal science.

**Mie Kikuchi** is a behaviourist and a dog trainer who works with veterinary practices and is a lecturer of companion animal behaviour at the University of Hokkaido, Japan. She has also been a journalist for Japanese media specialising in dogs and cats. She graduated from the University of Southampton with an MSc degree in companion animal behaviour counselling in 2004, and is currently studying cultural differences of public perception of human-directed aggressive behaviour in dogs for a PhD at the University of Lincoln. She has particular interest in cultural attitudes towards companion animals.

**Paul McGreevy** is a veterinarian and ethologist. He is a professor of Animal Behaviour and Animal Welfare Science at the University of Sydney's Faculty of Veterinary Science. The author of more than 180 peer-reviewed articles and six books, Paul has received numerous Australian and international awards for his research and teaching innovations. He has trained dogs for agility trials, film and television.

**Rachel Orritt** is a PhD candidate and teaching assistant at the University of Lincoln, where she is developing an evidence base for the assessment of human-directed aggressive behaviour in dogs. Rachel graduated from the University of Bristol, where she studied preclinical veterinary science and animal behaviour and welfare. Since then, she has investigated laying hen welfare while working as a research assistant at the Norwegian School of Veterinary Sciences in Oslo, and has also spent some time as a rehoming co-ordinator for the RSPCA. Rachel is also interested in public attitudes towards dogs and the political discourse on 'dangerous dogs'.

**Robert Christley** graduated as a veterinary surgeon from the University of Sydney (Australia) in 1991. Following periods in private and university veterinary practice he undertook a PhD in epidemiology in 1996–99. He has worked at the University of Liverpool since 2002. His work focuses on the epidemiology of a wide range of animal health-related issues and includes both research and teaching. He has conducted many studies of dog ownership and management, and of dog aggression. He has published more than 100 peer-reviewed scientific papers.

**Samantha Penrice** is an evolutionary paleozoologist with a BSc (Hons) in Zoology, an MSc in marine and fisheries science from the University of Aberdeen, and has lectured at Myerscough College. Samantha is currently completing her PhD at the University of Lincoln exploring the evolutionary history of stereospondyls, a large group of fossil amphibians alive from the late Carboniferous to the early Cretaceous. This research involves testing evolutionary models, and the analysis of shape and function. Samantha applies geometric morphometrics alongside quantitative palaeontology methods to solve questions on macroevolution and functional morphology.

**Simon Harding** is a senior lecturer in criminology at Middlesex University and a graduate of Edinburgh; South Bank; London; Bedfordshire; and Middlesex Universities. He previously worked as a Home Office regional crime advisor and director of community safety at Lambeth council. His four-year study into why young men use bull breed dogs to gain status was published in 2012 by the Policy Press as *Unleashed: The Phenomenon of Status Dogs and Weapon Dogs* and republished in 2014, leading to numerous media appearances both nationally and internationally. His latest book, *Street Casino: Survival in Violent Street Gangs*, was published in 2014.

**Susanne David** is a trained animal keeper (chamber of commerce, Hamburg, Germany) and a certified dog trainer (chamber of commerce, Potsdam, Germany), working for twenty years for the Hamburg Society for the Prevention of Cruelty to Animals (Hamburger Tierschutzverein e.V.). Based at the society's animal shelter, she is the head of the dog training sector and is responsible for the development and supervision of training programmes for dogs with behaviour problems.

**Tina Wagon** is the owner of Wheldon Law, a long-established firm of criminal defence solicitors that specialise in dog law cases. Tina has defended hundreds of dog law cases and has been involved in a number of high profile cases, including the landmark case of Sandhu in 2012. Her comprehensive knowledge of dog law and procedure, combined with her desire to achieve the best possible outcome for her clients, has helped to make Wheldon Law become one of the largest and best-known firms dealing with this area of law.

**Todd Hogue** is a professor in forensic psychology and a registered forensic and clinical psychologist with more than twenty-five years' experience working in prison and secure healthcare settings, mainly developing assessment and treatment services for those at high risk of future offending. In his current academic role, his research interests focus mainly on predicting future risk-related behaviour and developing systems to guide professionals in making risk decision-making. He is now applying these forensic psychology methods to developing an evidence-based system to assess and manage human-directed aggression in dogs.

**Tracey Clarke** was awarded a BSc (Hons) sociology, MSc psychology, and PhD life sciences. She has worked as a qualified social worker (CQSW) with children and families in deprived areas of Manchester and London for the last thirty years and currently working as an expert witness in child care cases. Tracey has always maintained a strong interest in the issue of discrimination, the welfare of domestic dogs and our relationship with them – the focus of her PhD research. In exploring this she was uniquely placed – drawing on both her professional and academic experience. She has three rescue Dachshunds.

**Wim Van de Voorde** is a forensic pathologist based at the University of Leuven, where he is professor and head of Forensic Biomedical Sciences and Head of the Department of Forensic Medicine at the University Hospitals Leuven. He is also president of the Belgium Royal Society of Forensic Medicine. In addition to having published widely in the area, he is co-editor of the text *Multidisciplinary Forensics: Legal and Scientific Aspects*, and published a key review on the forensic approach to fatal dog attacks.

# INTRODUCTION

*Carri Westgarth and Daniel Mills*

The subject of dog bites is an emotive one that can cloud the judgements of even those who are normally very rational. It is also an issue that impacts on many academic disciplines: it is a biological and psychological phenomenon; an informational quality issue; it has cultural connotations; legal implications; and is clearly a public health issue and matter of public interest in the media. Accordingly, it seems everyone has an opinion as to what the problem is (the dog, the owner or wider societal values) and how it needs to be fixed, such as some sort of legislative change or educational initiative. Despite much anecdote and enthusiasm, there has been little communication and debate between the different disciplines and groups that are affected by the issue, until now.

Here we present the first comprehensive resource outlining these issues from a wide range of perspectives. These are framed from the view of experts across a number of different disciplines relating to dog bites, and include a review of the evidential knowledge base and gold standard practical advice. Each author presents his or her own view, based on personal knowledge, experience and beliefs, as to the immediate urgent issues and current guidance relating to dog bites from within his or her own discipline. As editors we have tried to allow authors to keep to their own writing style, which varies due to their discipline. However, we have also tried to ensure that the text remains accessible to non-specialists and the wider public keen to make themselves better informed. Some readers will be discovering the topic of dog bites for the first time, perhaps as a result of an incident. This text should guide them through the complexity of the issues, and the need to avoid simple generalisations or the sometimes poorly grounded but impassioned opinions of advocates of one persuasion or another. We hope that you find it useful in this regard.

Due to the multidisciplinary nature of the topic, and newly emerging knowledge contained within, you should not be surprised to find that highly regarded experts may hold differing views on the problem, or even starkly contradict each other at times. There are still many matters of debate and we may accept different starting points for the conclusions we reach. It is only by informing ourselves of this that we can hope to reconcile these differences or agree to disagree until we have better evidence available. Please do not let this cloud your judgement and conclude that it is all simply a matter of opinion, as there are also many common perspectives that strengthen our position for moving forward. One thing is clear; we actually know very little about how to prevent dog bites effectively, although we know a bit about some of the measures that do not work. This book was borne out of a desire for better understanding of this most important of topics and is a starting point not only for future development and research but also current best practice.

**Section 1** therefore lays a foundation for what follows by considering some fundamental principles that should shape the way we think about the issues involved. In order to understand dog bites we need to be clear about what we know about the issue and how we know it. This might seem obvious, but when trying to understand the quality of our knowledge there is a big difference between personal opinions and beliefs (no matter how strongly held) and empirical information. As highlighted in this section, being clear on these matters is a major challenge to the study of dog bites. In order to study something, we need to be able to define it consistently, but in Chapter 1, Daniel Mills highlights the lack of consensus when we refer to aggressive behaviour and even bites in dogs. Perhaps if we can build a more consistent framework as suggested in this chapter, we will make better progress. In Chapter 2, Helen Zulch highlights how little we know about the meaning of signals produced by dogs and how much is based on opinion. The point is well made that if we can become more consistent in separating our descriptions of behaviour from our interpretations of it, then communications between those studying aggressive signals will be improved and we will recognise more clearly those areas where academic discussion and development should flourish in pursuit of knowledge. In Chapter 3, Kenton Morgan and colleagues present a refreshing and incisive view of the use and abuse of statistics in relation to dog bites. This is not about hard numbers or difficult statistical concepts, but rather it is about understanding uncertainty. It is essential to understand these principles if we are not to be taken in by those who may knowingly or unknowingly misrepresent dog bite statistics and the associated risks. Finally, in Chapter 4, Francine Watkins and Carri Westgarth highlight the value of learning from a public health theoretical perspective when considering the issue of dog bites. Public health is well-versed in dealing with the impact on human health of the complex interactions that exist between people and both their physical and social environments, and so provides an excellent framework for integrating all the information related to understanding why dogs bite. The chapters in this section not only highlight how complex the issue of dog bites is and how little we know, but also, and most importantly, provide a framework for making progress so we do not repeat the errors of the past.

**Section 2** of the text builds on the previous section by considering different aspects of our perceptions of dogs that bite. In Chapter 5, Mie Kikuchi and James Oxley introduce the topic of media representation of dog aggression. They present their findings about the inconsistency and unreliability of media reporting surrounding dog bite incidents. It is thus important that action and policy is not based solely on this biased media representation. In Chapter 6, Simon Harding uses humanities and social science methods to delve deeper into the societal perspectives surrounding the use of dogs for 'status'. He describes how he feels that some individuals of certain dog breeds, notably bull breeds, can be owned primarily for reasons of status and commodity, and linked with protection and aggression in gang-land culture. There is no doubt that these breeds are owned in high numbers in certain geographical locations and depicted to be aggressive in cultural media (as discussed further in Chapters 5 and 7). However, whether only these large, strong-looking dogs reflect the status and power of an owner requires deeper investigation. It could be argued that perhaps all types and breeds of dogs reflect the status of the owner in some way, for example the bejewelled 'handbag dogs' of the young model are as much a sign of status as the protection dog of the aggressive adolescent. Much more research is required into why people choose to own different breeds of dogs, and the impacts of these choices on the communities that they live in. In Chapter 7, Tracey Clarke explores specifically the issues of breed representation of aggressiveness and how this has been shaped by the popular media. She explains how the portrayal of the personality and behaviour of certain breeds is not always backed by clear evidence, and so comes to the conclusion that there are several reasons why breed-specific legislation should be repealed. Overall, this second section of the book illustrates that the societal perspectives surrounding risk of dog bites are based largely on cultural misperceptions and media perpetuation of these. It is a challenge to modify these views but it is a necessity if dog bite prevention initiatives are to be more evidence-based.

In **Section 3**, we consider the issue of dog bites and risk. As highlighted in the previous sections, the risk of a dog bite is commonly misunderstood or misrepresented. This includes both the absolute risk as well as the associated risk factors. In this section the issue of risk is considered from the perspective of a range of academic disciplines. In Chapter 8 Malgorzata Pilot and Fernanda Fadel consider the genetics of aggressive behaviour especially as it relates to dogs, but with a knowledge of what we can learn from the wider biological literature. A major theme identified throughout the text is the need for robust and biologically grounded definitions of aggression. To do this we need to appreciate the complexity of aggressive behaviour and understand the underlying mechanistic processes that regulate the likelihood of its expression, rather than consider it a simple entity that has simple genetic correlates. They conclude that there is still much to be done with the phenotyping (describing the key attributes) of aggressive behaviour. This point is developed further in the next chapter by Maya Braem Dubé, who examines the breadth of tests used to assess aggressive behaviour in dogs. The complexity of the task means that simple tests are often unreliable when examined in more detail. However, perhaps just as worrying is that for many forms of assessment we have no idea at all as to the predictive value of these tests. This is true even for tests that are used within the legal system to determine the fate of a dog, before or after any aggressive incident.

The identification of simple associations between a variable (risk factor) and the outcome of a dog bite is commonplace, but in Chapter 10 Rob Christley and colleagues illustrate both the danger and fallacy of this practice. Drawing on the most comprehensive review of the risk factors for human-directed aggressive behaviour in dogs, undertaken by co-author Jenny Newman, they show how weak the evidence is for many apparent associations. For even those associations where there is reasonable evidence, the causal nature of the relationship is unclear, and the reader would do well to refer back to Chapter 4 when considering this matter. Fatal attacks are rare but grab the headlines frequently because of their impact.

Again there is a danger of simplistic assumptions being made about these cases, such as fatal attacks being the inevitable extreme form of response from dogs with a tendency to bite. In Chapter 11, Wim Van der Voorde and Dingeman Rijken review dog bite–related fatalities in the scientific literature and highlight the error of this assumption, as well as how little we really know about these cases. These dogs are, understandably, often killed, but, perhaps less understandably, this often happens before an assessment is made of the dog to see what we can learn from the case. They emphasise the importance of a proper forensic investigation of the crime scene, so that no evidence is discarded, for example by destroying the dog or failing to examine it properly. This is a theme we return to in Section 4. Finally, Samantha Penrice and Marcello Ruta provide new data in Chapter 12 on how we might assess risk from a more detailed biomechanical consideration of jaw structure. It is often assumed that bite force is the primary risk factor to be considered in this regard, but this is shown to be a gross simplification, with different jaws equipped to deliver different types of bite and so posing different risks according to the circumstance.

In conclusion, this third section highlights the value of multi-disciplinary research into the risk of dog bites and the need to not make oversimplistic conclusions if we are genuinely interested in trying to manage the risk of dog bites effectively.

In **Section 4**, we move on to the investigative and legal issues surrounding dog bites. In the absence of clear guidelines in these areas, world-leading experts in their fields present best practice standards, sometimes for the first time. To introduce this subject, Fiona Cooke, in Chapter 13, guides us through the myriad of dog-related legislation in a range of countries and the key principles in which they connect and differ. She concludes that there is clearly no gold standard simple legislative mechanism in use, and a new trend towards repealing breed-specific legislation for being deemed ineffective.

When a dog bite incident occurs, a thorough investigation will provide evidence not only for any legal repercussions, but also to help society to understand why these occur in the first place. The quality of this investigation is varied, if it occurs at all. In Chapter 14, James Crosby presents a gold standard approach for investigating dog bite incidents and managing the scene for the purpose of gathering evidence. He points out clearly that when a bite occurs it is not a 'done deal' and the dog is in fact a crucial part of the evidence. This is further emphasised by Anna Maria Passantino in Chapter 15, who focuses on the specific forensic procedures used for investigating dog bites and suspects, in order to establish who has inflicted the bite. In Chapter 16, James Crosby takes a deeper look at the unique and identifying anatomy of dog bite wounds. This information can be critical to the rapid exclusion of the supposed perpetrator of a bite, who may not even be a dog, and it is for this reason that we include the chapter in this section. However, this information is also an essential primer for understanding some of the health- and medical-related issues that are discussed in the next section (Section 5). Continuing with the legal theme of this section, UK dog law expert, Tina Wagon, provides in Chapter 17 guidance on choosing a dog bite expert for the courts. Although the chapter is focused on the demands and needs of the UK legal system, the key messages are transferable to other countries. The best practice protocol for assessing 'dangerous dogs' for the courts is then presented in Chapter 18 by leading UK expert witness, Kendal Shepherd. She highlights the importance of a thorough behavioural examination if we are to understand why the bite may have occurred, and thus the risk of recurrence. This offers a humane and compassionate approach to risk reduction that considers the needs of both owners and victims in a mature way.

In **Section 5**, we consider the wider human health impact of dog bites. While many bites may be relatively innocuous, it is important to differentiate these from those requiring greater medical attention. In the first chapter of this section, Matt Burgess, in Chapter 19, provides an essential overview of first line assessment necessary for dog bite cases and the medical priorities for anyone encountering the victim of a bite. This theme is developed further in the subsequent chapters of this section. In Chapter 20, Lorna Lancaster reviews the infectious risks from dog bites and the microbiology of these injuries. Different bacteria may be associated with different types of wound, and while some of the infectious agents may come from the dog, others may come from the resident human flora. As in both the preceding and subsequent chapter, the importance of cleaning the wound effectively early on is emphasised. The routine use of antibiotics at a time of rising concern over the development of resistance is unwise, although there are special groups that fall outside this generalisation.

Only once the issues of potential infection have been addressed can surgical intervention be considered and in Chapter 21 Chris Mannion emphasises the importance of evaluating carefully both the patient and the wound to maximise the benefit of any surgical intervention. This is something that his data illustrates is routinely not done very well, and this chapter is a timely reminder of best practice. Reconstructive surgery is not just cosmetic, but it may play an important role in the mental rehabilitation of the patient. The special case of the risk of rabies is considered in Chapter 22 by Lorraine McElhinney. Rabies is a disease that strikes fear into many bitten by a dog where the disease is endemic. This is a global disease problem, but one which, she argues, need not cause high mortality in humans if the right measures are put in place by government for the management of dogs and bite victims. Indeed, if we understood dog bites as well as we understood rabies, then clearly the risks to society would be greatly reduced. Finally, Carri Westgarth and Francine Watkins highlight a much overlooked health consequence of dog bites; its psychological impact. Drawing on new data, they show how great this can be even for minor incidents. At the severe end of the scale is the potential for further complications such as post-traumatic stress disorder. Like all the authors in this section, they argue strongly for a much more joined up process to the management of victims, in order to minimise the risks involved.

In **Section 6** we consider issues relating to the handling of potentially aggressive dogs. Many professionals are handling such dogs on a daily basis; not only is this a risk to the person, but also it impacts on the welfare of the dog. In Chapter 24, Kevin McPeake guides us expertly through protocols for situations where we need to handle an aggressive dog, for example in the veterinary clinic, outlining physical and chemical restraint methods. With an emphasis on using the minimum restraint needed, he highlights the importance of avoiding the risk of making matters worse, increasing the risk of either the probability or severity of a bite in either the short or longer term. To this end, early chemical restraint should be considered. Strong physical handling and punishment are not recommended.

Many dog owners will also encounter a situation where their own dog becomes aggressive and a bite risk. In Chapter 25, Esther Schalke provides thoughtful counselling advice directed towards owners of dogs that have bitten as to the available options and short-term management. Her empathetic but realistic approach allows the stressful impact of owning an aggressive dog to be recognised and useful practical solutions employed. This chapter will be a useful first-line resource to manage the situation before specific professional behavioural help can be received. Knowledge of how to prevent and manage aggressive behaviour is useful to the pet owner and also to those working in shelters. In Chapter 26, Lynn Hewison and Graham Turton provide expert 'first aid' practical guidance as to the types of approaches that can be taken in order to prevent overtly aggressive behaviour, retrain a dog that is starting to show signs of an overt physical threat, and handle aggressive behaviour by dogs in everyday situations in the home or in kennels. Useful tips are also given as to what to do in the event of a dog fight. Again the central theme is to avoid confrontation where possible and show or teach the dog that alternative behaviour is preferable.

In summary, this sixth section contains many practical resources that should be of use to anyone owning or working with dogs, who wish to be informed of current thinking and best practice behind how to both prevent aggressive behaviour from developing, or how to minimise the risk to both human and animals when it is already present.

In **Section 7**, the two chapters provide practical examples of how we can reduce the risk of dog bites. Although we must acknowledge the many gaps in our scientific understanding of this issue, that does not mean we can, or should, do nothing to reduce the risks associated with dogs. Dog ownership, like many other pastimes, carries with it an inevitable element of risk. We must make best use of the available information and combine this with best professional practice to manage the problem effectively as far as is reasonably practical. This does not mean we eliminate risk, rather we wish to minimise the risk to a socially and societally acceptable level. In the first of these chapters, Barbara Schöning shows how the careful evaluation of dogs, combined with high standards of professional practice, can produce meaningful assessment with good prognostic value in real-life situations. While it is important to have a degree of standardisation, this is neither a simple nor prescriptive process. Each test, like each dog, is individual, and procedures need to be adapted to the circumstances according to the goal. This theme is very much repeated in the next chapter by Katharina Woytalewicz and Susanne David, who work in the rehabilitation of dogs that have bitten. In their chapter they draw on their experience to show how a solid understanding of scientific principles can be used to behaviourally rehabilitate many of these cases so they pose no greater risk than any other dog. With three case studies they illustrate the practical application of the principles and process they outline in the first half of their chapter. The effective application of science allows this process to be done in a compassionate, humane and reasonable way, which respects the needs of all involved. Clearly, as our knowledge and understanding of dog bites grow, so will the ability to more efficiently manage the risk associated with cases brought to our attention.

**Section 8**, is the final section and fittingly draws on what we know to critically appraise the wider options for dog bite prevention, in particular educational programmes regarding teaching signs that a dog is unhappy and may bite. In contrast, earlier chapters focused on prevention have considered the topic primarily in terms of an immediate practical perspective. In Chapter 29, Melissa Starling and Paul McGreevy provide a deep critique of the current dog bite prevention programmes and approaches. They find that, although such educational initiatives are designed with great intentions, evaluation of the effectiveness of such programmes is rare. They suggest there needs to be greater recognition that resources may also need to be directed into dog-related legislation and the supply of pet dogs that have a low inclination to bite. Nonetheless, it is well-established that there is no group more vulnerable to dog bites and in need of effective prevention than children. In Chapter 30, Kerstin Meints describes the Blue Dog bite prevention programme for children and shows how evaluations of this intervention, alongside her other research, has contributed to knowledge about how children's developmental psychology underpins why they are frequently bitten and so often on the face. She calls for interdisciplinary collaboration for further data collection into the contexts of dog bite incidents and how education of children and parents may change their behaviour around pet dogs.

Another key to dog bite prevention is often claimed to be the wider societal promotion of 'responsible dog ownership'. In Chapter 31, Heath Keogh presents a case study of multi-agency working in the London Borough of Sutton. Although, as highlighted in Chapter 29, hard evidence of the effectiveness of this initiative in preventing dog bites, like so many others, is lacking, nonetheless this scheme promoting 'responsible dog ownership' is well-regarded and serves as a model on which we can potentially build proper evaluation tools. It may also provide a framework for other locations where the value of cross-agency collaboration surrounding reporting and managing dog-related issues is recognised.

In summary, despite many programmes and educational initiatives being designed to prevent dog bites, there is often a lack of evidence that they are truly effective in changing both dog and human behaviour. Nonetheless, we are now in a much stronger position to identify those with the most promising characteristics and prioritise these for assessment.

Finally, in Chapter 32, Rachel Orritt and Todd Hogue draw on their combined expertise in forensic psychology and animal behaviour to reflect on an alternative way forward for assessing risk. This is based on methods used in other potentially high-risk situations for the public where there is a lack of clear scientific evidence but growing professional expertise. Forensic risk assessment using structured professional judgment allows the synthesis of scientific data with expert opinion in an organised way to allow best use of these resources. It may not be perfect but it provides a clearly traceable basis for both action and accountability.

As editors, we have learned a lot in the course of preparing this text and so we feel confident that you, the reader, will do likewise whatever your background. We hope this text will not only provide a source of reference of current knowledge and best practice to those interested in this subject whatever your discipline, but also provide a focus for future development and increased collaboration across the disciplines. This book provides a benchmark upon which we can build.

*Daniel Mills and Carri Westgarth, June 2016*

# Section 1
# Fundamental Principles

In Section 1 we lay a foundation for what follows by considering some fundamental principles that should shape the way we think about the issues involved. In order to understand dog bites we need to be clear about what we know about the issue and how we know it. This might seem obvious, but when trying to understand the quality of our knowledge there is a big difference between personal opinions and beliefs (no matter how strongly held) and empirical information. As highlighted in this section, being clear on these matters is a major challenge to the study of dog bites. In order to study something, we need to be able to define it consistently, but in Chapter 1, Daniel Mills highlights the lack of consensus when we refer to aggressive behaviour and even bites in dogs. Perhaps if we can build a more consistent framework, as suggested in this chapter, we will make better progress.

In Chapter 2, Helen Zulch highlights how little we know about the meaning of signals produced by dogs and how much is based on opinion. The point is well made that if we can become more consistent in separating our descriptions of behaviour from our interpretations of it, then communications between those studying aggressive signals will be improved and we will recognise more clearly those areas where academic discussion and development should flourish in pursuit of knowledge.

In Chapter 3, Kenton Morgan and colleagues present a refreshing and incisive view of the use and abuse of statistics in relation to dog bites. This is not about hard numbers or difficult statistical concepts, but rather it is about understanding uncertainty. It is essential to understand these principles if we are not to be taken in by those who may knowingly or unknowingly misrepresent dog bite statistics and the associated risks.

Finally in Chapter 4, Francine Watkins and Carri Westgarth highlight the value of learning from a public health theoretical perspective when considering the issue of dog bites. Public health is well versed in dealing with the impact on human health of the complex interactions that exist between people and both their physical and social environments, and so provides an excellent framework for integrating all the information related to understanding why dogs bite. The chapters in this section not only highlight how complex the issue of dog bites is and how little we know, but also, and most importantly, provide a framework for making progress so we do not repeat the errors of the past.

# Dog Bites and Aggressive Behaviour – Key Underpinning Principles for their Scientific Study

*Daniel Mills*

## 1.1 Problems with the study of dog aggression

Major challenges to the interdisciplinary study of dog bites include recognising the diverse academic disciplines that can contribute to our understanding of the subject but also, and perhaps more fundamentally, actually defining the key terms and concepts of interest. Dogs bite for many reasons; for example they may nip with their incisors as an enticement to play (Horowitz, 2009) or bite with their canines to protect a resource (Wright, 1991) or in self-defence (Wright, 1991); other bites might be purely accidental encounters, for example when getting in the way of the dog lunging at another target. Superficially the end product is a bite in all of these circumstances, but this is of very limited (if any) value on its own, since we generally want to understand either why the bite occurred or what should be done about it to prevent future bites.

### 1.1.1 What is aggression?

To do this we need to understand the biology of bites and associated processes, including the concept of aggression and the difference between an incident and a problem situation.

For example, we ask two questions to the same population of individuals:

- Has your dog ever bitten another individual?
- Is your dog aggressive?

We can expect a very different prevalence of 'yes' responses. Terms such as 'aggression' and many others associated with dog bites are value laden terms, with no consistent objective definition. Indeed, this problem is not unique to dogs and has been recognised for a long time in the human literature, with van Der Dennen (1980) identifying more than 100 definitions of aggression in the academic literature relating to human behaviour. Few studies of dog aggression appear to have recognised this problem, with the concept often poorly or subjectively defined, or not defined at all (e.g. see Polo et al., 2015). This leads to enormous variation in the prevalence of aggression according to the criteria used to define it. All of the following problems may be perceived as aggressive behaviour by owners and so present as aggression within the reporting of case series (e.g. Denenberg et al., 2005). This is illustrated by the findings of Mills and Mills (2003), who gathered descriptive data on the behaviour of 722 UK pet dogs within 502 families. It was found that 547 dogs (75.8%) from 399 households were reported to bark when visitors arrived, 339 dogs (46.9%) from 242 households were reported to bark at other dogs, 113 dogs (15.6%) from ninety-one households were reported to chase livestock, fifty-one dogs from forty-eight households chased cars, seventy-seven dogs from seventy households chased bicycles, sixty-eight dogs from seventy-eight households chased joggers, 411 dogs from 334 households chased cats, 216 dogs from 184 households chased dogs and 216 dogs from 213 households chased other items. Rabbits and hares were the most common of these (eighty-one) followed by wild birds (seventy-four), squirrels (sixty) with fewer than twenty reports of other items. Some 66% of dogs tended to chase two or more classes of objects. All of these are potential contexts in which a dog's response might be construed as aggressive, depending on how the term is defined or interpreted, but clearly this is not always the case; some dogs bark because they are alerting their owners to the presence of a visitor and some chase as a form of play with no intention of catching the target. The prevalence will clearly vary according to the definitions chosen, and also whether reporting and the owner or household level, and if comparisons are to be made between studies, e.g. to assess risk factors, then it must not be assumed that the term aggression is being used in the same way by different authors.

If we limit the definition of aggression to more direct signs of threat such as growling, snapping and biting, we obtain a very different picture. Forty-five (6.2%) showed one of these behaviours at least sometimes towards adult male household members, twenty-two (3.0%) towards male children in the household, thirty-one (4.3%) towards adult female household members, eighteen (2.5%) towards female children in the household, forty-eight (6.6%) towards familiar male adult visitors, twenty-five (3.5%) towards familiar male child visitors, forty-one (5.7%) towards familiar female adult visitors, thirty towards familiar female child visitors, 233 (32.3%) towards unknown male adult visitors, 106 (14.7%) towards unknown male child visitors, 191 (26.4%) towards unknown adult female visitors and 108 (15.0%) towards unknown female child visitors.

Overall, 48% showed growling, snapping or biting in three or more of the preceding contexts. One hundred and seventy-one (23.7%) dogs were said to growl to keep possession. Seventy-five (10.4%) would snap, bite or growl to protect their food bowl. One hundred and twenty (16.6%) growled and seventy-four (10.2%) snapped or bit to obstruct people from doing things; Seventy-eight (10.8%) would growl to stop people going somewhere and twenty-eight (3.9%) snap or bite at this time. Ninety-three (12.9%) dogs had attempted to or succeeded in biting an adult male, forty-six (6.4%) a male child, fifty-seven (7.9%) a female adult, forty (5.5%) a female child and 201 (27.8%) another dog, of whom eighty-seven of the targets were known to be male and sixty-six female. Seventy-nine incidents involving other animals were also reported, twenty-seven on cats, twenty on livestock, eighteen on wild mammals, nine on horses and the remaining on wild birds and other pets.

However, when asked to evaluate their dog's behaviour, 260 (51.8%) owners reported their dog had an annoying habit (primarily related to vocalisation or obedience problems, rarely including aggressive behaviour) and only 127 (25.3%) owners described their dog as having a behaviour problem. When asked to describe the problem, the most common response related to growling, snapping and biting or predation, with forty-eight (9.6%) recorded, but there was no obvious association between the context of the dog's growling, snapping and biting or its frequency and the likelihood that the dog would be described as having a problem in this regard. More recently, Westgarth and Watkins (2015) have even found disagreement over the perception of what a dog bite is, even though this might be thought to be more obviously definable on the basis of physical measures. The perception of participants as to whether a 'real' dog bite had occurred varied depending on whether or not the victim thought a dog 'intended' to bite for some. For others a bite received in play was a bite. Subjects also varied as to the need or nature of any skin damage, for some felt skin must be marked or broken for a bite to have occurred. Even within a single interview, a participant may contradict him or herself on such matters (Westgarth and Watkins, 2015). Clearly, there is little consistency in both an individual's perception of aggression and its component features, and this applies to those reporting on such events as well as victims. A clear definition of aggression is an essential prerequisite to any study, so the reader has a clearer idea of what is being reported on and is not left to his or her own ideas.

Nonetheless, one conclusion from this work is that incidents that might be described as aggressive are probably very common and perhaps a normal part of having a dog, and even bites may be far more common than is generally reported since most may not inflict serious injury. A second conclusion is that the prevalence of such behaviour will vary enormously depending on how it is defined, and if it is not clearly defined it is not really possible to compare different reports, since they may not be describing the same phenomenon. Thirdly, there is no clear consensus of the features of aggressive behaviour that lead to it being defined as 'problematic'. Certainly, owners do not appear to consider much of this behaviour problematic and, as reported in Chapter 23, perhaps victims might not either in some circumstances, although in others it might be more traumatic.

### 1.1.2 Is aggression a problem?

While this apparent lack of concern might be a cause for alarm, it perhaps also reflects a point that can easily be overlooked when a serious bite incident occurs, and receives significant media attention. People live with dogs and so have a lot of contact with them; there is an intrinsic risk associated with this, but serious injuries are not the norm, although these are the ones that attract the most attention and study. It is not logical to assume that non-injurious or minor dog bites reflect the fortunate avoidance of a more serious injury. To suggest this is to ignore the communicative function of most bites (see Chapter 2 and below). In many incidences it would be expected that a dog does not bite unless it has to, and it only inflicts the minimum damage necessary for it to convey its message. In support of this, we recently reported (Barcelos et al., 2015) that the bite incidents of dogs referred for being aggressive to the behaviour clinic at University of Lincoln had a number of commonalities when the dog was found to have a focus of musculoskeletal pain that had gone either unnoticed or unrecognised. Bites tended to be located on the extremities of the target, with incidents being of relatively short duration and easy to interupt, i.e they were brief incidents aimed at inflicting minimal damage in order to avoid further interaction. These features were not recurring themes in cases referred for similar reasons but without an identifiable pain focus, where the reasons for the behaviour were more variable, e.g. to control a valued resource.

As discussed elsewhere, if we really wish to manage the risk of significant harm, we need to also study the wider communicative context preceding dog bites. On the other hand, it is unwise to assume that dog bites, even serious ones, are always the prelude to a fatality. The latter are fortunately extremely rare (it has been reported that a child in the USA stands a greater chance of drowning in a 5 gallon bucket of water than dying from a dog bite (Bradley, 2014), even though they are exposed to dogs much more than buckets of water) and fatalities may have unique circumstances that require special consideration (e.g. see Chapter 11 and Patronek et al., 2013).

Good data are an essential prerequisite for good science and the usefulness of knowledge that we gain as a result. To get good data, we need to clearly distinguish what we observe from how we interpret it, and a failure to do this seems to be a recurring problem in this field. Chapter 2, describes the state of the art with regards to how we might interpret the aggressive behaviour of dogs, while this chapter focuses on the underlying principles and presents a framework for making inferences about the underlying motivation and emotion of a dog involved in an aggressive incident in a field rather than laboratory setting.

## 1.2  Aggression versus aggressive behaviour

### 1.2.1  The definition of aggression

The etymology of the noun 'aggression' stems from the Latin words 'ad' – 'towards' and 'gradi' – 'stride' or 'walk', and so implies the word was originally used to describe some form of active engagement with another. These words later became fused to create the Latin term 'aggredi', meaning 'an attack'. Interestingly, some popular texts describing dog body language (e.g. Abrantes, 1997) still appear to use the term in this way to some extent, distinguishing threats associated with 'aggression' at one end of a scale from those associated with 'fear' at the other end (Abrantes, 1997, p.110–111). 'Aggression', is defined by this author as: '1. The initiation of unprovoked hostilities. 2. The launching of attacks. 3. Hostile behaviour'. However, this is conceptually problematic, not least because the definition of aggression has elements of the subjectivity issues discussed in the preceding section but also because it places two different phenomena at opposite ends of a quantitative scale, when the two are qualitatively different. One is a perceived behaviour (aggression), the other an emotion (fear).

### 1.2.2  Forms of aggression

Other conceptual inconsistencies in relation to the description of aggression by dogs are also widespread. For example, Reisner (2002) reviewed the diagnostic categories used to define aggression in the veterinary behaviour literature. She identified twenty-six terms that were used by different authors, but only two were used by all authors (fear-induced and predatory), other terms were less consistently agreed upon, with some terms used by fewer than half the authors reviewed. So it seems that the form of aggression a dog shows – or perhaps the reason why it bit – depends on who is assessing the animal. This is clearly nonsensical from a scientific perspective, and indeed from a biological standpoint it might be argued that one of the 'forms' of aggression that they all agree on (predatory) should not be considered aggression at all, because it relates to a functionally different biological system (the acquisition of food, see Archer 1988). Closer inspection of this list reveals further problems both within and between authors, with some of the terms used related clearly to context, e.g. 'food- related', some to motivation e.g. 'dominance', and some to emotion, e.g. 'fear-induced'. Because the categories used are not conceptually consistent, it is not surprising that they are not mutually exclusive; so a dog that shows fear while protecting its food bowl, but is assumed to be doing this in order to gain dominance over the one trying to take the bowl, may be diagnosed as having dominance, food-related and fear-induced aggression.

Indeed, in the five years leading up to 2014 for the 'Animal Behavior Case of the Month' published by the leading *Journal of the American Veterinary Medical Association,* we (Barcelos and Mills, unpublished data) calculate that a dog-related aggression case has on average 2.4 aggression-related conditions assigned to it. Do these dogs have multiple forms of aggression? I would suggest it is more likely that these multi-diagnoses are a reflection of the conceptually poor terminology being used and the inconsistency of the framework we use to classify these cases.

In the first instance it reflects a failure to clearly distinguish between terms that qualify the behaviour in terms of its:

- Context – the circumstances surrounding the expression of the behaviour.
- Behavioural motivation – the biological goal of the behaviour.
- Emotional content – the processing of information relating to the personal significance of the circumstances to the individual (subjective importance). This serves to set the individual's strategic priorities, with regards to what goals to pursue at the current time, and can explain why two individuals in a similar objective biological state may respond differently to the same physical stimuli, i.e. because they make different personal evaluations of the situation.

The first of these can be defined objectively, but the latter two are inferences people make when observing animals and so cannot be measured directly. However, they still represent different biological phenomena that need to be distinguished and not confused (Reeve, 2014).

## 1.2.3 Definition of aggressive behaviour

There are other problems with the concept of 'aggression' that also deserve consideration. Aggression is a noun and, as such, describes something or a collection of things that are related; it is often implied that this defining feature is some form of behaviour.

However, **a fundamental principle of 'behaviourism' and the science of animal behaviour is that behaviours are objectively describable, but this does not appear to be the case when it comes to 'aggression'**, as there is no clear consensus on what behaviours make up aggression.

Instead, the noun 'aggression' refers to a wide range of behaviours in which there is a *perceived* risk of harm to another. It is *an interpretation of the behaviour,* which may or may not be an accurate assessment of the actual risk. It does not refer to an objectively definable behaviour in the normal scientific sense. It is perhaps because the term refers to a range of motivationally and emotionally disparate behaviours and not a single physiological entity that illogical inferences are often made about it, such as the classification error described above. The shared features of aggression are superficial and related to subjective characteristics within the reporter, not basic biology. Thus, it is not surprising that there is no consensus. The boundary between 'aggression' and 'non-aggression' is essentially arbitrary, even if we define it using objective terms. This is why it is essential that the definition used to identify aggression in any study is provided and not assumed.

**For this reason I prefer to use the term 'aggressive behaviour' to 'aggression'.** The use of the adjectival form of the term to qualify the noun, 'behaviour', emphasises that it is a form or style of behaviour that is being studied rather than a distinct unit of behaviour. This perspective stops us from making too many assumptions at the outset and highlights the need to gather more information about the behaviour and its context if we wish to understand what is happening.

## 1.3 Context motivation and emotion

In the previous section it was suggested that the contextual, motivational and emotional features of aggressive behaviour may not always be clearly differentiated. In this section we explain how each of these contributes to our understanding of animal behaviour, and especially a bite incident.

### 1.3.1 Context

The context of a bite defines the circumstances in which the behaviour arises, and should be considered a largely descriptive account of the situation and not a diagnosis. A diagnosis is the identification of the nature of the problem, not simply when the problem arises. The context may be used to help infer the reasons why the behaviour occurs, but it is not an explanation in its own right. To say a dog bit someone because there was food around does not really answer the question: why did the dog bite, from a biological perspective? All interventions aimed at controlling the problem need to take account of context, but if they are based on this alone, they are clearly going to be very broad and non-specific.

There are two elements to context:

- The general context, which refers to the prevailing conditions at the time (general risk factors – these increase the risk, but their onset does not have a close relationship in either space or time with the occurrence of a specific incident).
- The specific context, which refers to the triggers of the behaviour. To identify the latter we need to know what happened immediately before the dog bit. Contextual features relating to when the behaviour does and does not occur also provide one of the lines of evidence needed for making inferences about both the motivation and emotion under-lying the behaviour, but further information is also required too, as outlined below.

### 1.3.2 Motivation

Motivation refers to the biological function of the behaviour, and in a clinical animal behaviour setting cannot be assessed directly. Instead, the evidence from a range of sources is considered. In the author's opinion, one of the most rigorous ways of doing this is to undertake a functional assessment of behaviour, using the systematic approach described by Friedman (2007). This requires an identification and operational description of the focal **Behaviour** (in this case the bite), the identification of the immediate physical and environmental **Antecedents** to the focal behaviour and the **Consequences** that maintain or reinforce the behaviour. Thus, the event is described in terms of Antecedents, Behaviour and Consequences (ABC) and an inference can then be made about its motivation.

Motivation refers to the process that initiates, guides and maintains behaviour associated with a particular goal and it is often described by reference to intervening variables, e.g. hunger – the motivation to consume calories. When assessing motivation we need to consider both the immediate goal and also the biological value of the behaviour. The veracity of the hypothetical motivation inferred from the functional assessment process can be tested by predicting a range of other circumstances that should give rise or not give rise to the behaviour, as well as consequences that should terminate or prolong the response. The more the hypothesis is tested and predictions met, the more confident we can be in its accuracy, but the hypothesis may be rejected regardless of the amount of evidence supporting it, if one critical piece of evidence contradicts the prediction (falsification). In this situation it is necessary to generate a new hypothesis that fits all the data.

Motivational factors may be general or specific:

- General factors are perhaps best considered risk factors for the behaviour that create a predisposition towards a certain behaviour, and might include aspects of personality and learned associations as well as more proximate factors such as current hunger level or chronic pain
- Specific motivational factors are the potential immediate triggers (specific antecedents) to the behaviour.

Some motivational factors are extrinsic (i.e. come from outside the animal) and these can be either tangible (e.g. food) or psychological (e.g. praise); others are intrinsic (are generated from within), and these often involve some form of information acquisition and so include environmental exploration, increased control over the environment, or social learning (e.g. who are co-operators and who are competitors). Obviously, it can be much harder to identify internal motivational factors, and sometimes their significance only becomes apparent because a behaviour cannot be explained by reference to external factors. However, once inferred, their significance can be evaluated in the same way as any other motivational hypothesis.

### 1.3.3 Emotion

While motivation relates to the broad biological function of a behaviour, emotion relates to the subjective importance of the events to the individual and results in the individualised response, i.e. it explains why two animals may react differently to the same stimulus when all other biological factors are equal.

In the same way that the motivational predisposition of an animal can be described by reference to its arousal at the level of personality (e.g. a greedy dog), prevailing circumstance (hunger level) or the immediate situation (the overt availability of food), so too can emotional predisposition vary in a similar way (Mills, 2010). Temperament encompasses an affective style arising from the characteristics of the animal's early environment, and is largely dependent on genetics and early experience. Mood is a prevailing emotional state that arises in response to a series of events or pervasive changes that provides an adaptive bias in cognition, pre-attentive processes, accessibility to stored information and cognitive flexibility. By contrast, emotional reactions are normally a stimulus–bound response to spontaneous or unexpected events that have personal significance, but are relatively short lived (see Ekman and Davidson, 1994, for a discussion of these fundamental issues).

The key feature of emotional arousal is that it concerns the subjective value (rather than broader physical nature) of events and their associated responses, e.g. that person approaching is not just anyone, it is my mother. Thus, emotion relates to and influences the motivation to do a given behaviour, but also affects the perception of events, too. Emotional responses allow us to operate as an individual, with our own unique relationship with the world around us, and they create biases in our behaviour that are not simply due to learned experience. For an event to be emotional it must relate either unconditionally or through learned association to stimuli that are important at the personal individual level. For example, to a dog not all humans are equal; a given person may be the primary carer for one dog, but a threat or source of frustration to another. These stimuli are called *emotionally competent stimuli,* Emotional processes facilitate these distinctions.

In human psychology there are five components to human emotion that can be assessed and used to help infer it (Scherer, 2005) and it has recently been suggested that four of these (Table 1.1, excluding the subjective feeling experience) can be used to make similar inferences in the field (as opposed to laboratory) with companion animals (Mills et al., 2014).

**Table 1.1** Four components of emotion, their effects and function (adapted from Scherer, 2005)

| Component | Effect | Function |
|---|---|---|
| Cognitive | Appraisal | Evaluation of events and objects |
| Neurophysiological | Arousal and associated bodily sign | Preparation for action and associated regulation |
| Motivation | Action tendency | Strategic direction of activity |
| Motor expression | General and specific (e.g. facial) behaviour | Communication of reaction and intention |

These features provide four lines of evidence that must be consistent to test the hypothesis that a given emotional reaction is present:

1.  In relation to the cognitive component of appraisal it should be possible to consistently identify that the events relate to stimuli of specific definable personal importance to the individual (see below for the proposed list of emotionally competent stimuli associated with different reactions) and the response is associated with the anticipated or actual arrival or disappearance of these stimuli. In the case of aggressive behaviour, this might be a particular individual or a particular type of action, or a combination of the two.
2.  In relation to neurophysiological arousal, the response should be consistent (increase or decrease of sympathetic and parasympathetic nervous systems) with the emotional state

involved. Indirect measures of arousal include pupil dilation and pilo-erection consistent with activation of the sympathetic nervous system. This provides physiological support for what happens when the triggering event occurs.

3.  In relation to the motivational aspects of the emotional response, the range of behaviours observed should be consistent with a general change in behavioural tendency (e.g. the tendency to escape). However, the specifics of the behaviour may vary with the options available to the animal, i.e. the form of escape used varies with the circumstances. For example, a dog may try to flee but when this is not possible and the threat continues, it bites. A response that varies little may imply either an extreme reaction and/or the development of a conditioned habit.

4.  In relation to the motor expression of emotion, the event should produce consistent changes in behaviour associated with communication of this internal state, e.g. certain facial expressions (see also Chapter 2).

Critical to the systematic and reliable inference of emotion in non-human animals has been the identification of key emotional states of relevant biological value through a review of the affective neuroscience (e.g. Panksepp, 1998; Berridge, 1999; Zeki and Romaya, 2008; Kringelbach and Berridge, 2010; Panksepp and Biven, 2012) and in light of a knowledge of the neurobiology of the species of interest (Mills et al., 2013, 2014). As a result, the following emotionally competent stimuli and associated responses are proposed as the basis for the description of emotional reactions in the dog, i.e. triggers and the behavioural strategy they activate:

1.  Desirables: Things the animal wants at a given time lead to seeking out opportunities with them through activation of a desire/seeking system.

2.  Frustrations: Things the animal wants but cannot access or are less than expected lead to increased focused effort aimed at achieving the goal through activation of a rage/frustration system.

3.  General threats to the animal: Things that might harm the animal lead to self-preservation responses through activation of a fear system.

4.  Bodily damage: Things causing actual bodily damage lead to withdrawal and protection through activation of a pain system.

5.  Those with whom an affectionate playful bond is shared: Individuals that provide shared learning opportunities through playful social engagement including rough and tumble play through activation of a play system.

6.  Attachment figures and objects: Those that provide safety and protection lead to a strong dependence upon them at times of uncertainty and insecurity through activation of a panic/grief system.

7.  Offspring: Those that are dependent on an individual may invoke a range of caring behaviours directed towards them through activation of a care system.

8.  Potential sexual partners: Those with whom there may be breeding opportunities lead to the expression of courtship and reproductive activity through activation of a lust system.

9.  Undesirables: Those that are thought to be a threat to the benefits of the current social group, e.g. those who are predicted to take more than they give (social cheats), may

elicit responses associated with their expulsion and avoidance through activation of a hate system.

In the case of a report of aggressive behaviour by a dog, each of these needs to be considered in an initial list of differentials before further information has been gathered. For example:

1.  Stalking and chasing (predatory behaviour) often arise from activation of the desire/ seeking system.
2.  If the incident occurs within the context of the loss or denial of a resource, during restraint including touch, then it is possible that the rage/frustration system is active.
3.  If the incident occurs within the context of unexpected event or perceived threat of harm to the individual then the fear system may be active.
4.  In response to actual harm or the stimulation of a painful lesion, the pain system may be active. The anticipation of this event will result in activation of the fear system as well.
5.  Nips to entice play and in the course of rough and tumble exuberance relate to activation of the play system.
6.  Aggressive prevention of owner departure may arise because the dog finds it difficult to cope with his or her absence and so engages the panic/grief system.
7.  If the incident occurs in the context of a perceived threat to offspring or dependents (which can include humans) then the care system may be active.
8.  An incident involving a male around a bitch, especially in season, may relate to activation of the lust system.
9.  If the incident relates to a stranger who is not a physical threat but a potential drain on resources, and the dog is of otherwise sound temperament, then it might be that the hate system is involved.

As with the functional assessment process for inferring motivation, the inference of emotion begins with a systematic ABC evaluation. However, there is a different emphasis on the information being gathered, since it is used to answer the following four questions, based on the function identified for the four components of emotion described in Table 1.1:

1.  The preceding circumstances (antecedents) to the behaviour are consistent with which of the nine emotionally competent stimuli described above? (evaluation of events and objects).
2.  The level and fluctuations in arousal are consistent with that required to support which emotional states? (preparation for action and associated regulation).
3.  The observable behaviours, including attention focus, are all consistent with a strategic objective related to which emotional systems? (strategic direction of activity). Note that this has to be put in the context of the options available to the animal at that time. Certain experiences (e.g. previous punishment) may limit the perceived options, but these can be evidenced from a careful history.
4.  The signals that can be read are consistent with which emotions? (communication of reaction and intention) – see Chapter 2.

If the evidence from any one of these four lines of enquiry is inconsistent (as opposed to inconclusive) with any given emotional reaction, then it is unscientific to propose involvement of that affective state.

Using this approach we have found that we can improve the reliability and more rigorously defend the diagnoses we make, which are based largely on inferring the motivational and emotional state of the dog in a given context. This approach also has important practical value and implications for problem behaviour management, since many clinical behaviour problems, such as biting, relate to either a type of emotional arousal or an intensity of emotional arousal that the owner finds problematic. Given that an emotion may be expressed through a variety of behaviours, it is the emotional response that sets the overall strategy, while the specific behaviours that serve this have their own specific goals. Therefore, it is often more efficient to focus on controlling the emotion rather than the motivation of the behaviour, and useful to recognise which of these a given intervention might be targeting. For example, altering the specific target of the behaviour in the circumstances (redirection of behaviour), or training a behaviour with a different goal in the circumstances (operant counter-conditioning), are strategies that focus on the motivation and expression of behaviour – changes in emotion in the latter case are incidental. By contrast, controlling the intensity of arousal if the emotion being aroused is appropriate (e.g. through desensitisation or extinction methods) or changing the emotion if it is inappropriate (e.g. through emotional substitution/respondent counter-conditioning) are strategies with an emotional focus and it is the quality of the emotion that needs attention.

## 1.4 Conclusion

There is a need for a more critical evaluation of the concepts of aggression and aggressive behaviour in dogs if we are to make solid scientific progress in our understanding of these topics. This should involve greater recognition of the distinction between the context, motivation and emotion associated with a behaviour, and how these can be investigated. Although we cannot know for sure the motivation or emotional state of an animal (likewise another human – but we can make a reasonable interpretation), that does not mean we cannot be scientific in our approach to their investigation. Indeed, a rigorous approach, grounded in sound scientific theory and methodology, is possible and has been described in this chapter, which, if embraced widely, will undoubtedly help improve the progress of science, practical investigation, treatment and risk management associated with dog bites (see text box summary).

**Text box 1.1** Procedures for describing a dog bite incident

Extracting good quality information from available sources on which to make inferences is essential to the diagnostic process:

- What sources are available?
  - Observation

- History
- Clinical tests.

Information needed for making inferences:

- What the aggressive behaviour looks like, i.e.
  - What the animal did to deliver the bite/appear aggressive
  - Who was where, when it happened
  - What the injury looks like: location and severity, e.g. Dunbar Dog Bite Scale (undated)
  - What brought an end to the incident.

- What events predict it (when – antecedent trigger as well as eliciting contexts – broader circumstances)
- What the animal gains from expressing the behaviour (reinforcement)
- What inhibits/suppresses the behaviour (when did the behaviour stop – trigger for end of incident, as well as broader circumstance likely to defuse the situation)
- What was done after the event.

On the basis of this information it may then be possible to make inferences about:
- Biological function of the behaviour (<u>motivation</u> – e.g. protect food)
  - Inferences about the motivation are usually made on the basis of reflection of
    - The form of the behaviour and
    - Excitatory and Inhibitory motivational factors
      - General and Specific factors should be distinguished
- Personal significance to the dog of the situation (<u>emotional</u> state of the dog – e.g. frustrated by the potential loss of a resource)
  - Evaluation of underlying emotional reaction is made from the triangulation of evidence relating to the four components of emotion:
    - Appraisal
    - Arousal
    - Behaviour tendencies
    - Communication.

REMEMBER: Inferences are hypotheses and need to be constantly re-evaluated in light of new evidence that may challenge them.

- It is important to gather evidence to test all hypotheses to allow the exclusion of competing ideas, rather than just the evidence to support one of the many possibilities
- The amount of evidence in support of an idea is irrelevant. If there is a reliable piece of evidence that refutes it, the hypothesis needs to be rejected.

## 1.5 References

Abrantes, R. (1997). *Dog Language*. Dogwise Publishing.

Archer, J. (1988). *The Behavioural Biology of Aggression*. Cambridge University Press. Cambridge UK.

Barcelos, A. M., Mills, D. S., Zulch, H. (2015). Clinical indicators of occult musculoskeletal pain in aggressive dogs. *Veterinary Record*, *176*(18), 465–465.

Berridge, K. C., Pleasure, pain, desire and dread: hidden core processes of emotion, in *Well Being: The Foundations of Hedonic Psychology*. Edited by Kahneman D., Diener E., Schwarz, N. New York, Russell Sage Foundation, 1999, pp.525–557.

Bradley J. (2014). Dog Bites: Problems and Solutions (revised 2014) Policy Paper. Animals and Society Institute. Available from: http://nationalcanineresearchcouncil.com/uploaded_files/publications/541422429_Dog%20Bites%20Problems%20and%20Solutions%202nd%20Edition.pdf

Denenberg, S., Landsberg, G. M., Horwitz, D., Seksel, K. (2005). A comparison of cases referred to behaviourists in three different countries. Mills, D. et al. Current issues and research in veterinary behavioural medicine. Indiana: Purdue University, 56–62.

Dunbar bite scale: Available from www.dogtalk.com/BiteAssessmentScalesDunbarDTMRoss.pdf

Ekman, P. E., Davidson, R. J. (1994). *The Nature of Emotion: Fundamental Questions*. Oxford University Press.

Friedman, S. G. (2007). A framework for solving behaviour problems: Functional assessment and intervention planning. *Journal of Exotic Pet Medicine*, *16*(1), 6–10.

Horowitz, A. (2009). Attention to attention in domestic dog (Canis familiaris) dyadic play. *Animal Cognition*, *12*(1), 107–118.

Kringelbach, M. L., Berridge, K. C. (2010). *Pleasures of the Brain*. Oxford University Press.

Mills D. S., Mills C. B. (2003). A survey of the behaviour of UK household dogs. In: Seksel, K., Perry, G., Mills, D., Frank, D., Lindell, E., McGreevy, P., Pageat, P. (2003) *Fourth International Veterinary Behaviour Meeting Proceedings No: 352*. Post Graduate Foundation in Veterinary Science, University of Sydney, Sydney. 93–98.

Mills, D. S, Braem Dubé, M., Zulch, H. (2013). *Stress and Pheromonatherapy in Small Animal Clinical Behaviour*. Wiley Blackwells, Oxford. pp.294.

Mills, D. S., Karagiannis, C., Zulch, H. (2014). Stress and behavioural medicine – Veterinary Clinics of North America 44(3) 525–541.

Mills, D. S. (2010). Emotion, In Mills, D. (Ed in Chief) *The Encyclopaedia of Applied Animal Behaviour & Welfare*. CABI. Wallingford, 214–217.

Panksepp, J. (1998). *Affective Neuroscience: The Foundations of Human and Animal Emotions*. Oxford University Press.

Panksepp, J., Biven, L. (2012). *The Archaeology of Mind: Neuroevolutionary Origins of Human Emotions (Norton series on interpersonal neurobiology)*. W. W. Norton & Company.

Patronek, G. J., Sacks, J. J., Delise, K. M., Cleary, D. V., Marder, A. R. (2013). Co-occurrence of potentially preventable factors in 256 dog bite-related fatalities in the United States (2000–09). *Journal of the American Veterinary Medical Association*, *243*(12), 1726–1736.

Polo, G., Calderón, N., Clothier, S., Garcia, R. D. C. M. (2015). Understanding dog aggression: Epidemiologic aspects: In memoriam, Rudy de Meester (1953–2012). *Journal of Veterinary Behavior: Clinical Applications and Research*, *10*(6), 525–534.

Reeve, J. (2014). *Understanding Motivation and Emotion*. John Wiley & Sons.

Reisner, I. (2002). An overview of aggression. *BSAVA Manual of Canine and Feline Behavioural Medicine. British Small Animal Veterinary Association, Waterwells, England*, 181–194.

Scherer, K. R. (2005). What are emotions? And how can they be measured? *Social Science Information*, *44*(4), 695–729.

Van Der Dennen, J. M. G. (1980). Problems in the Concepts and Definitions of Aggression, Violence, and Some Related Terms: Pt.1. *Default journal*. Available from: https://www.rug.nl/research/portal/files/14532625/PROBLEM1.pdf

Westgarth, C., Watkins, F. (2015). A qualitative investigation of the perceptions of female dog-bite victims and implications for the prevention of dog bites. *Journal of Veterinary Behavior: Clinical applications and Research*, *10*(6), 479–488.

Wright, J. C. (1991). Canine aggression toward people: bite scenarios and prevention. *Veterinary Clinics of North America: Small Animal Practice*, *21*(2), 299–314.

Zeki, S., Romaya, J. P. (2008). Neural correlates of hate. *PloS one*, *3*(10), e3556.

# CHAPTER 2

# Reading Aggressive Behaviour in Dogs: From Observation to Inference

*Helen Zulch*

## 2.1 Introduction

Dogs communicate through visual, auditory and olfactory channels, and to help us decipher why a dog may have bitten, we can derive information to a greater or lesser degree from each of these. A dog's gross actions (such as running towards or away from, jumping up at or even lunging on the end of a lead) give limited information regarding its motivations and emotions as similar broad actions may occur in any one of a range of these states. Vocalisations can give additional information as they can usually be interpreted fairly well by people, if carefully guided about the need to attend to detail (Pongracz et al., 2005), but in much aggressive behaviour, especially the early stages, vocalisation is limited. Many dogs will also vocalise when excited in a manner that may be misinterpreted as aggressive.[1] We are denied the ability to read the majority of the chemical signals dogs may release, although it is likely that this will be of relevance to another dog and may help to contextualise or clarify visual signals. From a human perspective, the greatest opportunity we have for reading a dog's intentions is through body language cues and facial expression. The interpretation of this largely visual information forms the basis of the content of this chapter.

The literature categorises aggressive behaviour in a number of ways (Chapter 1) with some authors categorising by target (for example, stranger-directed), some categorising by emotion (fear aggression), some by environmental context (e.g. food bowl-related) and some by motivation (for example, to achieve dominance). A single literature source may utilise multiple levels of classifications for aggressive behaviour (for example, food aggression (contextual) and fear aggression (underlying emotion-related)) which can lead to confusion. For example, aggressive behaviour in the presence of food could be described in relation to a range of underlying emotions, e.g. as a form of 'fear-' or 'frustration-related' aggression, or

---

1   In this chapter, for simplicity and clarity, the term aggressive behaviour is used to refer to any behaviour that is intended to threaten or harm another individual, and excludes incidental injuries, etc.

in relation to motivation such as 'possessiveness', as well as by context, e.g. 'food bowl-related'. However, these are not different diagnoses, but merely different perceptions of the same thing (Chapter 1). This chapter will describe an aggressive response in terms of its underlying motivation and emotion as outlined in the previous chapter, in order to provide a consistent framework for this evaluation.

This chapter describes the process of what to observe in a dog presenting with aggressive behaviour within a specific context to determine its most likely intention, motivation and emotion. However, the majority of our interpretations regarding body language and facial expression in dogs are based largely on expert opinion with little support from empirical study in peer review literature. Although ongoing work at the University of Lincoln is currently using the framework described to validate these expressive signs of different emotional states, until these results are published all interpretations need to be made with caution. Any inference should be reviewed in light of evidence that might contradict the initial conclusions. A golden rule when evaluating dog behaviour is to look for evidence that allows you to exclude competing explanations rather than focus on supporting evidence for a particular belief about the cause.

## 2.2 The process of assessing aggressive behaviour

An aggressive response (excluding 'aggressive' behaviours such as bites seen in play and excluding predatory behaviour) is usually a distance increasing act. However, an exception to this would be where the behaviour is as a result of a redirected act due to frustration and the recipient of the action is not the trigger of the response (this is discussed in more detail later). The reason a dog may be motivated to increase distance can vary. It may be as a result of the dog trying to create distance for self-defence from a real or perceived threat, to protect itself from pain, either current or remembered, or it can be as a result of a desire to defend something of value to it. Different emotions are likely be involved in each of these cases, which, although possibly not of critical importance in avoiding an escalation of the aggressive response in the immediate term, will be of importance in the development of a treatment plan and avoidance of escalation of the problem in the longer term.

If overtly aggressive behaviour is seen, the first step is to examine the context before trying to understand the underlying motivation and emotion.

### 2.2.1 Context

Key points to note when examining the context of the aggressive response are:

1. **Is there a clear target of focus?** Can you see what the dog is looking at? Is the dog switching focus between two or more points (for example a possession and a person)?
2. **Is there something within the environment that may be of value to the dog?** For example, a space, food, a toy or another resource (such as a stolen item). The item may not be in close proximity to the dog for it to attempt to defend it, so a dog may defend a bone buried halfway across the garden, for example.
3. **Is there something in the environment that may be perceived as threatening to the dog?** This may not be something a person may consider frightening, but anything

that is different, novel or that may have scared the dog in the past may be perceived as a threat. In addition, gestures moving into a dog's space, particularly over its head, or rapid, accelerating or erratic movement in the dog's direction can all be perceived as a threat, even if, to a person, it is simply a friendly greeting.

4. **Is there a barrier or perceived barrier in place?** Doors, fences, gates and windows are easy to understand, however a lead can serve as a barrier, preventing a dog from accessing something it desires or moving away from something it chooses to avoid. Barriers can also be psychological. If a dog predicts from previous experience that a certain action may lead to a punishing consequence (being reprimanded by its owner from pulling away from something, for example) this can serve as a barrier to action. The presence of a barrier may give rise to frustration.

5. **Is the dog known or suspected to be suffering from any condition that may cause pain or discomfort or has the dog previously experienced such a condition in a similar context in the past?**

6. **Has the dog been exposed to any experiences or environmental changes that may have reduced its tolerance?** It is important to remember that stressors can accumulate and so a dog that is usually tolerant in a given situation may not be after a lifestyle change or series of interventions that have lowered its threshold to react.

Understanding fully the context of the aggressive behaviour will make assessing motivation and emotion easier.

### 2.2.2 Motivation

Most aggressive behaviour is distance increasing, however not all distance increasing behaviour is aggressive. For example, dogs may choose to actively avoid a situation by moving away or disengage from a situation by showing displacement behaviours such as sniffing the ground. Noting the presence of these behaviours in a dog is as important as paying attention to the overtly aggressive response as this may enable a person to intervene appropriately to diffuse a situation, thus removing the need for overt aggression.

Where the distance increasing behaviour is aggressive there may still be differences in the specific goal as well as the emotion and these may change during the encounter. Typical goals of aggressive behaviour include:

* Self-defence from threat, perceived threat or as a result of the presence of pain.
* Protection or possession of a resource such as food, a toy or a space.
* To take control of a situation where there is competition or conflict in relation to ownership or precedence.

It is important to note that it is possible for an observer to misinterpret the target of the behaviour and therefore make an erroneous inference regarding the motivation; for example if a dog is trying to make contact with an individual for a positive reason – e.g. wanting to greet them – but the lead is restraining them, behaviour interpreted as aggressive can be inferred towards the person as the dog gets frustrated, and the lead is a barrier to the dog acquiring what it wants. This is one of the reasons that a contextual assessment is also critical.

## *2.2.3 Emotion*

Chapter 1 described four lines of evidence that can be used to identify emotional responses and distinguish between them in a given situation:

1. The presence of a stimulus that has the capacity to cause an emotional response in the individual (emotionally competent stimulus).
2. The level and form of arousal associated with the stimulus.
3. Behaviour changes directed towards a common goal, e.g. self-defence or protection of a resource.
4. Communicative signals that are indicative of a specific emotional state.

However, not all aggressive behaviour has a clear emotional underpinning at the time that the behaviour is manifest. Although less common, it is possible for the behaviour to become an habitual response to a stimulus if the response gets a very predictable outcome, from the dog's perspective, each time the stimulus occurs (the initial response would have been emotional, but over time the emotional component of the behaviour has reduced until what is manifest is a learnt habitual response to the stimulus). An awareness of this is key for developing an appropriate treatment plan. Key factors to determine whether or not a behaviour has a significant emotional base are:

- Is there an identifiable emotionally competent stimulus in the environment preceding the behavioural response (something that is personally significant to the animal, such as something it wants or something the animal may be frightened of, or an individual with whom it has a special relationship)?
- Is there significant and changeable arousal noted? Arousal should co-vary with the emotion. However, it must be noted that arousal may not be manifest as action, a dog that is very fearful may freeze when aroused. Looking for signs of physiological arousal is therefore important – dilated pupils, increased respiratory rate and piloerection, for example.
- How long does the arousal take to dissipate? In individuals where there is an emotional component to the behaviour it is predicted that the arousal will outlast the physical presence of emotional trigger – in other words the dog does not return to a relaxed state immediately after the stimulus disappears.
- Does the response have a history of predictable outcome? As the outcome of a response becomes predictable, there is less demand for emotional engagement. For example, the postman will always leave after delivering the post, regardless of the dog's behaviour, but this is a very predictable outcome from the perspective of the dog's behaviour. The response, therefore, has the potential to become habitual.
- How variable is the response over repeated exposures to the stimulus? In an habitual response the behaviour seen is usually repetitive and invariant, (since it is a stimulus–response habit) whereas where there is emotional involvement the response is likely to be more varied depending on the perceived intensity of the stimulus.
- Do behaviours seen correlate with what is known about the expression of emotional states in dogs – in other words, is the dog communicating a specific emotion and is this linked reliably to the presence and proximity of the focus?

*For example*: A dog is barking aggressively at a person. If the dog is standing stationary with no evidence of changing levels of arousal during the encounter, no significant change in facial expression or posture between the stimulus arriving and leaving again and the bark is repetitive and monotonous, this is more likely to be a habitual response. If, on the other hand, there is evidence of arousal that changes with the intensity of the stimulus (proximity of the person) – raising of hackles, pupil dilation, fluctuating respiratory rate, the dog is moving back and forth, the posture and facial expression have changed noticeably (either demonstrating fear or frustration for example; see below) and the dog takes a while to relax after the person disappears, then it is more likely that the behaviour has an emotional base.

It is also important to remember that several emotions may be expressed to varying degrees at one time, for example there may be a mix of fear and frustration (a dog is fearful of an approaching person but is restrained by a lead and therefore experiences concurrent frustration as it cannot move to safety). For this reason it can be challenging to determine from body posture and expression a primary emotion underlying the behaviour, but exploration of how the behaviour has changed over time and how the behaviour is expressed in a range of situations can help prioritise the role of different emotional elements.

## 2.3  Reading dogs

To assess the motivation and emotion underlying an aggressive response we must infer from the behaviours seen. As dogs have a finite repertoire of muscular movements, for example a limited number of ways they can move their ears or their mouth, it is important that all aspects of the posture, expression and gestures are examined together, as each individual movement can correlate with a range of meanings. It is also important that the sequence in which behaviours occur is noted, as frequently this can provide vital information that enables the correct inference to be drawn. Interpretation is always underpinned by detailed observation, with evidence that contradicts the primary inference being of particular value, since it leads us to re-evaluate our hypothesis.

The next sections review the signs associated with particular emotional states, but it is important to appreciate that few if any signs are sufficient on their own to infer a given emotional state. The repetition of specific behaviours between emotions, once again, stresses the importance of assessing the whole dog, the context and the sequence of responses in order to make the most accurate inference from the four lines of evidence described above and in Chapter 1.

Please note, the descriptions below refer to dogs that are 'ideal' in the sense that they are behaviourally normal and can communicate using a full range of movements and expressions. Dogs that have severely modified features, for example due to breed conformation or as a result of surgery (e.g. tail docking or ear cropping where allowed), or who have serious behaviour problems, may not demonstrate this full range.

## 2.4  Early warning signs

Aggressive behaviour has a potential biological cost to the aggressor as embarking on this strategy means that he risks potential injury and damage to relationships on which he may depend. Dogs therefore have well-developed means of avoiding the need for aggression as well as well-developed means of reconciling with social group members after an aggressive incident (Horowitz, 2009). For this reason, dogs that are behaviourally normal will tend not to bite a person unless they feel that is their only option. There are therefore thought to be two main key factors to why people may get bitten by dogs showing aggressive behaviour:[2]

- They miss the early warning signs that tell of the dog's discomfort with their proximity.
- The dog has learnt over time that the early warning signs do not work and therefore they no longer exhibit these but move straight to the behaviour that (in their experience) works – the bite.

In general, dogs that are feeling uncomfortable with an encounter may show the following. As noted already, these behaviours may also be seen in other situations and contexts, and therefore the behaviour must be interpreted within the context. Of course, if there is doubt it is preferable to err on the side of caution to minimise risk.

In general, irrespective of the emotion, any of the following signs shown by a dog should encourage a person to calmly move away or freeze and avoid eye contact, if they wish to avoid the risk of a bite:

- **The dog becomes very still**. In some dogs it is easy to observe muscle tension through the body at this point, however, even if this is not visible, most dogs will show a tightening of the facial muscles, which may be seen as the muzzle becoming tense with the lips either pulled forward or elongated.
- **The dog's gaze may change – either to an averted gaze or to a fixed stare** towards the target.
- **The dog turns its head or body away or moves away** (note, if the dog does not have space to move away because of a physical barrier such as a wall or a lead, or a psychological barrier such as having learnt from past experience that this is a punishing option, it may not be able to/choose to show this).
- Whether or not the dog can move away, you may note a **lowering of the body towards the ground, either crouching on the spot or creeping away**. Only a slight backward shift of body weight and tucking of the hindquarters may be noticed, or the entire body may be lowered.
- **The dog rolling on to its back, usually with the hind legs splayed open**. To differentiate from a dog lying on its back to solicit attention, observe for signs of muscle tension in the face and note whether the tail is tucked in or relaxed. If the dog is unfamiliar, it is wisest to assume it is not doing this to 'get his tummy tickled'.
- **Movement forwards so that weight shifts over the forequarters and the dog appears to be standing taller**, perhaps positioning itself or its head between the

---

2    There are other reasons why people get bitten not related to aggressive behaviour as defined here, e.g. in relation to predation and predatory play and as an 'accidental' event.

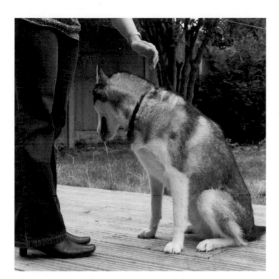

**Figure 2.1** A dog trying to avoid contact by averting the head. Additionally you can see the elongated lips with muscle tension around the mouth that indicates the dog is uncomfortable with the interaction. Photo: Peter Baumber

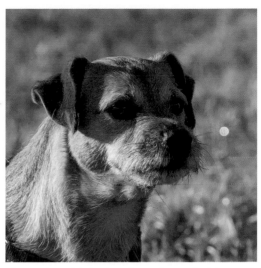

**Figure 2.2** This image shows lips pulled forward in tension as well as pricked ears and widened eyes focused on the object of interest. All the muscles in the face are tense. Photo: Peter Baumber

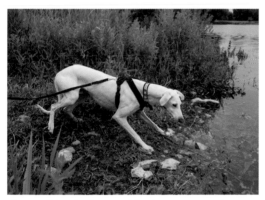

**Figure 2.3** The lowered body posture and tucked hindquarters with weight shifted backwards. Muscle tension is visible throughout the body and can also be seen in the face, with the corner of the lips pulled backwards. Photo: Peter Baumber

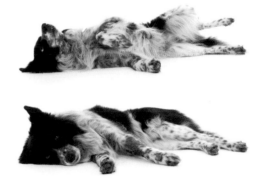

**Figure 2.4a–b** In the first image you can see the tension in the face (tense lips and focused eyes) and body, as well as the tucked tail. This dog is not comfortable with the person approaching. Compare this with the relaxation seen in the second image. Photo: Peter Baumber

person and a resource that it wishes to protect. Likewise, a dog lying down may place a paw on top of an object for which it wishes to keep hold.

- **Tension may be seen in the dog's tail and the tail carriage may alter, either moving the tail up over the back or tucking the tail down between the legs** (but it may be difficult to interpret tail carriage depending on the breed). Wagging, if it occurs, will be tight and with small deviation from the vertical.

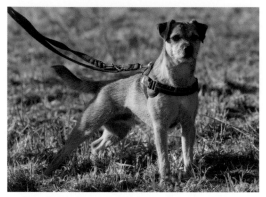

**Figure 2.5** This image shows the dog's body weight shifted forwards with the raised head, focused gaze and pricked ears. This dog may simply be interested in something in the distance, or be showing increasing levels of arousal that may lead to a reaction aimed at the focus of his attention. The context of the behaviour as well as the changes in the behaviour over time will enable an observer to better judge the dog's emotion and motivation. Photo: Peter Baumber

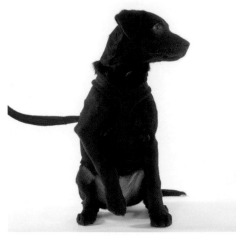

**Figure 2.6** Paw lifts can occur in multiple situations, so once again the context and behavioural sequence will give additional information regarding emotion and motivation. Here the rest of the dog's posture and expression indicate it is more likely to be interested in something in the environment rather than concerned about it. Photo: Peter Baumber

- **Specific actions such as yawning, blinking the eyes or nose licking** may all be signs that a dog is uncomfortable in a situation or that it is experiencing conflicting emotions or motivations. Each of these behaviours can be seen in a range of other contexts too, so it is important to view these in light of other postures and expressions. However, observing any of these should make one alert to the possibility that the dog is becoming distressed.
- **Some dogs may lift a paw** when they are uncomfortable or uncertain, and such a move, especially in a dog that is sitting, should cause a viewer to assess the situation carefully.

These postures, expressions and actions have not been listed in any specific order, although they have been assembled into a popular ladder of aggression (Shepherd, 2009). The order in which an individual dog expresses them when uncomfortable may differ between individuals, and certain elements may not feature in a given animal's repertoire, so it is key to view any of these signs as a reason to more fully assess the dog's emotional state and motivation.

## 2.5  Signs pertaining to specific emotions

### 2.5.1  Expressions of fear

#### 2.5.1.1  An anxious or mildly fearful dog

Anxiety or mild fear may manifest as body weight shifted backwards, hesitancy to approach or actually moving away or circling around to increase distance. The dog may approach

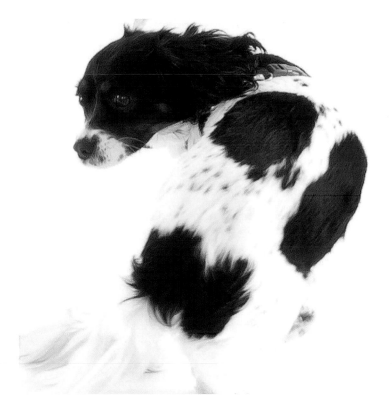

**Figure 2.7** This dog is showing mild fear. Note it is turning away from the stimulus on which it is focused with hindquarters and tail tucked under, ears pulled back, the muscles around the mouth tense and the eyes wide and staring. Photo: Peter Baumber

and back off again, or bark a few short barks. Usually the head is held low and the ears may move from pricked forward to pulled back, or may alternate. There will be tension in the muscles of the face with the eyes usually pulled into slits (the dog may have frown lines or a furrowed brow appearance) and the tail will be tucked under. If it is a person or another dog eliciting the response the tail may wag slightly, but the wagging movement is usually small, tight and may be slow.

In anxiety (the dog is worried about the possible fear inducing stimulus manifesting) as opposed to fear (the stimulus is present) it is likely to demonstrate vigilant behaviour where it scans the environment keeping a watch out for whatever it is anxious about.

### 2.5.1.2 A very fearful dog

All the above are likely to be seen, but additionally the dog is likely to attempt to freeze or try to run away. It may pant and tremble and its body will be very low to the ground with wide open eyes that appear black as a result of pupil dilation. Frequently its mouth will be open, but whether open or closed the lips will be pulled back so that the mouth opening appears long and the folds around the mouth are tight and tense. In some circumstances it may urinate or defecate.

Either of the above dogs may go on to demonstrate an overtly aggressive response, including a bite if the trigger does not move away or if they cannot remove themselves from the situation. An aggressive response as a result of fear is likely to show at least elements of the above, typically ears are pulled backwards (they may be during other aggressive responses too, hence the requirement to look at the display in its entirety), bodyweight is shifted backwards, tail is tucked and the mouth is pulled wide open. Vocalisations, if any, are likely to be of a higher pitch and variable.

*Note*: If a dog has no route to escape (including if it is on a lead) it may have to approach the individual proactively with a threat to get him or her to withdraw; this can reflect a combination of frustration (lack of easy access to safety) and fear.

### 2.5.1.3 A painful dog

Although the pain response may involve its own emotion, a dog in pain will often show fear in anticipation of painful interaction before it shows the emotion of pain. For this reason this scenario is considered here.

A dog that shows an aggressive response as a result of immediate pain may not show many warning signs, however a dog anticipating possible pain (fear of pain) may show any of the distance increasing signs listed above. Barcelos et al. (2015) recently described recurring themes in the aggressive responses of dogs with a pain focus compared to those where no pain underlies the response. Although this work does not discuss body postures or facial expressions, it was noted that dogs in pain routinely bite with less intensity at an area focused on the extremities and do not tend to undertake sustained attack, with bites frequently occurring when the dog is approached or when it is lying down. These were not consistent findings in dogs not in pain. The occurrence of these signs should not be taken to infer the animal is in pain, but rather they highlight that this possibility should be further investigated when these signs do occur.

### 2.5.2 Expressions of the desire to acquire something (emotional seeking)

#### 2.5.2.1 A dog that is attempting to control an interaction

Dogs can learn to use aggression to take control of situations, either where they feel uncomfortable or because they have learnt that the response has a positive consequence for them – through extrinsic or intrinsic reinforcement. For example, it is believed that dogs that experience approach avoidance conflict (a situation where it has a desire to move towards something and at the same time the desire to move away, e.g. it would like to greet an individual but is anxious about the consequences of an interaction) can be at risk for developing an aggressive display in these situations where it experiences the conflict (if it is not shown a more appropriate way to resolve it). It is thought that the aggressive response provides the dog with a sense of control over the situation and relief, both strong intrinsic reinforcers for the response. Additionally, as with any other behaviour, an aggressive response can be generalised across situations so once a dog has learnt that a response works to its advantage in one situation it is more likely it will evoke the same response in a novel situation.

The assessment of a dog using aggressive behaviour to take control proactively can be difficult but these dogs usually show little evidence of increased emotional arousal and will not show the preliminary warning signs indicating discomfort. Rather, they will go straight to the gesture that has worked in the past (possibly with other individuals), generally body weight forward, strong muscle tension and possibly a lowered head. It will probably stare with narrowed eyes and show lips puckered forward, possibly exposing its incisors and canines, growling, barking or snapping.

*Note:* Although dogs show non-aggressive postural signs of formal dominance and subordinance (largely based around high and low posture, van der Borg et al., 2015) in order to avoid conflict over resources, there is no evidence to indicate that a dog showing aggressive responses is motivated to do this in order to establish a hierarchy between the two for future benefit (i.e. as a demonstration of dominance now when there is no resource to compete over, so that a benefit may be gained at some later date). As far as we can tell, the dog simply finds that taking control of a specific situation pays more immediate dividends for it – either as it allows it to access something it desires, which might include a safer situation from its perspective, or because it creates a sense of relief that is reinforcing. Indeed, the expression of aggression in this context is more likely a sign that it is not clear who should take precedence.

### 2.5.2.2 A dog showing predatory behaviour

A key aspect that often differentiates bites associated with predatory behaviour from those occurring in many other circumstances is the silence of the action leading up to the attack, as the dog's aim is not to advertise its presence to its prey. In the stalk phase the body is held very still with tensed muscles, it may be slightly lowered but with weight forward. The facial expression will be tense with eyes focused on the target. If the stalking becomes a chase it will be very focused and silent, which contrasts with the usually looser body posture of a play chase, where there may also be barking.

### 2.5.2.3 A dog that enjoys chasing others

Chasing others may be a form of object or predatory play, both of which are linked to the same emotional system covered in this section. A defining feature of playful behaviour is that the signs are inherently inconsistent with the fully functional behaviour, and the dog may rapidly change behaviour spontaneously mid-sequence and turn its attention to something else. The body and face usually lack tension. Reciprocal social (rough and tumble) play is controlled by a different emotional system and its expression is discussed below.

## 2.5.3 Expressions of the emotion associated with social play

### 2.5.3.1 A dog intent on play with another individual

Although dogs appear to respond appropriately to many human gestures in playful interactions (Rooney et al., 2000, 2001), accidental bites and nips aimed at enticing play may occur in this context. There are a number of key indicators of social play. The most noticeable indication of playful intention is the presence of metasignals, such as the play bow where the front half of the body is lowered and the back half is raised. A non-visual signal known as the 'dog laugh' may also function to entice play (Simonet et al., 2005), including a playful nip. Other key signs are behaviours that are mixed into 'non-functional' sequences, i.e. they are not the complete act. For example, the dog may stalk, then run away, or chase then roll over, and finally during reciprocal play there should be swapping of roles (Bauer and Smuts, 2007) – when this occurs in humans it is easy for an accident to occur. Body postures during play are variable, in fact dogs can express virtually every posture and behaviour in their repertoire during a bout of play. So while it is common to see the relaxed open mouth expression sometimes known as a play face, it is also possible to see wrinkled lips

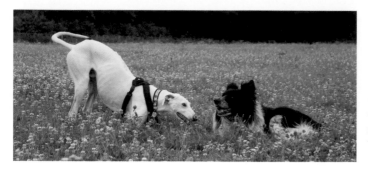

**Figure 2.8** The lurcher is exhibiting a play bow as well as showing a relaxed play face as it tries to solicit the collie to play. Photo: Peter Baumber

and snarling following a play bow, although the latter may go unnoticed and so be misinterpreted. While dogs may lope in a relaxed manner, they may also show muscle tension. They may growl and snap and bite (inhibited bites only) during play and they can also hurt one another inadvertently. Hence the importance of documenting the observations made of the encounter carefully to ensure that the correct assessment is made, with interpretations from third parties replaced by fully descriptive data wherever possible.

## 2.5.4 Expressions of emotional frustration

### 2.5.4.1 A dog defending a resource (threat of loss of a resource)

Dogs defending something they want to keep (for example, food, a possession or their space) usually start with increased muscle tension and fixed staring with their body weight shifted forward and their tail very tense and frequently raised. Ears are frequently pricked forward or rotated laterally and eyes may be narrowed, with tension seen in the muscles surrounding them. If this posturing is not successful at moving the other individual away, the dog is likely to lift its lips in a snarl, exposing the incisors and canine teeth. This is a different

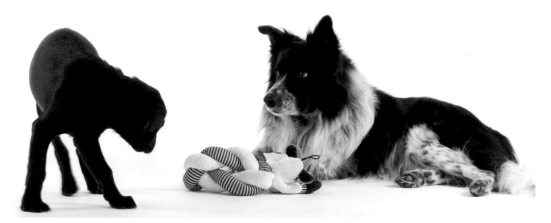

**Figure 2.9** The collie is defending the toy from the puppy. Note the direct stare with the ears pricked forward. The puppy is showing body language indicative of a desire to avoid conflict with the lowered head and averted gaze. Photo: Peter Baumber

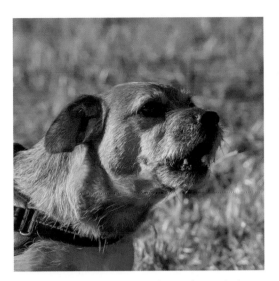

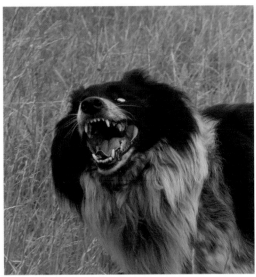

**Figure 2.10** These images shows the typical expression of an aggressive response related to frustration with the lips pulled forward and only the canines showing as the dog barks. In some cases the lips will be wrinkled up so that an overt C shape is formed, with the incisors and canines showing. Photo: Peter Baumber

**Figure 2.11** The collie in this image is showing all its teeth, however the lack of muscle tension in the face as well as the narrowed eyes tell you that this is an expression seen in play, rather than a dog that is acting defensively. Photo: Peter Baumber

expression to the mouth fully open expression where fear is the underlying emotion. A growl may accompany this. If this is unsuccessful a lunge, snap or bite may follow. Barking, if it occurs, is likely to be lower pitched.

### 2.5.4.2 A dog prevented from accessing what it wants (denial of a resource, or less than expected resource forthcoming)

The barrier to a resource may be real or perceived. In general, dogs that are demonstrating aggressive behaviour in this context will not show the early warning signs discussed above but will, in addition to the aggressive behaviours they show, exhibit a range of other responses. These dogs usually show high arousal, especially if the resource they are trying to access is very valuable to them (or the stimulus they are trying to move away from or remove from their proximity is inducing high levels of fear). They may bark (and the bark may be very variable in pitch and volume), they may pace or bounce back and forth or jump at or towards the target they are trying to access. They may show displacement behaviours such as circling or urinating. In addition, frustrated dogs may redirect their behaviour to another individual or object in the environment and for this reason can bite innocent bystanders. It is therefore key to assess the entire situation to identify the real trigger of any emotional response as well as those inadvertently caught up in the situation.

The actual aggressive response shown by these dogs may have variable ear position, tail carriage, facial expressions and vocalisations, but there will often be an immediate focus on the resource that it wishes to acquire. A prevalence of one type of posture and expression may help to understand better whether the frustration stems from the inability to move towards safety and away from an aversive stimulus (in this case fearful posturing will also be seen, this may take the form of flicking of ears between a backward and forward posture) or the inability to access a desired stimulus (in which case, fearful postures and expressions are likely to be absent, ears will not be laid back).

## 2.6 Conclusion

Thus far there are no empirical studies that characterise aggression using a consistent framework for inferring the motivational and emotional state of the animal, although a recent model has been proposed (Chapter 1 and Mills et al., 2013). Terminology is often used very loosely and confusingly without a consistent theoretical basis. Studies in this field are also hampered by a lack of empirical evidence concerning the key postures and expressions that should be attended to, with descriptions often being general (e.g. nose lick) or interpretive (e.g. worried expression), reducing their precision. Nonetheless, improvement is possible and with a rigorous scientific approach it is to be hoped that much more will become evident in the near future as interest in this field grows.

## 2.7 References

Barcelos, A. M., Mills, D. S., Zulch, H. (2015). Clinical indicators of musculoskeletal pain in aggressive dogs. Veterinary Record.

Bauer, E. B., Smuts, B. B. (2007). Co-operation and competition during dyadic play in domestic dogs, Canis familiaris. Animal Behaviour 73(3), 489–499.

Horowitz, A. (2009). Disambiguating the 'guilty look': Salient prompts to a familiar dog behaviour. Behavioural Processes 81(3) 447–452.

Mills, D., Braem Dube, M., Zulch, H. (2013). Stress and Pheromonatherapy in Small Animal Clinical Behaviour. Wiley-Blackwell, Oxford.

Pongracz, P., Molnar, C., Mikolsi, A., Csanyi, V. (2005). Human listeners are able to classify dog (Canis familiaris) barks recorded in different situations. Journal of Comparative Psychology 119(2) 136–144.

Rooney, N. J., Bradshaw, J. W., Robinson, I. H. (2000). A comparison of dog–dog and dog–human play behaviour. Applied Animal Behaviour Science, 66(3), 235–248.

Rooney, N. J., Bradshaw, J. W., Robinson, I. H. (2001). Do dogs respond to play signals given by humans? Animal Behaviour 61(4), 715-722.

Shepherd, K. (2009). Chapter 2 BSAVA Manual of Canine and Feline Behavioural Medicine Second Edition. Ed: Horwitz, D. F., Mills, D. S. 13–16 British Small Animal Veterinary Association, Gloucester.

Simonet, P., Donna, V., Storie, D. 'Dog-laughter: Recorded playback reduces stress related behavior in shelter dogs'. In Proceedings of the 7th International Conference on Environmental Enrichment, vol. 2005.

Van der Borg, J. A., Schilder, M. B., Vinke, C. M., de Vries, H. (2015). Dominance in domestic dogs: a quantitative analysis of its behavioural measures. PloS one, 10(8), e0133978.

# CHAPTER 3

# Dog Bite Statistics – Where do They Come From and What Can They Tell Us?
## *'Life is denominator based'*

*Kenton Morgan, Amy Curtis, Nicky Goodson, Libby Wilson, Laura Potts, Clare Pritchard*

## 3.1 Introduction

If you are not reading this book from cover to cover, it is likely that you have turned to this chapter to get some figures. You may not have even bothered to read this far and have already scanned the chapter for the relevant table. It isn't there! To find what you are looking for in this chapter you are going to have to read it. At the end you may feel you don't need the figures, perhaps because they don't support your argument or because you don't believe them. You may have even decided to look somewhere else – this would be a mistake – we can say with some confidence that this chapter is your best source. Read it and these figures, indeed all figures, will mean much more to you.

Stats, statistics, figures; we are seduced by them! But are they helpful? Is it of any comfort to the grieving mother of a badly mauled child to know that her tragedy is one of ten thousand or ten million? To her, one is important enough! In rich countries her heartbreak may be communicated by a disaster-hungry press to amateur dog connoisseurs keen to promote their pet theory on the control of dog aggression (see Chapters 5 and 6), and to legislators with the will and wherewithal to adopt these theories and power to change the laws. In poor countries the grief may be confined to an extended family and the relief of survival may be tempered by the threat of a lingering death from rabies, a preventable disease (Chapter 22).

## 3.2 Making sense of statistics?

So, why do we need figures? Is a report of one case of dog aggression less important than one hundred thousand? Emotionally and psychologically you may ponder this but mathematically the answer is, 'You can't tell!' These figures are meaningless. In the first case, if there were only two people in the country and one experienced dog aggression this would be fifty per cent, or one in two of the population. In the second case there may be ten million people in the country and in this case one per cent, or one in a hundred, of the population would experience dog aggression. You will note at this stage that we are expressing figures as text. This not only prevents scanning of the chapter to look for a numerical quote but it also serves to reinforce how meaningless numbers can be. The key question when presented with a number is to ask, 'What fraction or percentage of the population does this represent?' We can only estimate this by knowing the total number of the population at risk, i.e. the number of those below the line in the fraction – *the denominator*. Do not be seduced or impressed by a number again. *Life is denominator based – always ask for it.* This can be illustrated by the statistic that most pedestrians are knocked down at zebra crossings (a UK institution); this does not mean that they are dangerous places, just that a large number of people *use* them to cross the road. The proportion or fraction of people knocked down at zebra crossings is quite small.

### 3.2.1  Life is denominator based!

So, next time you see or hear any number in the media or in a scientific journal whatever the topic, you should always ask, 'What is the denominator?' Let us now explore why this is important. When we make the statement, for example, 'There are one hundred thousand cases of dog bites each year in a population of ten million,' we are expressing a probability. If we take a moment to write out the fraction one hundred thousand over ten million, and cancel out the zeros, we are left with one in a hundred. This is a probability or risk. In statistical terms, they are the same thing. Currently, society thinks of risk in a negative way, but historically, and possibly in the future, its use was and will be synonymous with probability. Knowing that the denominator allows us to state the risk that a particular dog breed should be banned because it is responsible for most bites, we can recognise the importance of asking, 'How many individuals of that breed are there in the population?' Using this as the denominator, we could estimate the risk of a particular breed biting someone, and perhaps get surprising results. A major practical problem is the lack of an accurate census that provides the total number of dogs and dog breeds.

## 3.3  What is the risk from dog aggression?

We hope that you recognise that you want to know about risk, not numbers, so you might well ask, 'What is the risk of a person experiencing dog aggression?' Unfortunately the answer is, 'No one knows.' But we can try to answer other relevant questions such as, 'What is the risk of a person attending a hospital accident and emergency unit because of a dog bite?' It is one in three hundred and eighty five; or two point six per thousand per year.

### 3.3.1  How confident can we be in these figures?

'How do we know?' This is an average figure for all the reports published in peer review journals up to 2012 from all over the world for which the population at risk is given (Edwards 2012a). 'Are we certain?' 'No!' This single figure combines data from different countries, and is influenced by factors such as differences in access to emergency care, population age structure, ratio of dogs to people, etc., and social and housing variability, etc.. It homogenises data from very heterogeneous countries into one number representing risk. But, given these caveats, we are ninety five per cent confident that the figure lies between one point four and three point eight per thousand per year (Edwards, 2012a). This is called the confidence interval and every percentage you ever see has one in its shadow; we will discuss how important confidence intervals are, and why they are rarely seen, later in this chapter.

So, in a city with a population of five hundred thousand we would expect between seven hundred and nineteen hundred cases a year, about two to five per day. Dog bites are not an uncommon phenomenon at accident and emergency units.

So, it might seem we have some reliable global summary statistics for the risk of being bitten by a dog. But do we? Next time you are with a group of friends, pose the question, 'Have you *ever* been bitten by a dog?' The answers may surprise you. Follow this with, 'Did you go to the doctor?' and you will immediately become aware of the difficulty in estimating the risk of dog bites. Many more people are bitten than those reporting to a GP or hospital accident and emergency unit. If the cases are never recorded they cannot be used to estimate risk. So, the best estimate we have is the risk of attending an accident and emergency unit because of a dog bite. By their very nature these are the most severe bites or those that become infected.

Let us imagine what might happen if someone gets bitten by a dog; the bite may be painful but not penetrate the skin or it may cause superficial injury that is treated by washing and the application of antiseptic. What fraction, proportion or percentage of bites is in this category? We can only guess, but your casual survey of friends may suggest that it is quite high, possibly more than fifty per cent, one half! We can consider the decision as to whether to go to a doctor or not like a fork in the road with left and right turns representing the decision to seek medical help or not. This is shown in Figure 3.1. Let us say, for example, that twenty per cent of people who are bitten seek medical assistance, as suggested by one study (Sacks et al., 1996) So eighty per cent of bites are treated at home. The probability of seeking medical attention is zero point two. If the bite is severe the victim may immediately attend a hospital accident and emergency unit. If it is mild he or she may wait for evening surgery and see a GP. Let us assume that forty per cent attend hospital accident and emergency unit. We can now calculate the percentage of total bites seen at a hospital by multiplying the probabilities; it is eight per cent! So the real risk of bites may be more than twelve times greater that the estimate obtained by our diligent attempts to review every published paper, reporting bites presented at hospital accident and emergency units, in which the denominator is mentioned.

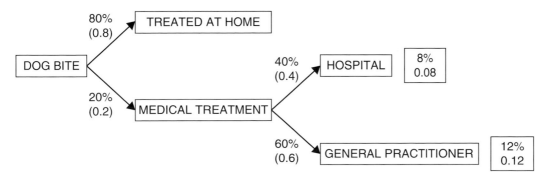

**Figure 3.1** Hypothetical probability of a person who has been bitten ending up in a hospital accident and emergency unit.

## 3.3.2  Confidence intervals

We hope that by this point we have convinced you of the dangers of being swayed by figures, and the importance of asking for denominators and the confidence intervals that lurk in the shadow of every percentage. Let us look at these important shadows more closely.

The only way the results of a survey can be scientifically extended or generalised to the whole population is by using confidence intervals. Unless the whole population is surveyed, using a census, no percentage value whether for a bite, a viewpoint or disease is exact. It is an estimate. If the sample is random and reasonably large, this percentage can be used to estimate what the real value is in the whole population. Unfortunately this is not one figure; it is a range of figures lying between a high and low percentage. This is the confidence interval. The range of these percentages will depend on how confident you want to be about this estimate – it is important to appreciate that in science we can never be 100 per cent confident. Usually ninety-five per cent is used, but this is just a convention. So, the next time you see the results of a poll that indicates that fifty-five per cent of people are going to vote for a political party, think about the confidence interval. If it is forty-five to sixty-five, it means that the poll is ninety-five per cent certain that the real voting pattern lies between these figures. So, the predicted winner might lose; confidence intervals are rarely mentioned in politics!

## 3.4  Do dog bite reports relate to dog bites?

### 3.4.1  Hospital populations

So now, armed with the dictum that *life is denominator based* let us re-examine the figures on dog-related incidents that result in people going to hospital. Of course, they are important. If two thousand people present with a dog bite injury at hospital accident and emergency units each year (we sneaked in a denominator – time) then the doctors and nurses staffing these departments need to be trained in how to deal with these cases. If the figure is two every ten years it is a low priority. Hospital statistics are useful for hospital management, training and prioritisation but they tell us little about the risk in the population. Nevertheless, a number of estimates of the dog bite problem are based on cases seen in hospitals. So what proportion of cases seen in a hospital accident and emergency unit are dog bites? A review of all published data in which the denominator is mentioned (the rest is unusable) indicates that the proportion of patients attending hospital accident and emergency units who have dog bites is six point seven per thousand. 'And the 95 per cent confidence intervals?' From three point eight to nine point five.

But this is not the whole story, and we cannot simply quote this figure as a matter of fact and leave it at that. We are only halfway through our search for value in this sideways look at dog bite accounting.

We need to consider what we mean by a dog bite (see also Chapter 1). What are they? Why do they happen? Although this book aims to increase our understanding of dog bites, in many chapters, the authors talk about dog aggression. These are not synonymous. Is the child that gets bitten when playing tug with an energetic pup a victim of dog aggression? Is the owner who gets bitten because he or she tried to break up a fight between two dogs a victim of dog aggression towards people or, in military terms, just collateral damage?

Definitions are important. Here we focus on 'reports of dog bites'. Getting an estimate of the frequency of dog aggression in a population is almost impossible; finding it for dog bites is hard enough. Definitions are important because they influence the way in which dog bites are recorded on official statistics. In UK accident and emergency data, dog bites are categorised and recorded among 'Bites, Strikes and Stings'. An audit of this category in one major UK hospital revealed that fewer than half (forty three per cent) were dog bites, nineteen were insect stings and twenty-one per cent were human bites. And the shadow? The confidence interval for dog bites was thirty-seven to fifty per cent. (Edwards, 2012b). It is important to note that in the UK hospital admission data for 'dog bites', often quoted in the media, actually relate to 'being bitten or struck by a dog'; it includes being knocked over by a dog.

People may be bitten by dogs for a multitude of reasons. Many people have a pet theory as to how they can be prevented but the evidence that any of these interventions work is at best slim (see Chapter 29). But what about the bites themselves; can they be classified in any way? Is the dog that has its owners hand playfully between its teeth biting? Is a bite to the leg different to that to the hand? Is a bite that penetrates the skin different to one that results in teeth mark bruises? Are bites that involve children different to those that involve adults?

The location of the bite on the body and the age and sex of person are recorded at hospital accident and emergency units; what do they tell us about the physical location of dog bites and the age and sex of the person who has been bitten? Let us start with gender or sex; our systematic review of the literature revealed a percentage split of about sixty–forty in favour of males. We hope you didn't just accept this figure! The percentage of males was sixty-two with a tight confidence interval from sixty-one to sixty-three.

What about the location of bites? If we classify bites into those to the head, trunk upper and lower limbs we find that thirty-seven per cent of dog bites that involve children affect the head, this is about one in three. The confidence interval? Between twenty-four and forty-eight per cent of the total. This is very different to adults, where only eight per cent of bites affect the head (confidence interval zero point five to twenty-one per cent) (Edwards, 2012a).

A plausible explanation of this difference is the relative height of children and adults compared to dogs (but see Chapter 30 for greater discussion of this point).

So can we conclude that the risk of a bite injury to a child being on the face or head is between zero point two four and zero point four eight? Sadly not, our conclusion can only be that this is the risk of a bite injury to a child *that results in hospital attendance* being on the face or head. Similar caveats apply to the risk of injury to the torso, upper and lower limbs. The prevalence of injury to the lower limbs is forty-six per cent for adults (confidence interval: twenty-six to sixty-six per cent) and thirty per cent for children (confidence interval: twenty to thirty-nine). Here we see that the confidence intervals overlap. So while we might be tempted to conclude that the statistics provide support for the conclusion that the anatomical location of serious bite injuries reflects the relative size of dog and person, these percentages may not be statistically different. This is why confidence intervals are so important. If we always ask for them when presented with a percentage it will indicate whether the percentages are different without using complicated statistical tests.

## 3.4.2 The wider population

The above data are from hospital populations and, as we have seen, this probably represents a limited proportion of the total number of bites. Is there any way we can get data from the general population … what about social media? Is it possible that a being bitten by a dog is such a marked event in someone's life that they would tweet it or post to Facebook or Instagram?

Using #dogbite to search Twitter, Facebook and Instagram produced around 13,000 images in Instagram (Statigram) and about two-thirds of these were dog bite injuries; eighty-four per cent (confidence interval: seventy-nine to eighty-eight) were of adults and nine per cent (confidence interval: six to thirteen) children (Potts, 2014). Seventy-three per cent (confidence interval: fifty-seven to eighty-six) of bites to children in this population were to the face, compared with seventeen per cent (confidence interval: thirteen to twenty-three) for adults. In adults, around half the bites (confidence interval: forty-three to fifty-six per cent) were to the finger, hand and lower arm with approximately equal distributions to each. This compares with thirty-six (confidence interval: nineteen to fifty-three) per cent from hospital data. Are these percentages different? You decide. The most common type of injury was superficial but penetrated the skin. These accounted for almost two-thirds of injuries (confidence interval: fifty-four to sixty-six) per cent. Fewer than twenty per cent of injuries were non-penetrative.

The wealth of photos on Instagram provide a hint of the way in which 'big data' gathered by scraping the internet may be used to gather statistics about health issues in future. But who are these individuals who post traumatic images of themselves for public view and epidemiological analysis? At the time of our study Instagram had eighty million users; from this we can estimate the proportion of Instagram users who report dog bite injuries to be one in ten thousand.

This is an estimate of the risk of dog bites in the general population, but this is less than our estimate of risk based on the proportion of the population visiting hospital accident and emergency departments.

* Is this because our systematic review was incorrect?
* Is it because not all the Instagram population report dog bites?
* Is it because Instagram users are less at risk because they don't go out, preferring to play virtual games with dogs rather than confront the real thing?

Who knows, but what these figures demonstrate is that **just because the data are big and easily available they may not be representative of the general population**.

## 3.5 Breed-related risk

And now to the final question, the big question, the legislative question, the headline grabbing question. Which breed of dog is most frequently involved in dog bite injuries? This is perhaps easier to answer: German shepherd dogs!

You don't believe us? You should want the data, so that you can assess the evidence yourself. Let us look at it. A review of all the papers in which the breed of dog is described provides data on almost one thousand five hundred dog bite injuries (Edwards, 2012a). Ignoring for the moment the ability of people to recognise different breeds, German shepherds are responsible for just over a third of these with the next most common breeds – Doberman, Jack Russell, Pit Bull and Chow Chow – accounting for just seven per cent each. These represent the combination of nineteen published studies. But since 'life is denominator based', we need to know which dogs are most common? In the absence of a world dog census we really have no accurate figure on this.

We can find data on the internet relating to registration numbers with kennel clubs for many countries or microchip data. But what do these data mean? Are they really representative of the popularity of dog breeds or do they reflect value, breeding potential or socio-economic status of the owner? These data indicate that one of the most common breeds of dog is the German shepherd! The most common culprit is also one of the most common dogs. We are back at the zebra crossing again.

So, does this mean breed is not important? By no means! It's just that the evidence that incriminated breeds rather than individual animals is non-existent. There may be a breed effect. Labradors are the most common breed worldwide in almost all surveys but in the hierarchy of published dog bite data they come tenth, accounting for just three per cent of bites – seen in hospital accident and emergency units. There have been just three studies that have tried to relate the number of bites by each breed to the number of that breed in the population. Rottweilers had the highest Breed Risk Index in one study and German shepherds in another. In the third 'terriers' were the most common group associated with bites (Edwards, 2012a).

## 3.6 Conclusion

If dog bites are so important why aren't figures collected in the correct way? This is a challenge to epidemiologists and requires a concerted effort from a number of different researchers, agencies and research funders.

But what would happen even if we had a result? Let us pretend for the moment that we carry out this study in the UK and we demonstrate that German shepherds and Jack Russell Terriers pose the greatest threat of being bitten. Would these breeds be banned or is their social status such that they would get away with a reprimand or with carefully collected data being discredited because they produced the wrong answer?

'Life is denominator based' and it is our concluding request that in future the opinions of those seeking to understand and manage issues relating to dog bites, will be too.

## 3.7 References

Edwards, A. R., (2012a). The Dog Bite Problem: A Meta-Analysis and Systematic Review of Existing Dog Bite Literature. Dissertation submitted under requirement for MRes. University of Liverpool.

Edwards, A. R., (2012b). A Clinical Audit of Dog Bite Information Recorded at Two Liverpool Hospitals. Dissertation submitted under requirement for MRes. University of Liverpool.

Potts, L., (2014). #Dogbite: Analysis of reporting human dog bite injuries using social networking websites. Dissertation submitted as part of BVSc degree, University of Liverpool

Sacks, J. J., Kresnow, M., Houston, B. (1996). Dog bites: how big a problem? *Injury Prevention* 2:52–4.

# CHAPTER 4

# Dog Bites From a Public Health Perspective

*Francine Watkins and Carri Westgarth*

## 4.1 Introduction

Dog bites have come to represent a significant public health problem in the United Kingdom and other western countries. In addition to how much the physical consequences of dog bites can cost to the health system, even those not requiring medical attention can still have a significant impact on physical health and also on mental health due to the psychological distress experienced by victims (Chapter 23).

## 4.2 What is public health?

The World Health Organisation defines public health as, 'The organised measures (whether public or private) to prevent disease, promote health, and prolong life among the population as a whole.' The WHO activities aim to, 'provide conditions in which people can be healthy and focus on entire populations, not on individual patients or diseases'. Public health is therefore concerned with the total health system and how it operates at all levels – local, regional and national. The three main public health functions defined by the WHO are:

- The assessment and monitoring of the health of communities and populations at risk to identify health problems and priorities
- The formulation of public policies designed to solve identified local and national health problems and priorities
- To ensure that all populations have access to appropriate and cost-effective care, including health promotion and disease prevention services.

WHO 2015

Public health is therefore the study of health and well-being at the community and population levels especially as monitored, regulated, and promoted by the state. The UK's Faculty of Public Health defines public health as:

*The science and art of promoting and protecting health and well-being, preventing ill-health and prolonging life through the organised efforts of society.*

The faculty's approach is that public health is population-based; it emphasises collective responsibility for health, its protection and prevention and the key role of the state, and there is a link to the underlying socio-economic and wider determinants of health and disease.

## 4.3 The current approach to dog bite prevention

Most bites are considered by experts to be preventable (De Keuster, Lamoureux et al., 2006; Mills and Levine, 2006) and most people are bitten by dogs familiar to them (Voith, 2009). Experts are increasingly turning their attention to *how* bites occur and implying that a major (if not the main) reason is because people misinterpret or cannot read dog behaviour (Overall and Love, 2001, Chapter 2). As such, intervention programmes have been developed to target the education of children and adults about reading the signs that a dog is unhappy and may bite; strategies are then provided about how to interact safely with dogs (Wilson, Dwyer et al., 2003; Duperrex, Blackhall et al., 2009; Schwebel, Morrongiello et al., 2012, Chapter 29). Intervention materials therefore have been designed to educate people on how they can prevent a dog bite by assessing the body language of dogs in high-risk situations in order for them to recognise the risk and take appropriate action (Chapter 30). These preventions are based on the perception that the dog is only biting because it has to and therefore implicit to this approach is that it is the victim who is therefore considered largely at fault. This is despite the view in the media that it is the dog that is to blame rather than the victim, especially in the case of child bites (Chapter 5).

However, this perspective and the approaches that follow from it, i.e. that dog bites can be largely prevented (apart from those sustained from an 'attack' dog) by education in dog body language, does not appear to have been challenged intellectually to any great degree. As dog bites are thought to be increasing (BBC, 2011), it poses the question of whether this traditional 'victim blaming' approach to dog bite prevention is working as well as it should. There has also been little research on the circumstances surrounding a dog bite. In particular, little is known about the socio-economic circumstances of those who are bitten as well as the experiences of being bitten by a dog, in particular how victims thought the incident could have been prevented and why the dog bit them.

## 4.4 The social determinants of health and health inequalities

Wilkinson and Marmot (2003) have argued that even in the most affluent countries people who are poorer will have a substantially shorter life expectancy and be prone to more disease and ill health than those who are better off. This is due to the specific social, environmental and economic conditions within which people are born, grow, live, work and age, and these can be shaped by the distribution, or uneven distribution, of resources at a local, national and international level. These differences in health can be attributed to the social determinants of health (Department of Health, 1998; Marmot and Wilkinson, 2006; World Health

# The Main Determinants of Health

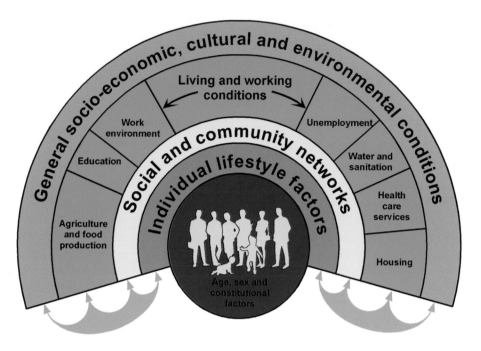

Source: Dahlgren and Whitehead, 1993

**Figure 4.1** Determinants of Health. (Source: Dahlgren and Whitehead, 1993)

Organisation, 2013). These social determinants do not exist in isolation but are interlinked, as clearly demonstrated in the representation of the wider social determinants of health by Dahlgren and Whitehead (1993) (see Figure 4.1).

This model provides a clear representation of how these determinants of health are related and are interlinked. Individuals can be exposed to multiple determinants of health at any one time. So, for example, where people lives can impact on their access to education and then later to work opportunities and, if they are then in long-term unemployment because of their poor education, this can then impact on their access to affordable housing and access to resources. The interlinking of these social determinants can also impact on an individual's resilience and their ability to change their situation. Researchers have also identified a relationship between health inequalities and the social determinants of health (Marmot, 2006; 2010; Graham, 2007; Wilkinson and Pickering, 2010):

> *'The weight of scientific evidence supports a socio-economic explanation of health inequalities. This traces the roots of ill health to such determinants as income, education and employment as well as to the material environment and lifestyle.'*
>
> *(Acheson et al., 1998)*

To really understand dog bites, and therefore understand how to prevent them, there is a need to examine the impact of the social determinants of health on the prevalence of dog bites and dog aggression, and consequently the role of health inequalities. See Figure 4.2 for a hypothesised model of determinants of dog bites.

However, there is still not enough evidence about the social determinants of health and health inequalities in relation to dog bites and dog aggression. The Black Report in 1980 (Townsend and Davidson, 1982), the Whitehead Report in 1987 (Whitehead et al., 1992), the Acheson Report in 1998 (Department of Health, 1998) and the Marmot Review (Marmot, 2010) have all highlighted the existence of disparities in health across the population and demonstrated a clear link to social class and economic disadvantage. Therefore it may not be surprising that geographical locations with high dog bite incidents in the UK are also locations with high deprivation (HSCIC, 2014). Although these types of findings may be explained in part by higher rates of dog ownership in low socio-economic areas (Westgarth et al., 2013), there may also be a conducive mixture of environments, knowledge, social norms and dog breed types, which combine to increase the risk of serious dog bites requiring hospital treatment. However, in a similar manner to making individuals more responsible for their own health through initiatives such as Change 4 Life, the emphasis is often placed on the responsibility of the dog owner, or the bite victim, and an assumption that if dog owners were more responsible, or bite victims behaved appropriately around dogs, there would be a reduction in dog bite incidence, without addressing the social determinants of their behaviour (see Chapter 31).

## 4.5 Understanding the evidence in relation to dog bites

### 4.5.1 Traditional approaches

As Christley and colleagues argue (Chapter 10) numerous studies have adopted an epidemiological approach to investigate issues related to dog bites in order to identify patterns of occurrence, and whether the pattern varies in individuals with different characteristics. The type of evidence produced through epidemiological studies is underpinned by positivist philosophical epistemology. Positivist epistemology is based on the principle that there is one concrete 'truth' that exists and this truth can be measured and observed using quantitative research methods (Bruce and Watkins, 2008).

### 4.5.2 Getting a more complete picture

In public health there has been a historical privilege of epidemiological studies over other types of research paradigms but other researchers have critiqued this approach and argued that this approach does not always reveal the full picture (Petticrew and Roberts, 2003). Researchers can adopt a different approach to gathering and understanding evidence. These more qualitative approaches have been influenced by social constructivism and instead argue that there is not one truth but multiple 'truths'. Human beings actively construct and interpret knowledge as a result of the historical, social, political processes and interactions they experience. These constructions are made in relation to our own biographies and through shared understandings, and modified in the light of new experiences. For that reason there cannot be one universal truth but rather multiple meanings and understandings that are

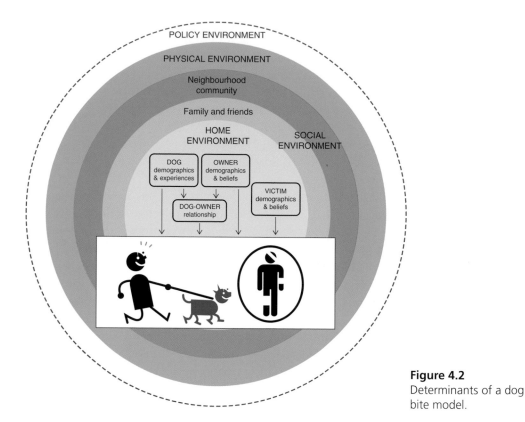

**Figure 4.2**
Determinants of a dog bite model.

therefore socially constructed and coexist (Nettleton, 2006; Green and Thorogood, 2014). These 'truths' will change and shift over time, and between different contexts. Therefore, to only look for 'one factual truth' and not look at the 'multiple truths' surrounding a dog bite incident means that critical parts of the issue may be missed. This links to the discussion in Chapter 1, where it has been argued that there is not one 'truth' of how a bite occurs but multiple circumstances and emotions that can result in a bite. Each of these will therefore require different prevention strategies and not just one universal prevention strategy.

There is a significant paucity of qualitative work exploring the perspectives of people bitten by dogs and the context within which they live and work. What has not been understood clearly is how social determinants may restrict an individual's ability to prevent being bitten within the constraints of their circumstances. To really understand dog bites, and understand how to prevent them, there is a need to examine the impact of the social determinants of health on the prevalence of dog bites and identify the health inequalities associated with dog aggression.

For example, the effectiveness of an educational interventional approach, and therefore successful prevention, is dependent on whether the victim believes that he or she requires this knowledge, can make sense of the knowledge and has the ability to implement it within his or her own context and take action. Before interventions can be tailored, greater understanding of the specific circumstances surrounding how dog bites happen is needed in order to know how to target interventions that will tackle the underlying issues.

**Table 4.1** Key themes identified and their parallels with common beliefs recognised as impediments to injury prevention (Westgarth & Watkins, 2015).

| Identified theme concerning perception of dog bites | Common beliefs recognised as impediments to injury prevention (Hemenway, 2013) | Description |
|---|---|---|
| "It will never happen to me" | It will never happen to me | Optimism that nothing bad will happen |
| "Just one of those things" | Accidents happen | A fatalistic view than nothing could be done to prevent it |
| "Don't blame the dog" – Victim or owner at fault instead | Victim blaming | When bad things happen the person probably deserved it |

A recent qualitative in-depth study into the perspectives of dog bite victims as to why the bite occurred (Westgarth and Watkins, 2015) has begun to elucidate the complexity in trying to prevent bites in a real-life context. It suggests that there may be constructed beliefs and perceptions that act as barriers to successful injury prevention, regardless of how knowledgeable the victim is in reading the signs that a dog is unhappy and may bite. These barriers include: the perception of the victim that he or she does not 'blame the dog' and is more likely to blame the owner; the perception that dog bites are 'just one of those things'; and a perception that 'it wouldn't happen to me' (See Table 4.1).

## 4.6 Conclusion

A public health approach to dog bite prevention should focus not on blame, whether that is 'victim blaming' or 'owner blaming', but instead on the creation of a society where dog bites are less likely to occur in the first place, by tackling the societal determinants of dog bites from a public health perspective. This includes individual human and dog behaviour, but also family and physical environments, access to resources, and policies impacting dog ownership and breeding. If bites are to be prevented, far more research into the contexts and circumstances of dog bites is required.

## 4.7 References

BBC. (2011, 11 August). 'More people admitted to hospital after dog injuries'. BBC News, from www.bbc.co.uk/news/health-14489360

Bruce, N., Watkins, F. (2008). Philosophy of Science and Introduction to Epidemiology. In Bruce, N., Pope, D., Stanistreet, D. (2008). Quantitative Research Methods in Public Health: A practical, interactive guide. J Wiley & Sons: London.

Dahlgren, G., Whitehead, M. (1993). Tackling inequalities in health: what can we learn from what has been tried? Working paper prepared for the King's Fund International Seminar on Tackling Inequalities in Health, September 1993, Ditchley Park, Oxfordshire.

De Keuster, T., Lamoureux, J., Kahn, A. (2006). Epidemiology of dog bites: a Belgian experience of canine behaviour and public health concerns. The Veterinary Journal, 172(3), 482–487.

Department of Health (1998) The Acheson Report. Independent inquiry into inequalities in health. Accessed at https://www.gov.uk/government/uploads/system/uploads/attachment_data/file/265503/ih.pdf

Duperrex, O., Blackhall, K., Burri, M., Jeannot, E. (2009). Education of children and adolescents for the prevention of dog bite injuries. The Cochrane Library.

Graham, H. (2007). Unequal Lives: Health and Socioeconomic Inequalities. Open University Press.

Green, J., Thorogood, N. (2014). Qualitative Methods for Health Research. 3rd Edn. Sage: London.

Hemenway, D. (2013). Three common beliefs that are impediments to injury prevention. Injury prevention, 19(4), 290–293.

Health & Social Care Information Centre (2014). Provisional monthly topic of interest: admissions caused by dogs and other mammals. http://www.hscic.gov.uk/catalogue/PUB14030/prov-mont-hes-admi-outp-ae-April%202013%20to%20January%202014-toi-rep.pdf

Marmot, M. (2006). Health in an unequal world. Lancet 368 (9552) 2081–2094.

Marmot, M., Wilkinson, R., (2006). Social Determinants of Health (2nd Edition). Oxford University Press.

Marmot, M., (2010) Fair Society, Healthy Lives: A Strategic Review of Health Inequalities in England Post-2010. The Marmot Review.

Mills, D. S., Levine, E. (2006). The need for a co-ordinated scientific approach to the investigation of dog bite injuries. The Veterinary Journal 172(3): 398–399.

Nettleton, S. (2006). The Sociology of Health and Illness. Plity Press: Cambridge.

Overall, K. L., M., Love. (2001). 'Dog bites to humans – demography, epidemiology, injury, and risk.' Journal of the American Veterinary Medical Association 218(12): 1923–1934.

Petticrew, M., Roberts, H. (2003). Evidence, hierarchies, and typologies: horses for courses. Journal Epidemiology Community Health 57: 527–529

Schwebel, D. C., Morrongiello, B. A., Davis, A. L., Stewart, J., Bell, M. (2012). The Blue Dog: Evaluation of an interactive software program to teach young children how to interact safely with dogs. Journal of Pediatric Psychology 37(3): 272–281.

Townsend, P., Davidson, N., (1982). Inequalities in Health: The Black Report.

Voith, V. L. (2009). The Impact of Companion Animal Problems on Society and the Role of Veterinarians. Veterinary Clinics of North America-Small Animal Practice 39(2): 327–345.

Westgarth, C., Boddy, L. M., Stratton, G., German, A. J., Gaskell, R. M., Coyne, K. P., Bundred, P., McCune, S., Dawson, S, et al. (2013). 'Pet ownership, dog types and attachment to pets in 9–10 year old children in Liverpool, UK'. BMC Veterinary Research 9(1): 102.

Westgarth, C., Watkins, F. (2015). A qualitative investigation of the perceptions of female dog-bite victims and implications for the prevention of dog bites. Journal of Veterinary Behavior: Clinical Applications and Research, 10(6), 479–488.

Whitehead, M. (1992). The Health Divide. In Townsend, P., Whitehead, M., and Davidson, N. Inequalities in Health: New Edition. London, Penguin, 1992.

WHO. World Health Organisation, 2013. Review of social determinants and the health divide in the WHO European Region: final report. WHO http://www.euro.who.int/__data/assets/pdf_file/0004/251878/Review-of-social-determinants-and-the-health-divide-in-the-WHO-European-Region-FINAL-REPORT.pdf?ua=1

Wilkinson, R., Marmot, M., 2003. The Social Determinants of Health: The Solid Facts. Available at: http://www.euro.who.int/__data/assets/pdf_file/0005/98438/e81384.pdf

Wilkinson, R.G., Pickering, K. (2010). The Spirit Level: Why Equality is Better for Everyone. Penguin: London.

Wilson, F., Dwyer, F., Bennett, P. C. (2003). Prevention of dog bites: Evaluation of a brief educational intervention program for preschool children. Journal of Community Psychology, 31(1), 75–86.

# Section 2
# Perceptions of Dogs that Bite

In Section 2 we consider different aspects of our perceptions of dogs that bite. In Chapter 5, Mie Kikuchi and James Oxley introduce the topic of media representation of dog aggression. They present their findings about the inconsistency and unreliability of media reporting surrounding bite incidents. It is thus important that action and policy is not driven solely by this biased media representation. In Chapter 6, Simon Harding uses humanities and social science methods to delve deeper into the societal perspectives surrounding the use of dogs for 'status'. He describes how he feels that some individuals of certain dog breeds, notably bull breeds, can be owned primarily for reasons of status and commodity, and linked with protection and aggression in gang-land culture. There is no doubt that these breeds are owned in high numbers in certain geographical locations and depicted to be aggressive in cultural media (as discussed further in Chapters 5 and 7). However, whether only these large, strong-looking dogs reflect status and power of an owner requires deeper investigation. It could be argued that perhaps all types and breeds of dogs reflect status of the owner in some way, for example the bejewelled 'handbag dogs' of the young model are as much a sign of status as the protection dog of the aggressive adolescent. Much more research is required into why people choose to own different breeds of dogs, and the impacts of these choices on the communities that they live in. In Chapter 7, Tracey Clarke explores specifically the issues of breed representation of aggressiveness and how this has been shaped by the popular media. She explains how the portrayal of the personality and behaviour of certain breeds is not always backed by clear evidence, and so comes to the conclusion that there are several reasons why breed-specific legislation should be repealed. Overall, this second section of the book illustrates that the societal perspectives surrounding risk of dog bites are based largely on cultural misperceptions and media perpetuation of these. It is a challenge to modify these views but a necessity if dog bite prevention initiatives are to be more evidence based.

CHAPTER 5

# The Representation of Human-Directed Aggression in the Popular Media

*Mie Kikuchi and James Oxley*

## 5.1 Introduction

Human–directed aggressive dog behaviour (HDAB) is considered to be the most serious behaviour problem of dogs in a worldwide context (Overall and Love, 2001; Messam et al., 2007; Hsu and Sun, 2010) and so it is not surprising that it receives a lot of media attention. The public acquire their knowledge through a variety of sources such as books, magazines, newspapers, television, family/friends, breeders, pet shops, and the internet. Oxley et al. (2012) conducted an online and face to face survey of 459 UK dog owners. They found that 361 (78.6%) could name at least one type of banned dog listed under the Dangerous Dogs Act 1991, of these, 48.7% sourced their information from either the internet or television, 12% by word of mouth and a further 7.6% were from newspapers.

As technology improves, public media is becoming increasingly accessible (through the internet, mobile phones, tablets, etc.), providing current information almost instantaneously, anywhere and on demand (Semiocast, 2013). For example: the National Readership Survey (2014) found 90% (46.5 million/52 million) of those aged fifteen or over in Great Britain read news brands via hardcopy and/or digital format. Some 71% of those aged fifteen or over read hardcopy, while 69% read online news brands. The Japanese Ministry of Internal Affairs and Communications (2014) found that 93% of survey participants (N=1,500) sourced general information from television, 71.1% from newspapers, 66% from the internet and 25% from magazines. This means that people can easily select a wide range of online information that, as with hardcopy, may be inaccurate, and often biased. Therefore, the media and its representation of canine aggression has an important role in delivering information about both risk and prevention to the public as it influences their perception/belief and knowledge about these subjects. Further, it needs to be recognised that the content provided is often adjusted to cater for the interests of the target audience and so the way in which the message is delivered is also important in shaping public attitudes (Tanaka, 1998; Orritt and Harper, 2015). Overall, there exists only a small number of studies into what information regarding dog aggression, attacks and bites is covered in popular media (Podberscek, 1994;

Oxley and Tibbott, 2012; Kikuchi et al., 2014). However, it is clear certain breeds of dog can have their popularity altered rapidly as a result of their portrayal by the popular media (Chapter 7, Ghirlanda et al., 2014).

In this chapter, we review how the popular media represents aggressive behaviour, attacks and bites in dogs and what factors influence public perception of HDAB, including possible cultural effects.

## 5.2  Previous research relating to dog bites and the media

Newspaper and online media articles related to dog bites have been collated previously in the United States, Canada and the UK (see Table 5.1).

For example, Pinckney and Kennedy (1982) collected information on seventy-four individual dog attack newspaper cases in the United States, from 1966 to June 1980. These resulted in sixty-four deaths, twenty-three of which were babies under the age of one and therefore unlikely to be accused of teasing a dog. Of the 106 dogs involved in reported fatal attacks, the majority (seventy-nine) were stated as being of a recognisable breed, most often the German shepherd, with just twenty-two noted as mixed breeds. Although the authors conclude that German shepherds were the most popular breed associated with reported attacks, they note that breed-related information may be unreliable and interpretation needs caution. Nonetheless, in the UK, as a result of intense media coverage and speculation in relation to the role of certain breeds in dog attacks, breed-specific legislation in the form of the Dangerous Dogs Act 1991 was introduced without scientific evidence to support this risk (Brooman and Legge, 1997). Podberscek (1994) investigated dog attacks and associated breeds in newspaper articles two years before and two years after the implementation of this highly controversial law and concluded that the legislation was an overreaction in response to media articles that were biased in relation to specific breeds such as the pit bull. Orritt and Harper (2015) have recently described a cycle of events involving behaviour reported in media articles, public risk/perception and legislative change (see Figure 5.1.) that may initiate and perpetuate the implementation of a controversial law instigated by increased media coverage, as seen with the Dangerous Dogs Act 1991. Orritt and Harper (2015) also discuss similarities between UK media articles covering aggressive dogs and that referring to sex offenders, noting specific commonalities in the terms used, themes concerning the

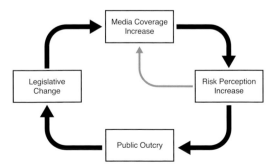

**Figure 5.1** The Cyclical Model by Orritt and Harper (2015) displays the repeated media coverage of a risk such as dog bites that results in an increased perceived risk by the public, which results in swift legislative change (similar to the Dangerous Dogs Act 1991). However, the swift, and often inaccurate, legislative change does not address the initial problem, resulting in continued recycling of dog bites in the media and heightened perceived risk to the public as a result. (Diagram reproduced courtesy of Rachel Orritt)

**Table 5.1** A summary of scientific research articles in newspapers and online media that review dog bite related fatalities (DBRF) (see also Chapter 11).

| Source | Country | Study Period | No. DBRFs | Typical Age of Victims | Location / ownership of dog | Most popular Breeds involved |
|---|---|---|---|---|---|---|
| Winkler (1977)* | US | 1 year | 11 | 8 were 6 years or under | 4 victim-owned, 7 neighbour-owned | St Bernard, 'shepherd' |
| Pinckney and Kennedy (1982)* | US | 1966 – 1980 (15 years) | 74 | 80% were 6 years or under | Majority occurred on owner's property | GSD, Husky and St Bernard |
| Podberscek (1994)+ | UK | 1988 – 1992 (5 years) | 7 | 3 were 11 years or under, 4 were 58 years or over | - | Rottweiler, APBT, GSD |
| Lockwood (1997)* | US | 1995 – 1996 (2 year) | 25 | 80% were 11 years or under | 80% on owner's property | Rottweiler, Pit Bull, Multiple |
| Sacks et al. (1996)* | US | 1989 – 1994 (6 years) | 109 | 57% were < 10 years | 77% on owner's property | Pit Bull, Rottweiler, GSD |
| Sacks et al. (2000)* | US | 1979 – 1998 (20 years) | 238 | - | 75% on owner's property | Pit Bull, Rottweiler, GSD |
| Raghavan (2008)+ | Canada | 1990 – 2007 (18 years) | 28 | 85.7% were < 12 years | 60.7% occurred on private property | Crossbreeds, Husky, Rottweiler |
| Oxley and Tibbott (2012)+ | UK | 12/2011 – 01/2012 (6 weeks) | 2 | 2 weeks, 52 years | Both on owner's property | Neapolitan Mastiff and Husky |
| Patronek et al. (2013)* | US | 2000 – 2009 (10 years) | 256 | 45.4% were < 5 years | 74.2% on owner's property | - |

+ Figures were from newspapers/media articles only

* Figures were gathered from multiple sources including newspapers/media articles

2

individuals involved (victim/offender), and focus on extreme cases resulting in politically driven, rather than evidence-based, legislative change.

## 5.3 Media inconsistency and inaccuracy

The media undoubtedly has a story to sell, and while some aspects of reporting are faithful and accurate, others are more open to opinion and bias. A frequently referred to misconception is dog bite figures from the Health and Social Care Information Centre (HSCIC), which provides figures of people who have been admitted to hospital as a result of '*being bitten or struck by a dog*' (HSCIC, 2014). However, the media commonly refers to the HSCIC figures purely as 'dog bites or attacks' in headlines but generally fails to mention those that have been struck by a dog, which could include something as simple as someone injured by tripping over their dog or another dog-related injury (see Orritt, 2014). Delise (2007) and Orritt and Oxley (2015) have highlighted additional inaccurate figures, which have also been recorded in the media and within academic literature, some of which relate to a dog's biting force and the number of dog bites that occur per year.

Newspapers may provide detailed photographic evidence of an injury (e.g. before and after stitches) noted to be as a result of a dog bite that is difficult to gain through other avenues (e.g. hospital records are protected as a result of patient confidentiality), but the circumstances leading to the bite are often more refutable. A brief report of the incident may be given that may provide some insight into why the bite occurred (e.g. teasing a dog or playing near it while it was eating), but the level of corroboration of the story often falls below what might be expected in the case of a serious assault by one person on another. Accordingly, such descriptions need to be treated with caution as they may be biased towards specific breeds (such as pit bulls), inaccurate and/or inconsistent in their reporting (Mills and Levine, 2006; Delise, 2007; Voith et al., 2009; Voith et al., 2013; Hoffman et al., 2014). Certain cases attract a lot of attention and it is easy for the public to seriously overestimate the risk associated with dogs. Indeed, in the USA it has been estimated that an individual is half as likely to die from a dog bite as from a lightning strike and a child under ten is three times more likely to drown in a 5 gallon bucket than die from a dog bite injury (Bradley, 2014).

It is difficult to track the true number of dog 'attacks', especially in a rabies-free country that does not require mandatory reporting for public health reasons. However, there are multiple sources such as medical records, local authority reports, newspapers, etc. that can be used to triangulate the quality of information being produced by the media. Such records can be compared and contrasted to determine accuracy and consistency. Such an approach was adopted recently by Patronek et al. (2013) in the USA, who concluded that media articles were factually incorrect after interviewing law enforcement individuals with first-hand experience of the event. Media articles often refer to second-hand accounts of the incidents that are difficult to validate.

Furthermore, Patronek et al. (2013) made comparisons of the description of dogs described in more than one media article and between media articles versus animal control reports of breeds. They found frequent inconsistency between sources. This study used criteria based on strict and expanded concordance (i.e. agreement) for assessment of reliability of reporting. Strict concordance was defined as '*an exact match in the reported breed descriptor between two*

**Table 5.2** Breed discrepancies noted in comparisons between multiple media articles and reports and animal control reports in the US (Patronek et al., 2013).

| | Not in Strict Concordance* | Not in Expanded Concordance* (i.e. part of breed correct) |
|---|---|---|
| Different Media Accounts | 124/401 (30.9%) | 62/401 (15.5%) |
| Media Accounts v Animal Control Breed Reports | 139/346 (40.2%) | 42/346 (12.1%) |

*Legend: **Strict concordance** was defined as *'an exact match in the reported breed descriptor between two accounts'*. **Expanded concordance** was defined as *'have an overlap of one breed descriptor and so are concordant by the expanded definition'*. The above table shows figures that were not concordant with these categories (i.e. breeds differed between sources).

*accounts'* (e.g. Staffordshire Bull Terrier and Staffordshire Bull Terrier cross would not be in agreement and regarded as 'discordant'). Expanded concordance was defined as a rough match in the breed descriptor. In this case, the Staffordshire bull terrier and Staffordshire Bull Terrier cross would be in agreement (concordant) under the expanded definition (*'have an overlap of one breed descriptor and so are concordant by the expanded definition'*) (Patronek et al., 2013). Either type of concordance was low enough to cast doubt on breed reporting within new articles (see Table 5.2). Furthermore, 90.1% of media articles stated the dog as being of a specific breed and not as a cross-breed, which does not accord with published population figures (Patronek et al., 2013). As a result, Patronek et al. (2013) question the reliability of previous articles using newspapers for breed identification (e.g. Sacks et al., 1989), although it might also be used to argue that purebreds are more likely to bite than cross-breeds.

## 5.4 A survey of popular books, magazines and the internet in the UK and Japan

Kikuchi et al. (2014) reviewed how popular books, magazines and internet sites describe the classification of aggressive behaviour by dogs in the UK and Japan. This focused specifically on whether there were differences with regard to the context, motivation and emotion underlying the animal's behaviour. This was selected since within the field of veterinary behavioural medicine there is no accepted standard method for classifying aggressive dog behaviour (Chapter 1, Mills et al., 2007; De Keuster and Jung, 2009; Mills and Zulch, 2010; Mills et al., 2013). The literature selected comprised of ten books in print in 2012 and listed on Amazon, that were sorted by 'popularity' in both the UK and Japan; ten articles from each of the three popular dog-related magazines from UK and four from Japan over the period 2010–12; and the first ten sites listed by the search engines Yahoo and Google that were studied during the last week in March 2012, when the search terms 'dog aggression' and 'dog bite' were entered. The descriptions for HDAB in the three different media inferred territorial/protective and fear underlying motivation and emotion in both countries, but there was a smaller range of classifications for HDAB in the Japanese media referring more often to dominance as a motivation, in addition to territorial and fear-based forms. It was often implied that the dog was challenging the person, which was a form of 'dominance aggression'. In contrast, in the UK the primary focus was on the emotion of 'fear'. Some descriptions were clearly confused. For example, one internet site explains 'territorial aggression' as being motivated by 'dominance', suggesting the term 'dominance' can be used whenever a dog attempts to take control of an area. However, this is not an accepted scientific interpretation, with researchers suggesting that the motivation for territorial aggression may be defensive or an emotion related to fear or frustration depending on the context (Bradshaw et al., 2009; Mills and Zulch, 2010; Mills et al., 2013).

A marked difference between the countries' descriptions was that in the Japanese media there was little if any mention of possible explanations for the behaviour; with the emphasis being placed on solutions. By contrast, in the UK articles appeared to be more technical and theoretical, tending to follow a scheme: the problem is stated, potential causes identified, and solutions suggested. Therefore it seems that in the UK greater emphasis is given to public understanding of the issue.

## 5.5 A review of newspaper articles in the UK and Japan

To help further understand dog bites in popular media the authors recently reviewed a wide range of articles to identify newspaper reports and if these differ between countries and cultures. To do this, the authors examined articles of significant dog-related incidents and how the dogs involved were represented for the period 01/2013 – 12/2014 in the UK and Japan. In the UK, three national newspaper websites (*Daily Mail/Mail Online*, the *Guardian* and the *Mirror*) and the BBC news website were reviewed, whereas in Japan, four major national newspaper websites were chosen (*Asahi, Yomiuri, Mainichi* and *Sankei*). The newspapers and websites were chosen based on their popularity as national newspapers, and open accessibility. The newspapers' websites were searched directly and via Google search engines with the key terms 'Dog bite', 'Dog attack' and 'Dog aggression'. If there was the same news article in the different newspapers, the longest single article was selected. Seventeen aspects of the report were noted per article (Table 5.3).

Overall, the search identified thirty-five incidents reported in the UK and seventeen in Japan relating to human bite incidents for the years 2013 and 2014. In the UK, thirty-five reports involved a single dog (thirty-one; 88.6%) or multiple dogs (four; 11.4%) attacking a person. Twenty per cent (seven out of thirty-five) of the latter were noted to

**Table 5.3** The human, dog and situational factors that were recorded for each newspaper article of significant dog-related incidents for the period 01/2013–12/2014 in the UK and Japan.

| Human-Related Factors | Dog-Related Factors | Situational Factors |
|---|---|---|
| Age | Age | Circumstances |
| Number of victims | Breed | Location |
| Gender | Size | Cause |
| Victims action before the incident | Gender | Further information post-incident |
| Owner management of the dog | Dog's action before incident | |
| How the dog showed aggressive behaviour | What happened to the dog after the incidents (e.g. destroyed) | |
| Level of injury | | |

**Table 5.4** A comparison of content between newspaper articles reviewed in the UK (n=35) and Japan (n=17).

|  | UK (n=35)<br>n (% of total ) | Japan (n=17)<br>n (% of total ) |
|---|---|---|
| **Dog-related factors reported** | | |
| Dog's Age | 3 (8.6%) | 2 (11.8%) |
| Dog's Size | 2 (5.7%) | 9 (52.9%) |
| Breed/'Type'* | 31 (88.6%) | 15 (88.2%) |
| Most popular breed reported | American Pit Bull Terrier/<br>Pit Bull/Pit Bull Type (7) | Dalmatian (2) |
| The dog's action before the incident | 7 (20%) | 2 (11.8%) |
| What happened to the dog (e.g. destroyed, caught) | 14 (40%) | 7 (41.2%) |
| **Human related factors reported** | | |
| Number of victims | 31 (88.6%) | 17 (100%) |
| Age of the victims | 31 (88.6%) | 13 (76.5%) |
| Gender of victims | 34 (97.1%) | 17 (100%) |
| The victims action before the incident | 13 (37.1%) | 3 (17.6%) |
| Owner management of the dog | 3 (8.6%) | 15 (88.2%) |
| How the dog showed aggressive behaviour | 10 (28.6%) | 17 (100%) |
| Level of injury | 29 (82.8%) | 17 (100%) |
| Further information post incident | 12 (34.3%) | 2 (11.8%) |
| **Situational Factors** | | |
| Location of bite | | |
| *Victims home, but not their dog* | 1 (2.9%) | 0 |
| *Dog/owner's home, but victim visiting* | 8 (22.9%) | 0 |
| *Dog/owner's/victims home* | 7 (20%) | 0 |
| *Public* | 15 (42.8%) | 17 (100%) |
| *Unknown* | 4 (11.4%) | 0 |
| Cause of the bite | 22.9% | 0 |

* The Pit Bull Terrier in the UK is referred to as a 'type' not a breed according to the Dangerous Dogs Act 1991

be dog bite–related fatalities. Two articles referred to severe infections from the bacteria *Capnocytophaga canimorsus* resulting in the loss of limbs due to a minor dog bite. Two articles were related to police dog attacks. In Japan, eleven (64.7%) articles stated that a single dog was involved, whereas four (23.5%) stated multiple dogs and two (11.8%) it was unknown if there were single or multiple dogs. Most of the articles described the breed/type (fifteen; 88.2%) with the most commonly reported breed being Dalmatians (two reports). A full review and comparison of findings can be seen in Table 5.4.

In general, similarities were found between the UK and Japanese incidents as articles were short and they only covered the breed of the dog and the age, gender of the victim, location, how the incident occurred and the level of injury. However, in Japan there was no mention of cause clearly in any of the articles. In contrast, in the UK the surrounding factors of a bite were often described but in most cases not the actual cause or unjustified inferences were made as to why a dog attacked. The breed, and in some cases the size of the dog, seem to be described in order to make the public consider how serious the incident was or label the breed. In the UK two articles noted the weight of the dog, which may also reflect the size of the dog. There was an obvious difference between the breeds mentioned in the articles in the UK compared to those mentioned in Japan. The UK articles were consistent with a biased opinion of specific breeds such as bull breeds, as found in previous research (Podberscek, 1994) despite no evidence to suggest that these breeds are responsible for more dog bites in the UK than any other. By contrast, most Japanese articles emphasised the size of the dog more than the breed. In Japan, all articles described aggressive behaviour without any mention of the victim's reaction/behaviour or details of the circumstances and seemed to blame the dog and owner's management. This also appeared to be the case for the majority of articles in the UK, although the victim's behaviour was mentioned in a number of articles. Furthermore, in the UK, two articles focused on police dog attacks and three on the compensation received as a result of a bite.

The difference in popularity of breed reports in UK and Japan is likely to reflect the individual country breed popularity and lack of breed-specific controversy in Japan compared with the UK. Given the track record of the UK media as reviewed by Podberscek (1994), it is no surprise that the majority of breeds described in the UK were pit bulls, followed by Staffordshire bull terriers. However, the inaccuracy and potential bias of such reports needs to be taken into account. A recent high profile incident in the UK involving four dogs and a teenager (Jade Anderson) was reported as follows: The *Mail Online* (26 March 2013) noted the dog breeds included a bull Mastiff, Two Staffordshire bull terriers and an American bulldog; whereas, the *Mirror* (27 March 2013) stated two bull Mastiffs and two Staffordshire bull terriers. There is also evidence to suggest that a media report may initially guess the type of breed and then change it upon police confirmation. For example, the *Mirror* initially noted the breed that was involved in the death of Lexi Branson was a French Mastiff (*Mirror*, 6 November 2013; 8:17am), but later noted it to be a bulldog upon police confirmation (*Mirror*, 6 November 2013; 22:11pm). Such poor verification of information in relation to dog 'attacks' would not be acceptable in other aspects of journalism relating to the harm of others and any research that uses media reports as a basis for data analysis should take this problem into account.

In both Japan and the UK the majority of bites occurred in public. In 2012 in Japan, the official report by the Ministry of Environment indicated that 4,198 dog bite incidents were reported by victims (Ministry of Environment, 2015). 3,987 (94%) of these were human-directed incidents. A total of 1,130 (28%) were reported to occur while walking or playing on a lead, 1,063 (27%) while leaving the dog, not on a lead, in a public place and 901 (23%) occurred when the dog was left in a kennel/cage and escaped as the door was unlocked or the dog opened it. This brings into question the initial cause of bites in a public location. Furthermore, the media reports in this study mainly noted incidents where a dog was not on a lead. However, the incidents may have been caused by the owner's reaction or attitudes towards the dog's or victim's behaviour. Moreover, if we assume public perception of risk follows from media reports, as proposed by Orritt and Harper (2015), then the Japanese public are being presented with a distorted view of the risk posed by dogs and may inadvertently underestimate the primary risk situations as these are not commonly reported. By contrast, in the UK there seems to be an equally unhelpful emphasis on breed type (Clarke et al., 2013; see Chapter 7).

There is no doubt that media headlines attempt to be eye-catching to influence an individual to read an article. This study also found that common reference/words are used in the UK to label dogs such as 'devil dogs', 'mauled' or 'savaged'. Such words have been used for many years and continue to the present day (Podberscek, 1994; Delise, 2007). These may help emphasise the contrast and polarity between the portrayed innocent victim and guilty dog (similar to that of human offenders, Wardle, 2007). Furthermore, as with previous research, this study found articles that refer to dog attacks generally include pictures of unrepresentative imagery (e.g. an aggressive dog baring its teeth) (Orritt and Oxley, 2015).

In Japan, there is no law relating to aggressive dogs like the 'Dangerous Dogs Act' in the UK and the only regulation relating to injury caused by a dog results in a fixed fine that an owner must pay (except in a serious case such as the victim's death). This may reflect the public's general view towards animals (e.g. they do not take responsibility for a dog's behaviour), and as a result it is perhaps not surprising that articles may not cover much legal information. By contrast, in the UK several articles have focused on the legal implications of dog bites: two articles were associated with the cost of legal fees as a result of a postman being bitten, which has been a topic of recent debate (see CWU, 2014) and one article noted the legal settlement as a result of a police dog bite to a student.

## 5.6 Conclusion and future research

In conclusion, it seems the popular media are an inaccurate and unreliable source of information on dog bites, with country- and possibly culture-specific styles and traditions (Tanaka, 1998). This might reflect or affect public interest in the subject. There are inconsistencies across countries in both the description of the cause of a dog bite and its context. However, if the report is inaccurate, includes bias or subjective labelling of the dog and its behaviour, it affects the public perception of dogs, their behaviour and perceived risk. In the interest of responsible reporting, the media should deliver information to the public as accurately and honestly as possible, following normal journalistic standards of reporting, even if it only reports the incident briefly. Police, owner family members or the local authority may be more accurate sources, whereas, neighbours, eye witnesses and other media sources are less likely to be reliable. It might be useful if dog behaviour experts produced guidelines that can be specifically referred to by journalists. An obvious and common error in the UK relates to the reporting of NHS statistics that generally do not describe dog bites, such as the HSCIC (code W54) '*bitten or struck by a dog*' (HSCIC, 2014), and so should not be reported in the media as such. Furthermore, media journalists could take a proactive approach to help inform the public about prevention methods and the schemes available (See Chapters 29, 30 and 31).

There is a range of other important information the media could also help highlight such as potential concerns and issues relating to the welfare of dogs that have been seized by police or euthanised directly after a bite.

Frequent reviews of the media are of importance as the media is highly influential in shaping public perceptions on specific issues such as dog bites, and so may have the power to affect legislation, as occurred with the Dangerous Dogs Act 1991. How informative or inaccurate is the media is useful to monitor and types of articles and the associated time frames for reporting (e.g. directly after a dog bite, several versus months after a dog bite as a result of a court case or legal dispute) are important to know.

It is also important to acknowledge that a wide range of media sources have yet to be examined, such as the growing forms and potential influence of social media. It is relatively easy to aggregate a number of tweets using specific key words such as 'dog bite' (see Oxley and Ellis, 2015). Furthermore, it is also possible to collect photographic content from social media sites that are assigned to specific key words. This would help identify potentially useful information on less publicly reported dog bites (See also Chapter 3).

## 5.7 References

Bradley, J. (2014). Dog bites: Problems and solutions (revised 2014). Animal and Society Institute.

Bradshaw, J. W., Blackwell, E. J., Casey, R. A. (2009). Dominance in domestic dogs – useful construct or bad habit? *Journal of Veterinary Behaviour: Clinical Applications and Research.* **4,** 135–144.

Brooman, S., Legge, D. (1997). *Law relating to animals.* Cavendish Publishing Limited: London.

Clarke, T., Cooper, J., Mills, D. (2013). Acculturation – Perceptions of breed differences in behavior of the dog (Canis familiaris) Human-Animal Interaction Bulletin, 1, 16–33.

CWU (Communication Workers Union) (2014) Dangerous Dog – Bite Back. Available at: www.cwu.org/dangerous-dogs-bite-back.html (Accessed on: 5 March 2015).

De Keuster, T., Jung, H. (2009). Aggression toward familiar people and animals. In: D Horwitz and D Mills (eds.) *BSAVA manual of canine and feline behavioural medicine*: 2nd Edition: 182–210.

Delise, K. (2007). The pit bull placebo: The media, myths, and politics of canine aggression. Anubis Publishing: Ramsey.

Ghirlanda, S., Acerbi, A., Herzog, H. (2014). Dog Movie Stars and Dog Breed Popularity: A Case Study in Media Influence on Choice. *Plos One.* E106565.

Hoffman, C., Harrison, N., Wolff, N., Westgarth, C. (2014). Is that dog a pit bull? A cross-country comparison of perceptions of shelter workers regarding breed identification. *Journal of Applied Animal Welfare Science.* 17, 322–339.

HSCIC (Health & Social Care Information Centre) (2014). Provisional monthly hospital episode statistics for admitted patient care, outpatients and accident and emergency data – April 2013 to January 2014. http://www.hscic.gov.uk/searchcatalogue?productid=14625&q=dog+bites&infotype=0%2fOfficial+statistics&sort=Most+recent&size=10&page=1#top

Hsu, Y., Sun, L. (2010). Factors associated with aggressive responses in pet dogs. *Applied Animal Behaviour Science.* 123, 108–123.

Japanese Ministry of Internal Affairs and Communications (2014). The survey of how the public use time for media. Available at: http://www.soumu.go.jp/main_content/000357570.pdf (Accessed: 24 June 2015).

Kikuchi, M., Oxley, J., Hogue, T., Mills, D. S. (2014). The representation of aggressive behavior of dogs in the popular media in the UK and Japan. *Journal of Veterinary Behavior: Clinical Applications and Research.* 9 e9.

Lockwood, R. (1997). Dog-bite-related fatalities – United States, 1995–1996. *Morbidity and Mortality Weekly Report.* 46, 463 – 466.

Messam, L. M., Kass, H. P., Chmel, B. B., Hart, L. A. (2007). The human–canine environment: A risk factor for non-play bites? *The Veterinary Journal.* 177, 205–215.

Mills, D., Levine, E. (2006). The need for a co-ordinated scientific approach to the investigation of dog bite injuries. *The Veterinary Journal.* 172, 398–399.

Mills, D., Millman, S., Levine, E. (2007). Applied animal behaviour: assessment, pain and aggression. In *Animal Physiotherapy: Assessment, Treatment and Rehabilitation of Animals.* C. McGowan, L. Goff, and N. Stubbs, ed. Blackwell Publishing, Ames, IA, 3–13.

Mills, D. S., Zulch, H. (2010). Appreciating the role of fear and anxiety in aggressive behaviour by dogs. *Veterinary Focus.* 20, 44–49.

Mills, D., Braem Dube, M., Zulch H. (2013). Principles of Pheromonatherapy. *Stress and Pheromonatherapy in Small Animal Clinical Behaviour*, West Sussex. Wiley-Blackwell. 127–145.

Ministry of Environment (2015). A number of dog bites incidents from 1996–2012 Available at: www.env.go.jp/council/14animal/ext/2-3-1.pdf (Accessed: 24 June 2015).

National Readership Survey (2014). National Readership Survey. Available at: www.nrs.co.uk/training-2/helpful-tools/useful-chart/ (Accessed: 24 June 2015).

Orritt, R. (2014). Dog ownership has unknown risks but known health benefits: we need evidence based policy. *British Medical Journal.* 349: g4081.

Orritt, R., Harper, C. (2015). Similarities between the representation of 'Aggressive Dogs' and 'Sex Offenders' in the British news media. E-book: www.inter-disciplinary.net/probing- the-bound aries/wp-content/uploads/2014/05/orrittahpaper.pdf

Orritt, R., Oxley, J. A. (2015). The history of dog bite misinformation in UK news media and public policy. ISAZ Conference: Significance in History and for the future. Saratoga Springs, New York, USA. 7–9 July 2015.

Overall, L. K., Love, M. (2001). Dog bites to humans – demography, epidemiology, injury, and risk. *Journal of the American Veterinary Medical Association.* 218, 1923–1934.

Oxley, J. A., Ellis, C. F. (2015). Dog bites: What can social media tells us? AWSELVA conference: Bristol. 29–30 September 2015.

Oxley, J. A., Farr K. J., De Luna, C. J. (2012). Dog owners' perceptions of breed-specific dangerous dog legislation in the UK. *Veterinary Record.* 171, 424–427.

Oxley, J. A., Tibbott, A. R. (2012). A brief review of dog-related articles in British newspapers and associated factors. ISAZ Conference: Arts and Sciences of Human-Animal Interactions. Murray Edwards College, Cambridge, UK. 11–13 July 2012.

Patronek, G. J., Sacks, J. J., Delise, K. M., Cleary, D. V., Marder, A. R. (2013). Co-occurrence of potentially preventable factors in 256 dog bite–related fatalities in the United States (2000–2009). *Journal of the American Veterinary Medical Association.* 243, 1726–1736.

Pinckney, L. E., Kennedy, L. A. (1982). Traumatic deaths from dog attacks in the United States. *Pediatrics.* 69, 193–196.

Podberscek, A. L. (1994). Dogs on a tightrope: the position of the dog in British Society as influenced by the press reports on dog attacks (1988–1992). *Anthrozoos.* 7, 232–241.

Raghavan, M. (2008). Fatal dog attacks in Canada, 1990–2007. *Canadian Veterinary Journal.* 49, 577–581.

Sacks, J. J., Lockwood, R., Hornreicht, J., Sattin, R. W. (1996). Fatal dog attacks, 1989–1994. *Pediatrics.* 97, 891–895.

Sacks, J. J., Sattin, R. W., Bonzo, S. E. (1989). Dog bite-related fatalities from 1979 through 1988. *Journal of the American Veterinary Medical Association.* 262, 1489–1492.

Sacks, J. J., Sinclair, L., Gilchrist, J., Golab, G. C., Lockwood, R. (2000). Breeds of dogs involved in fatal human attacks in the United States between 1979 and 1998. *Journal of the American Veterinary Medical Association.* 217, 836–840.

Semiocast (2013). Geolocation and activity analysis of Pinterest accounts by Semiocast. Available at:

http://semiocast.com/en/publications/2013_07_10_Pinterest_has_70_million_users (Accessed: 15 March 2015).

Tanaka, K. (1998). Japanese Women's Magazines: The Language of Aspiration. *The Worlds of Japanese Popular Culture: Gender, Shifting Boundaries and Global Cultures*. Ed. Martinez, D. P. Cambridge, University Press: 100–132.

Voith, V. L., Ingram, E., Mitsouras, K., Irizarry, K. (2009). Comparison of adoption agency breed identification and DNA breed identification of dogs. *Journal of Applied Animal Welfare Science*. 12, 253–262.

Voith, V. L., Trevejo, R., Dowling-Guyer, S., Chadik, C., Marder, A., Johnson, V., Irizarry, K. (2013). Comparison of visual and DNA breed identification of dogs and inter-observer reliability. *American Journal of Sociological Research*. 3, 17–29.

Wardle, C. (2007). Monsters and Angels. Visual press coverage of child murders in the USA and UK, 1930–2000. *Journalism*. 8, 263–284.

Winkler, W. G. (1977). Human deaths induced by dog bites, United States, 1974–75. *Public Health Reports*. 92, 425.

# CHAPTER 6

# Aggressive Dogs and Public Image

*Simon Harding*

## 6.1 Introduction

So-called aggressive dogs, (dogs that are widely viewed as being aggressive to other dogs, to humans, or to both) remain a high profile issue for the media and public (see Chapter 5). This issue is widely reported as combining concepts and debates around dangerous dogs, illegal or proscribed dogs, breed-specific legislation (BSL) (see Chapter 13), status dogs and weapon dogs. In the public mind these issues are conflated with or associated to violence, criminal activity, anti-social behaviour and dog fighting, and are indicative of the subterranean or anti-establishment values of an emergent underclass (Harding, 2012; 2014). While this topic touches upon or engages each of these elements, it remains a complex subject that releases many emotions and generates strong views among the numerous headlines. However, despite this widespread interest, it remains surprisingly under-researched.

This chapter therefore attempts to explain the topic and disentangle the key elements while attempting to explain the links between seemingly aggressive dogs, their owners and an increasingly negative public image.

## 6.2 Banning of 'aggressive' dogs

Throughout the 1980s in the UK an increasing number of dog attacks upon humans were reported avidly in the British press (see Chapter 5). There was also concern that 'Pit Bull-type' dogs were being introduced into the UK for criminal activity (dog fighting and drug dealing), (Hood et al., 2001; Lodge and Hood, 2002). Home Secretary Kenneth Baker argued in favour of regulation of proscribed breeds, claiming that it would reduce breeding and ownership, which would result in their eventual disappearance from the UK (Baker, 1993). The Conservative government came under intense pressure from a highly agitated media to address these concerns and in 1991 passed (in only one day) the Dangerous Dogs Act 1991 (Radford, 2001) (See Chapter 13). The Act banned four types, namely the Pit Bull Terrier and three dogs rarely if ever seen in the UK: the Dogo

Argentino, Fila Brasileiro and the Japanese Tosa. The law banned importation, buying, breeding or selling of such animals. Notably German shepherds and Rottweilers were excluded as they were widely argued to have a significant role in the security indus-try. From the outset this legislation was contested and controversial, (Kasperson, 2008; Hallsworth, 2011). Simultaneously, the Act was criticised for failing to tackle the issue of dog bites occurring on private property. While the Act is rarely out of the British media even twenty five years later, Oxley has shown that few members of the public fully understand it (Oxley, 2012).

The DDA 1991 established the proposition of breed-specific legislation (BSL) with its presumption that certain breeds, or types, of dog were inherently more aggressive than others. Such views remain widely contested (see Casey et al., 2013 for recent debates). Associated to this was the view that certain owners of these animals were either criminally oriented or aggressive themselves (Barnes et al., 2006; Dunne, 2009; Harding, 2013). In other countries, similar assumptions have been made to justify the introduction of breed-specific legislation, so that this has now become a global phenomenon, although some countries, e.g. the Netherlands, have reconsidered their position and repealed such statutes (see Chapter 13).

## 6.3  So why is this an issue today?

The DDA 1991 is widely assumed to have failed in its goals, e.g. the All-Parliamentary Group for Animal Welfare (2008) has indicated that Pit Bull Terriers are now present in greater numbers than before the Act – a view widely supported by animal welfare agencies and charities. In 2010 this was reported as a 'dramatic rise' in dangerous dogs, (BBC News, 2010). Consequently, the issue of dangerous dogs remains high on the public agenda. Post-1991 the UK government has recorded increases in dog attacks, in dogs processed through the courts, in kennelling costs, in aggressive and dangerous dogs arriving at rehoming centres and consequently greater difficulties in rehoming large bull breed dogs. Such issues have recently focused the government to develop a number of initiatives to improve law enforcement (Defra 2009; 2010b; 2012; 2014).

Since the introduction of the DDA in 1991, several significant events have contrived to retain the high public profile of this issue and to generate a negative public image of bull breed dogs:

- **An increase in dog bites**
  Injuries from 'bites and strikes' from a dog incident requiring hospital admission rose rapidly from 2,915 (1997–98) to 6,118 (2010–11) indicating a rise of 210%. The cost of NHS treatment for the most serious cases in 2009 was estimated at £3.3 million (Defra, 2012).

- **Dog bite fatalities**
  Between 1989 and 2015, media and court reports in the UK have reported there have been thirty fatal dog attacks on humans in the UK with ages ranging from six days old to ninety years (Harding unpublished data).

- **Widespread media ridicule and public complaints about the DDA 1991**
  The DDA has generated acres of print headlines and commentary over the past twenty five years, along with frequent radio debates. See Harding (2012; 2014) Appendix A for a more in depth coverage of this topic. See also Cuddy (2014), who has described the Act as 'Pit Bull genocide by government order'.

- **High profile public campaigns**. For example the Bite Back campaign by the Communications Workers Union. The CWU reports 5,329 attacks on Royal Mail, Parcelforce and BT staff in 2007–08, falling to around 3,000 attacks in the year April 2011–April 2012 (www.parliament.uk 2012). A total of 70% of attacks on Royal Mail staff occurred on private property with 313 RIDDOR (Reporting of Injuries, Diseases and Dangerous Occurrences Regulations) reportable (Defra, 2012).

- **Media debates re dangerous dogs, microchipping and dog licensing**
  Many of the themes of such debates are evident in the following headlines:

  *'Calls grow to set up death courts for dangerous dogs', Evening Standard, 14 May 2010*
  *'The owners are just as dangerous as the dog that attacked me', The Observer, 14 March 2010*
  *'A young man's best friend is his fashion statement', The Guardian, Williams, Z., 11 March 2010*

- **Increased visibility of large bull breed dogs**.
  Media headlines such as *'Armed to the teeth: the problem with Pitbulls* (*The Telegraph* 15 April 10) summarised popular anxieties about increased visibility.

In 2010 Harding (2012; 2014) undertook research site visits to forty London parks and identified large bull breed dogs/Pit Bull -type dogs/PBT cross-breeds in thirty-four (85%) of the parks, indicating an apparent high degree of visibility and presence.

In addition, there have been reports of significant increases in the number of admissions of bull breed dogs at local animal rescue centres and rehoming centres, (Dogs Trust Surveys 2010–13). In 2012 Battersea Dogs and Cats Home received a total of 3,357 dogs in its 2012 intake, of which approximately two–thirds were identified as bull breed dogs (both pure breeds and cross-breeds). Of these, 150 were Pit Bulls, 1,682 were Staffordshire Bull Terriers, 114 were Mastiffs, 127 were bulldogs and 125 were Rottweilers, (Battersea Dogs and Cats Home, 2012).

## 6.4 Stigma and status dogs

By 2008 the deteriorating public image of certain breeds and types (and one might say of their owners) found a new outlet in a new vocabulary of stigma. Speaking in 2010 following government consultation on the issue, Animal Welfare Minister Lord Henley said:

*'The issue of dangerous dogs is not just a problem of dangerous breeds but also one of bad owners. They need to be held to account and stopped from ruining people's lives. Dangerous dogs are a major issue affecting many people.' (Defra, 2010a).*

However, by now the debate had moved beyond 'dangerous dogs', as defined by the 1991 Act, to now include a variety of bull breed and cross-breed dogs (including the Staffordshire bull terrier) with owners widely denounced as 'chavs', 'hoodies', 'soap-dodgers', 'thugs' and the criminal underclass. This clearly links a stigmatisation of certain 'other' demonised societal groups now with specific breeds of similarly stigmatised dogs. The media quickly created a new sensationalist and melodramatic vocabulary for those dogs involved, including, 'land sharks', 'devil dogs', 'trophy dogs', and, of course, 'status dogs' (see Harding 2010; 2012 for a fuller account of this media coverage, including a critical discourse analysis of the coverage of status dogs in UK media).

Though the term 'status dog' is almost exclusive to the UK, definitions vary as to what exactly a status dog is, however, the opening statement of the Defra Public Consultation on Dangerous Dogs (2010b) states the issue quite clearly,

> *'There has been growing concern over public safety issues relating to dangerous and status dogs. The term 'status dog' describes the ownership of certain types of dogs which are used by individuals to intimidate and harass members of the public. These dogs are traditionally, but not exclusively, associated with young people on inner city estates and those involved in criminal activity. In recent years, incidents, attacks and fighting of these dogs has increased and some of these incidents have involved children resulting in tragic fatalities. This is an issue which the Government takes very seriously.'*
>
> *(Defra Public Consultation on Dangerous Dogs, 9 March 2010, Defra)*

While for years the term 'status dog' might have referred to rare and expensive lap dogs used by the rich and upper class, the term is now a pejorative label used, in the UK at least, to describe large and often aggressive bull breed dogs, (including proscribed or Dangerous Dogs) used by young men to generate or project a hyper-masculine image of aggression among their peer group, (Rollins, 2014). Although there is no clear definition of breeds included as 'status dogs', they are often portrayed as now including any overtly well-muscled medium to large-sized dog. This rather spurious commonly held perception favours Mastiffs, Malamutes, Staffies, cross-breeds and Akitas over other large dogs, such as German shepherds, Newfoundlands and retrievers, which the general public have essentially classified as being family dogs.

By 2009 press reports indicated certain dogs were being used as weapons, either to intimidate and cause fear or to cause actual bodily harm: *'Demands grow for "weapon dogs" to be brought to heel'. (The Independent*, 10 November 2009). The use of bull breed dogs as weapons was identified in the brutal murders of sixteen-year-olds, Kodjo Yenga (2007) and Seyi Ogumyemi (2009). Later in 2009 the Greater London Association (GLA) published a report entitled 'Weapon dogs: the Situation in London'. It reported young men aged 20–24 'causing fear and intimidation by having a powerful looking dog'. It introduced the concept of weapon dogs as those 'used in crime as weapons for intimidation' and noted a link to street gangs and anti-social youth.

Among widespread media reporting, distortion and exaggeration lies a need to locate data that defines accurately what the public witness, or what ultimately becomes a generalised perception, namely,

a)   There are more dangerous dogs on the streets than ever before, and

b)   The owners are as aggressive as the dogs themselves.

In the absence of accurate data, some writers, (notably Hallsworth, 2011, and Kasperson, 2008) have concluded the whole topic is more urban myth than urban fact. This topic does suffer from a deficit of research. The work by Cardiff University (Hughes, Maher and Lawson, 2011) and Harding (2010; 2012; 2014) evidences that there is abundant media coverage but little verifiable data; nor indeed can the public be relied upon to identify breed type accurately.

Despite a lack of research it is believed that a social or cultural shift has taken place whereby certain breeds or types once considered ill-suited, unfashionable or inappropriate, are now commonplace in our high streets and parks. Furthermore, it appears that many owners of such dogs fail to socialise their dogs effectively, or in some cases purposefully socialise them to be aggressive (Hughes, Maher and Lawson, 2011; Harding, 2012. In the BBC Three production, *My Weapon is a Dog* (broadcast 21 May 2009) Interviewer Rickie Hayward-Williams asked one young man why he would want to train his dog to attack people? The young respondent replied:

*'It was a challenge; makes me feel I've got control over my dog. She's more like a bodyguard. I can use her as a weapon if I wanted to.'*

For some the malleability of Pit Bulls was a key issue:

*'If you are an aggressive person, then the dog is like a sponge, it will become aggressive with you.'*

While another youthful owner of a French Mastiff reported that:

*'If someone tries it with you, you're going to feel happy when you see your dog doing damage to somebody.'*

So with such views being stated openly by some young men, the question to ask is, does this represent a cultural shift in our attitude towards dogs, and if so what lies beneath this cultural shift?

## 6.5  Commodification and brand values

One theory to explain this cultural or social shift is that these owners treat their dog as a commodity, rather like a pair of trainers or a mobile phone, or meat producing animal in some contexts, (Gunderson, 2011; Harding, 2014). Nast (2006) theorises that that in our post-industrialised world, dogs are both anthropomorphised and commodified, while Power (2008) contends that humans project behavioural and personality expectations on to their animals to ensure they fit within their family domain. The conclusion of this argument is that where an individual seeks to replicate the violent and aggressive environment in which they live, they may seek out, or seek to develop through mal-socialisation and cruel training techniques, a dog that will mirror and replicate this. While such theories require further research, the interviews with young owners of so-called status dogs conducted by Harding (2012) certainly identified that these views were held and resonated for some owners. In this world, the dog may be something that can be traded up or down depending on requirements. This process may be made easy by emotional detachment brought about by viewing items as disposable, tradable or exchangeable and not of intrinsic, but of passing, value.

One London paper (*London Evening Standard*, 6 September 2013) noted that dogs were being traded for mobile phones and games consoles. Quoting the Pet Advertising Advisory Group, it revealed that one seller was offering a 'fighting dog with big teeth', while another south London-based seller offering a Staffordshire Bull Terrier for £120 wrote online, 'I don't mind swapping for a PS3, Xbox 360, Nintendo, Wii, laptop or moped.' The key significance is that the dog is no longer viewed as a sentient being and family member – but shifts to a less valued 'thing' whose value depends upon its currency in the current market. Brand values are now sought out and buyers/owners determine their position by asking '*what can this dog do for me? How much will it make for me?*' Brand values are driven by market reputation. For Pit Bulls in particular there may be several perceived brand values that are theoretically attractive (see Chapter 7):

*   Pariah social status
*   Reputation
*   Malleable nature
*   Aggressive nature
*   Fierce loyalty
*   Violence and strength
*   High pain threshold
*   'Ultimate warriors'
*   Powerful
*   Won't let go.

Despite the widespread nature of these phenomena there remains a lack of research in the UK into issues of human-animal relations and more specifically a lack of research into what attracts certain young people to certain dog breeds.

## 6.6 The making of a public image

While some of these values are suggestive of urban mythology, that matters not as these are examples of globally recognised values linked to and representing the Pit Bull-type dog (see Chapter 7). Dogs provide secondary but implicit associations conveying concepts of animalism, loyalty, alpha male superiority, unpredictability, illegality and ability to confer or even 'unleash' sexual prowess (Harding, 2012). Such attributes appeal and endure in gang mythology, where Pit Bull types in particular have become more than new bling – they are elevated into gang hierarchies, eulogised and lionised. Of key importance is that some of these are the same brand values that members of urban street gangs seek to apply to themselves: loyal, violent, aggressive, an urban survivor. In this way, for some young gang–affiliated men in particular, a Pit Bull dog that has been trained to become aggressive and vicious takes on the mantle of avatar: an animalistic representation of the self. For them the dog becomes a mirror of who they believe they are and also a projection of who they would like to be, or perceived to be – a totally fearless, adaptive urban warrior who will fight to the death if required. Such views may perhaps link into counter-culture values of a class fight between the underdogs of society against the government and the establishment. The pariah social status of the Pit Bull thus both echoes and references this simultaneously, further adding to its valourisation and acceptance within gang culture.

While both values and image are socially constructed and products of socialisation and environment, they nonetheless ring very true for those operating in street worlds. Thus, members of urban street gangs create a perfect match with the Pit Bull, sharing the same pariah status, life trajectory and social fate. This creates a bond of belief and affection that may view the Pit Bull not as an 'addition' to the urban street gang, but as an actual bona fide member in its own right. Although there are likely cultural differences that require investigation, this perspective is now globally acknowledged by street gangs from Brazil to South Africa and from Los Angeles to London (Harding, 2014).

The Pit Bull is reflected as a full gang member in cultural depictions of ghetto life, or 'Thug Life', largely through Hip Hop music. Depicted as active gang members, lyrical devices are used to:

equate the lethal capacity of Pit Bulls to bullets:

> *If my glocks on safe that means my dogz on the leash*
> *Twenty shells in the clip, each bullet's the teeth (Sticky Fingaz)*

demonstrate Pit Bulls as weaponry:

> *Let all your Pit Bulls off the leash (Big Pokey)*

illustrate the centrality of the Pit Bull to gang life:

> *Where the f***** Hood At? It's all good, the dog IS the hood! (DMX)*

Dogs are central to photo images (see Chapter 7), videos and musical lyrics as well as the gang-land neighbourhood and what French sociologist Bourdieu (1977) calls the 'habitus' of the community. Through such cultural expressions and representations the Pit Bull became representative and then symbolic of the urban street gang and by the early 1990s, in the USA, was viewed widely by many as a 'gangster's dog'. As Allen (2007: 41–49) notes, media coverage increased the association of Pit Bulls with gangs and criminal activity, ensuring the Pit Bull began, 'its transformation into a threatening outsider' or 'ghetto monster'. This further signalled the Pit Bull's declining favour in the eyes of the wider public, while similarly raising its pariah social status that became so appealing to global youth. **Stigmatised dogs such as the Pit Bull fit with stigmatised communities**.

This hard urban warrior image was sealed from the 1980s onwards when new legislation in the USA brought to light the widespread use of Pit Bulls in the underground dog fighting scene. Early empirical data (Randour and Hardiman, 2006) was soon supported by research from the Humane Society of the US (HSUS) that identified approximately 40,000 people were involved regularly in dog fighting in the USA (Peters, 2008; Smith-Spark, 2007). Dog fighting is not new, nor is the involvement of Pit Bulls in this so called 'sport', however, the movement of the Pit Bull from its traditional role of 'frontier dog' to urban ghetto dog also sealed the fate of many individuals within the breed as they became increasingly used in new forms of dog fighting located in urban warehouses and underground garages (Evans, Kalich and Forsyth, 1998; Evans and Forsyth, 1998; Harding and Nurse, 2015). Again, evidence of this sensationally surfaced with the indictment of NFL star quarterback Michael Vick in 2007 for his involvement in an interstate dog fighting ring (Strouse, 2009); Vick served twenty-one months in prison for his involvement. Increasingly, over the past twenty five years, police raids on US dog fighting matches now focus on urban and suburban warehouses and deprived housing projects as well as the rural farmyards of the southern states of America, traditionally associated with dog fighting (Evans and Forsyth, 1998). More recently, such raids have exposed a world of firearms, illegal gambling, prostitution and violence that consolidate the negative public image of Pit Bulls and their owners. Some critics, however, argue that the shift in public image of the Pit Bull is more closely associated with racism as the widespread ownership of the dog has moved from white rural farmers and frontiersmen to black and Hispanic occupants of deprived housing projects (Delise, 2007; Allen, 2007).

Although it is likely that cultural changes in representation of the Pit Bull in the USA has similarities and effects on the UK, this requires independent scrutiny. Similar changes appear to be occurring in the UK as illegal dog fighting in deprived housing estates is reported increasingly with debates expressing these views voiced routinely in radio talk shows. Hughes, Maher and Lawson (2011) confirmed that among the young men interviewed in Cardiff, many used their dogs for casual fighting. They also noted that the 'size, colour and potential of the dogs' was more important than breed type when selling puppies – suggesting 'potential' links to violence, aggression and intimidation. Abuse is often central to the training of dogs for fighting (RSPCA, 2009; Harding, 2012, 2014; Maher and Pierpoint, 2011). Training will include multiple match fights but also cruel treatment including hanging the dog for hours from tree branches, beating the dog with sticks, injecting it with steroids or building its muscles on a treadmill, (RSPCA, 2009; Merck, 2013; Harding, 2014).

Aside from the brutalisation of dogs used for fighting, it is clear that the public image of the Pit Bull and other bull breed dogs has undergone a transformation in the public mind, however this does not fully answer the question as to why people might then wish to own one, and in particular non-gang members.

## 6.7 Motivations for owning a status dog

All of us who own a pet animal receive some form of companionship (Ormerod, 2008) and this is particularly so with dogs. For many there are explicit therapeutic benefits of animal–human relationships (Fawcett and Gullone, 2001) that offer opportunities for social and family bonding, to experience and develop caring and nurturing skills or to increase social capital and physical activity through dog walking and companionship (Harding, 2012; Hughes, Maher and Lawson, 2011; Nast, 2006; Power, 2008). Improved self-control, decreased hostility and greater pro-social behaviour are also evidenced benefits of dog ownership (Ascione, 2005).

Recent research into status dogs by University of Cardiff (Hughes, Maher and Lawson, 2011; Maher and Pierpoint, 2011) noted that companionship was one important element in why young men choose to have status dogs. However, as this is a factor for most of us who own a dog, I believe the real motivations for ownership of a status dog lie much deeper.

To explore this more deeply, from April 2009 to April 2011 I undertook extensive research into the motivations of owning a status dog; this research was published in Harding, S. (2014) *Unleashed: the Phenomena of Status Dogs and Weapon Dogs*. During this time I successfully completed 100 qualitative interviews with professionals working with dogs, police, probation, residents, gang-affiliated youth and owners/handlers of supposedly aggressive breeds. Professionals were sampled by snowballing methods and youths were sampled by convenience sampling in a variety of different locations. Interviews were conducted outside RSPCA hospitals, in parks, high streets and on public transport. I also undertook the UK's first ever focus group specifically with young status dog owners actively involved in breeding and fighting dogs. The research identified four major motivational categories for ownership of status dogs. In ascending priority they are:

### 6.7.1 Fashion

Owners here view themselves as anti-establishment and will 'play outside society rules'. Large aggressive dogs may become fashionable, anti-fashion statements by those seeking a talking point; those following trends or those seeking to be different and demonstrate their 'urban cool'. David Grant, director of the RSPCA's Harmondsworth Animal Hospital in north London, has sought to distinguish between 'fashion dogs', which he views as part of a craze, and 'status dogs', which he believes are bred for offence and defence. Offering a statement on this he continues:

> 'Fashion dogs tend to be staffie crosses that are naturally good-natured, turning nasty only when they suffer abuse, or neglect when their owners get bored. Status dogs, on the other hand, are bred to intimidate. At the worst level, gangs will use them for mascots, muggings, safeguarding territory, and fighting enemies and other dogs.' (Davis, 2010)

### 6.7.2 Protection

Those owners motivated to use the dog for protection are perhaps the most traditional of owners. This category usually contained older more mature men and young women living in inner city areas. Here the dog is used for the traditional role of pet/guardian. It is likely that twenty to forty years ago German shepherds may have been used by this group for the role.

As author Justin Rollins noted in his book, *Status Dogs and Gangs* (2014):

> '*I myself have lived on a small housing estate in a south London town where crime, drugs and alcohol abuse are rife … Living in this environment is enough to send anyone over the edge and that is why a minority of status dogs are really not for social status, they are simply guard dogs, bought out of fear of the environment one happens to find themselves living in.*'

Some, however, view protection in other ways with the dog effectively substituting another weapon such as a knife. In the BBC Three production, *My Weapon is a Dog* (Broadcast 21 May 2009) one respondent claimed:

> '*Nowadays you know that (a dog) is just as good as having a knife. The damage that (dog) can do to a person if used in the right way, it can inflict more pain than the knife, cos it's going to be crushing bones and piercing skin.*'

### 6.7.3  Making money (entrepreneurship)

Undoubtedly some people are motivated to make money from their dog as their prime motivational reason for ownership. Three sub-categories are evident, including income generation from breeding; dog fighting; and use of dogs in crime, for example using the dog as a 'heavy' to collect drug debts. Breeding dogs, and in particular backstreet breeding, can act as an income generator for some as they seek to meet the increased demand for large bull breed dogs or status dogs with increased supply. Some of the increased supply will be met by importing dogs from Eastern Europe, while others will be supplied by backstreet breeders who both over-breed and hybridise their animals for profit. A pair of Pit Bulls with two litters per year can generate up to £7,000 untaxed income for a family in one year. As one seventeen-year-old breeder revealed (Harding, 2012) when discussing breeding his pair of Pit Bulls:

> '*Three of them died out of [a litter of] 16. All the rest got sold. I sold two to my cousin and I sold the rest to my mates, no advertising, just sold them off privately. I sold some for £600 and some for £400. Girls were £600 and the boys £400. Girls are more 'cos they are the ones for breeding. And the rare ones I sold for £650, the rare boys, if the colour is good.*'

Separate from this are those owners who utilise large aggressive bull breed dogs to act as a 'heavy' in the collection of drug debts. Here dogs provide a 'credible threat of violence', offering silent but effective intimidation that facilitate money making exercises.

> '*I've set my dog on people in the past, but nobody who didn't deserve it. Dogs become more legendary than their owners. One dealer on this estate had a Pitbull which was so tough a gang set out to assassinate it.*' (Francis, 2010).

Lastly, money can be generated by dog fighting. Dog fighting can occur between youths in the street in impromptu 'street rolls', in converted garages and houses by hobbyists or in specially constructed pits by professional organised Dogmen, or within the traveller community in the UK:

> *'Pitbulls are big in the Travellers' community. It's fighting, and to make money, you've always got to make money. But it's tradition, you've got to have a dog, to protect you or the pitch. But a pit will bring in the money, travellers also breed 'em.' (Professional dog fighter quoted from Harding, 2014)*

### 6.7.4 Image enhancement among peers

The largest motivational category by far, however, is that of image and identity. Within this category are groups of largely working-class young men who have been 'typically denied masculine status in education and employment'. In seeking to define themselves as men they embrace global images of gangsters, urban cool and violence. They strive to build local reputations for violence and to generate respect among peers. This in turn generates street capital, which can elevate their status among street-based hierarchies or groups. A fast track way to achieve this is to acquire a large bull breed dog that shows aggressive displays and then permits them to control public space, to control conversations and to determine group actions. In such ways young men become the centre of the peer groups and rise in popularity, and achieve superiority in group status. As one young man articulated in Harding's research (2012):

> *'I have it [the Pitbull dog] 'cos when I walk her people move out of the way. I like that. It makes me feel good.'*

An interviewee from the Hughes, Maher and Lawson (2011) research responded when asked what kind of people own large bull breed or status dogs:

> *'People that think they're big and they're not. They just want their dogs to make them look big. They try to get a rep [reputation].'*

Looked at from another perspective, author and reporter Graham Johnson was quoted as saying:

> *'If a gang member has a weapon dog with him he instantly becomes the most feared person in that group. Vicious dogs give people power and status on estates that have been sucked dry of aspiration and esteem by deprivation.' (Francis, 2010).*

## 6.8 Limitations of the Harding research (2012)

The research conducted by Harding included thirty-seven qualitative interviews of professional staff; thirty interviews in the London borough of Lambeth related to gang membership; and 138 interviews of owners of status dogs (of which thirty-three were completed successfully). One focus group was also conducted with four young men involved in fighting and breeding their dogs for money. Interviews were aimed solely at those involved with, (i.e. owning or handling) large bull breed dogs or so-called status dogs and did not include or indeed seek to include interviews with owners of other dogs. The purpose of the research, which was conducted between April 2009 and April 2011, was to explore the issue of status dog ownership and in particular to uncover the motivations underlying ownership and desire for ownership.

It is likely, indeed highly probable, that breeds other than large bull breed dogs are used for the purposes of fashion, protection or for generating money and that for many these motivational categories will apply to them and their circumstances. However, the breeds favoured by the public will change and alter over time as trends change. What is clear from the research is that, in the UK at least, currently, large bull breed dogs are the breeds that offer the best fit for all three motivational categories for many people and for a significant number these breeds become their first choice. Moreover, it appears that this match between motivations and breed type is not limited to London or urban metropolitan areas but is recognised widely and extensively across the UK.

## 6.9  Brand values and public image

It appears that the physical and brand attributes of large, seemingly aggressive dogs and bull breeds in particular are therefore sought out by different owners to match their requirements. Those motivated by fashion seek a bull-breed dog to give a sense of rule-breaking and non-conformist lifestyles, while those using such dogs for protection utilise the traditional canine attributes of protection/defence and ability to instil fear of attack. For those using the dogs to generate income, the canine attributes shift again to marketable stock and bloodlines.

It is therefore in the motivational category of image and identity where the crux of this issue lies. In multiply deprived environments, young men seek to bolster or supplement perceived fragile masculinity and identity by utilising large bull breed dogs to generate reputation. Street reputations, or street capital, is manufactured by being in control of breeds commonly perceived to be difficult to control. This perception is enhanced by training the dog to be human-aggressive and adorning the dog in ghetto-warrior harness, chains and spikes.

Motivations naturally depend upon the owners' functional requirements, or how they intend to use the dog. Essentially people seek the right dog for the right purpose, i.e. they have a purpose in mind and then seek out the brand values and breeds that match this. Some functional requirements are overt or open and manifest while others, such as using a dog to boost image, are likely to be latent or at least not openly discussed.

What is clear is that if we live in a world where dogs are increasingly commodified, the brand values or breed reputational values will become dominant in the purchasing decisions of prospective owners. In the Pit Bull-type dog these brand values are so universally recognised and adopted they now act as symbols of the dog itself. In this way the Pit Bull 'brand' represents not just a powerful dog but a pariah social status, an aggressive force of nature demonstrating fierce loyalty and a determination to 'never let go'. Combined with a high pain threshold and dog-on-dog aggression, they have become viewed as the gangster's dog. Such values are a perfect match for street-oriented or gang-affiliated youth who also view themselves with the same attributes and brand values, i.e. being tough, aggressive, ultimate warriors who are looked down upon by society.

The canine attributes of bull breed dogs used for image amplification are power, aggression, hyper-masculinity, alpha male superiority and ability to control space. Sadly, the purported malleable nature of Pit Bulls and Staffordshire Bull Terriers make them ideal for owners seeking to utilise these branded values or simply to create them in the dog through mal-socialisation (Harding, 2012).

## 6.10 Implications for the public

The increased prevalence of aggressive and bull-breed type dogs leads to increased public visibility, which in turn leads to increased public anxiety over public safety, notably in parks and open spaces. Here dogs are paraded or exercised and while many pose no problem to the public, they often generate complaints from park users. If dogs are being trained to be aggressive by their owners they can be used to chew tree bark to strengthen jaws and teeth. In 2009 the London Tree Officers Association reported £100,000 of damage to trees in Islington borough alone due to dogs attacking trees (2010). Other boroughs reported dogs being 'trained' by chewing children's swings in playgrounds (BBC News, 2009). Media reports are also common regarding supposed Pit Bulls and aggressive behaviour in bull breeds or bull breed crosses resulting in the attack and injury of working dogs and guide dogs for the blind, as well as children.

In an attempt to address some of these issues new legislation has been introduced (see Chapter 13). In 2012 the Government began consultation on tackling irresponsible dog ownership, and published new, tougher sentencing guidelines for those involved in dangerous dogs offences. In 2013 the Government announced its decision to introduce compulsory microchipping of all dogs from April 2016. Also, in 2013 the Government published draft legislation for scrutiny by Defra. In 2014 the Government introduced the Antisocial Behaviour, Crime and Policing Act (2014), which extended dangerous dogs legislation to private property and increased the powers relating to dogs and antisocial behaviour. In addition, in Scotland, the Control of Dogs (Scotland) Act 2010, requires all owners to keep control of their dogs in private and public places, regardless of their breed. Dog microchipping was made compulsory in Northern Ireland in 2011 and in Wales in 2015. Police and local authorities can also demand that owners take action to prevent a dog attack. Failure to do so can lead to a fine of up to £20,000 (Defra, 2013).

While legislation changes attempt to address widespread public concerns (Defra, 2014), it also reinforces perceptions that dangerous dogs and their dangerous owners must require exceptional or even draconian legislation to keep them in check. The line between 'responsible' and 'irresponsible' owner–dog partnerships within these breed types is also muddled, as clearly not all owners of these dogs are gang-linked youths. Nevertheless, so long as the public image of 'aggressive' bull-breed dogs and their owners as overtly negative, dangerous and a real public safety concern remains co-joined and sealed in the public mind, it is likely to be an issue with us for a long time to come.

## 6.11 References

Allen, I. (2007). 'Petey and Chato: the Pitbulls transition from mainstream to marginalised masculinity', Unpublished thesis, University of Southern California.

Ascione, F. R. (2005). *Children and animals: Exploring the roots of kindness and cruelty,* West Lafayette, IN: Purdue University Press.

Baker (1993). The Turbulent Years: My Life in Politics, London: Faber and Faber.

Barnes, J., Boat, B., Putnam, F., Dates, H., Mahlman, A. (2006). Ownership of High-Risk ('Vicious') Dogs as a Marker for Deviant Behaviours: Implication for Risk Assessment, *Journal of Interpersonal Violence* 21: 1616.

Battersea Dogs and Cats Home (2012). Best of British: Annual Review 2012. London: BDCH.

BBC News (2009). http://news.bbc.co.uk/go/pr/fr/-/1/hi/northern_ireland

BBC News (2010). Law change call after 'dramatic' rise in dangerous dogs, BBC news: Politics 29 December 2010.

Bourdieu, P. (1977). *Outline of a Theory of Practice.* Cambridge: Cambridge University Press.

Casey, R., Loftus, B., Bolster, C., Richards, G., Blackwell, E. (2013). Human directed aggression in domestic dogs (Canis Familiaris): Occurrence in different contexts and risk factors, Applied animal Behaviour Science 2013: DOI 10.10.1016/j.applanim.2013.12.003.

Cuddy, B. (2014). *'Pit Bulls, Witchhunts, Genocide and Dogifestos'* The Huffington Post 8 October 2014.

Davis, R. (2010). Are dogs the new weapon of choice for young people? *The Guardian* 17 February 2010.

Defra (2009). Dangerous Dogs law guidance for enforcers, London: Defra.

Defra (2010a). Press release, Dangerous dogs consultation responses published. 25 November 2010. https://www.gov.uk/government/news/dangerous-dogs-consultation-responses-published

Defra (2010b). Public Consultation on Dangerous Dogs, 9 March 2010, Defra.

Defra (2012). Annex A Promoting more responsible dog ownership. Proposals to tackle irresponsible dog ownership (April 2012) www.defra.gov.uk

Defra (2013). Dangerous Dogs Act 1991. Proposed Changes to maximum Penalties for Dog Attacks: Summary of Responses and Way Forward. www.gov.uk/Defra

Defra (2014). Dealing with irresponsible dog ownership: Practitioner's Manual. www.gov.uk/Defra

Delise, K. (2007). The Pit Bull placebo: The media, myths and politics of canine aggression, Manonville, NY: Anubis Press.

Dogs Trust (2010–13). Stray Dogs Survey (various by year), London: GFK NOP Research.

Dunne, P. (2009). The Rise of the urban status dog, www.animalwardens.co.uk

Evans, R. Kalich, D., Forsyth, C. (1998). Dogfighting: Symbolic Expression and Validation of Masculinity, in *Sex Roles* 39 (11–12): 825–832. Plenum Publishing Corporation/Springer.

Fawcett, N. R., Gullone, E. (2001). Cute and cuddly and a whole lot more? A call for empirical investigation into the therapeutic benefits of human–animal interaction for children. *Behaviour Change*, 18(2), 124–133.

Forsyth, C., Evans, R. (1998). Dogmen: The Rationalisation of Deviance, *Society and Animals*, Vol 6, No. 3.

Francis, N. (2010). My dog could kill a man in minutes, *The Sun*, 11 March 2010.

Gunderson, R. (2011). From cattle to capital: exchange value, animal commodification, and barbarism. *Critical Sociology*, 0896920511421031.

Hallsworth, S. (2011). *'Then they came for the dogs',* Crime, law and Social Change, vol 5: 391–403.

Harding, S. (2010). 'Status dogs and gangs', *Safer Communities*, vol 9, no 1, pp.30–35.

Harding, S. (2012). *Unleashed: The phenomena of status dogs and weapon dogs*, Bristol: The Policy Press.

Harding, S. (2013). 'Bling with Bite' – the rise of status and weapon dogs, Veterinary Record 173: 261–263.

Harding, S. (2014). *The Street Casino: Survival in the violent street gang*, Bristol: The Policy Press.

Harding, S., Nurse, A. (2015). Analysis of UK Dog Fighting, Laws and Offences: A Research Working Paper, Middlesex University.

Hood, C., Rothstein, H., Baldwin, R. (2001). *The Government of Risk: Understanding Risk Regulation Regimes*. Oxford University Press.

Hughes, G., Maher, J., Lawson, C. (2011). *Status Dogs, young people and criminalisation: towards a preventative strategy*. RSPCA and Cardiff University.

Kasperson, M. (2008). 'On *treating the symptoms and not the cause, reflections on the Dangerous Dogs Act'*, papers from the British Criminology Conference, vol 8: 205–25.

Lodge, M., Hood, C. (2002). Pavlovian policy responses to media feeding frenzies? Dangerous Dogs regulation in comparative perspective. *Journal of Contingencies and Crisis*, 10, 1–13.

LTOA (London Tree Officers Association) (2010) Bark better than bite: Damage to trees by dogs, London: LTOA.

Maher, J., Pierpoint, H. (2011). Friends, status symbols and weapons: the use of dogs by youth groups and youth gangs. Crime, Law and Social Change, 55(5), 405–420.

Merck, M. (2013). Veterinary Forensics (Second Edition): Animal Cruelty Investigations, Sussex: Wiley-Blackwell.

Nast, H. (2006). Loving …Whatever: Alienation, neoliberalism and Pet-Love in the Twenty-First Century. International Studies Program, DePaul University, Chicago, USA.

Ormerod, E. (2008). Companion animals and offender rehabilitation – Experiences from a prison therapeutic community in Scotland. Therapeutic Communities, 29(3), 285–296

Oxley, J. A. (2012). Dog owners' perception of breed-specific dangerous dog legislation in the UK, *Veterinary Record*, DOI: 10.1136/vr.100495.

Peters, S. (2008). A fight to save urban youth from dogfighting, USA Today, 29th September 2008.

Podersbeck, A. L. (1994). Dogs on a tightrope: the position of the dog in British society as influenced by the press reports on dog attacks (1988–1992) *Anthrozoos* 7, 232–241.

Power, E. (2008). 'Furry families: making a human-dog family through home', *Social and Cultural Geography*, vol 9, no 5: 535–55.

Radford, M. (2001). *Animal Welfare Law in Britain: Regulation and Responsibility*. Oxford University Press.

Randour, M. L., Hardiman, T. (2006). Creating Synergy for Gang Prevention: Taking a Look at Animal Fighting and Gangs, Proceedings of Persistently Safe Schools: The 2007 National Conference on Safe Schools.

Rollins, J. (2014). Status Dogs and Gangs. Self-published.

Smith-Spark, L. (2007). Brutal Culture of US Dog fighting, BBC News, Washington. 24 August 2007.

Strouse, K. (2009). Badd Newz: The Untold Story of the Michael Vick dog fighting Case, Dog fighting Investigations Publications LLC. USA.

www.parliament.uk (2012). Early day motion 822: Tackling Dog Attacks on Postmen and Postwomen (Session: 2012–13; Date tabled: 12 May 2012). www.parliament.uk/edm/2012-13/822

# CHAPTER 7

# Public Perceptions of Breed-Related Risk – Fact or Fiction?

*Tracey Clarke*

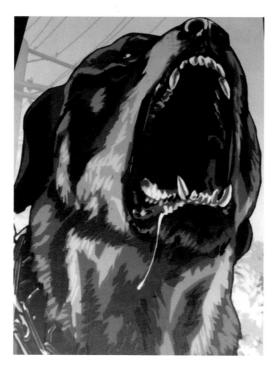

**Figure 7.1** Image from promotional poster of computer game Grand Theft Auto, Spring 2013.

## 7.1 Introduction

The branding and symbolisation of dog breeds/types (e.g. Figure 7.1) through the media has proven to be potent and enduring for not just selling newspapers and merchandise, but more worryingly in shaping public perception of the risk they pose. For effective social policy that safeguards the public and promotes canine welfare it is, however, important to separate fact from fiction.

Public perception of 'risk' is subject to cultural and historical variations, and so it needs to be placed within a socio-political context. This chapter focuses primarily on the United Kingdom, which was at the forefront of the introduction of breed-specific legislation – Dangerous Dogs Act, 1991 (DDA, 1991). It is suggested that this legitimised the public's perception of certain dog types as inherently 'dangerous' and a risk to the safety of the public, including globally as many other countries followed suit, although some are now recoiling from their initial reaction (see Chapter 13).

The media representation of supposedly dangerous dog breeds/types, statistical data of dog – bite incidents, and research evidence are examined within this chapter. The usefulness of statistical data is undermined by there being no official figures available for breed populations in the United Kingdom. Furthermore, official dog bite statistics cannot alone provide us with an accurate representation of breed-specific aggression, as not all dog bites are recorded (i.e. many victims do not seek medical treatment or otherwise register the incident) and, like statistics for dog bite fatalities, as kept by the Office of National Statistics (ONS), breed is not necessarily recorded. Nonetheless, the ONS (UK) maintains a record of all registered dog bite fatalities and the ages of victims, cross-referenced against media reporting of highly publicised cases. This reveals trends in media reporting of dog bite fatalities that, it is suggested, would have likely informed public perception of particular dog breeds/types and the risk they pose. Drawing on sociological and psychological research, this chapter also offers an explanation for the endurance of the public's misconceived perception of breed/dog type as a major predictor of aggressive behaviour.

## 7.2 Fear and public perception of risk in the UK

In safeguarding the public, fear serves a valuable evolutionary function and may be a 'duty' when it assists reason. Without reason, its purpose may be to serve a more insidious role, which should be challenged. As the eminent English writer and literary critic, Samuel Johnson (1751) put it,

> *'Fear is implanted in us as a preservative from evil: but its duty, like that of the other passions, is not to overbear reason, but to assist it; nor should it be suffered to tyrannize in the imagination, to raise phantoms of horror, or beset life with supernumerary distresses.'*

While the use of the word '*evil*' is contentious, there are perhaps few who would challenge the importance of separating fact from fiction in assessing risk to better assist reason and social policy. Regrettably however, fear and the '*phantoms of horror*' it raises are powerful marketing tools in the sale of newspapers, media headlines and merchandise, and powerful political tools in the hands of politicians, informing public perception of risk, responsibility and action required. This is no more evident than in media reporting of supposedly 'dangerous dogs' in the UK (see Chapter 5).

The genesis of the public's fear of particular dog breeds/types can perhaps be found in an increasingly risk aversive society, particularly if it relates to child safety. A search of UK newspapers by Furedi (2006) found that in 1994 the term 'at risk' was mentioned 2,037 times. This escalated to 18,003 in 2000. This perception of risk is further

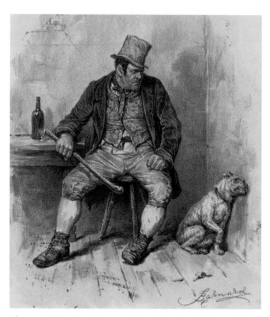

**Figure 7.2** Fred Barnard's 1878 depiction of the characters Bill Sykes and Bullseye from Charles Dickens' novel *Oliver Twist* (1838).

amplified by a 'culture of fear' driven by the media's use of sensationalism to drive a narrative or sell a brand (Altheide, 2002; Furedi, 2006; Ericson et al., 1991; Goode and Ben-Yehuda, 2010). An increasingly risk aversive society with a focus on child safety, and the powerful imagery afforded by the representation of particular dog breeds/types to drive a highly accessible narrative offers an explanation for the public's increased anxiety and perception of risk concerning particular dog breeds/types.

This process dates back centuries, including notable examples such as the bull terrier's association with the criminal underworld in *Oliver Twist* (Dickens, 1838, Figure 7.2) and more recent depiction in films such as *No Country for Old Men* (2007) and *Julia (*2008), or symbolic of some British underclass, for example in films such as *Tyrannosaur* (2011).

In the case of the Rottweiler, this breed is often represented in the media as a malevolent force, with their appearance in the now iconic graveyard scene of the *The Omen* (1976) soon followed by starring roles in films – *Devil Dog, The Hound of Hell* (1978) and *Dogs of Hell* (1982), and more recently in *Rottweiler* (2004). In marked contrast, other breeds such as golden retrievers and Labradors are typically depicted in film as 'safe' and 'family-friendly', e.g. *Poltergeist* (1982), *Fatal Attraction* (1987) and in the Disney franchise, *Air Bud* (1997). This misconception of safe dogs, which also arises from the idea that there are dangerous dogs, can also lead to the equally disastrous events, as individuals may feel these dogs will tolerate any amount of inappropriate handling. The media's use of breed images and the assumptions they engender in the public consciousness concerning expectations of dog behaviour is a much under-researched area of study.

## 7.3  Media reporting of 'dangerous dog' breeds/types

An exploration of the nature of the UK print media's reporting of dog attacks over the period 1988–92 by Podberscek (1994) reveals:

- In 1989 and 1990 German shepherds and Rottweilers were the most commonly reported breeds in headlines involving dog bite incidents.
- In 1989–91 a total of seven dog bite fatalities were reported. Of this total, three were children (under fifteen years) and four were older adults (aged fifty-eight years plus). The attacks on children were more widely reported (60% or more of reports).
- Of the eleven dogs (comprising seven breeds/types – Rottweiler, German shepherd, Staffordshire Bull Terrier, Bull Terriers, Great Dane, Lakeland Terrier)

involved in dog bite fatalities – just one individual dog was identified as a 'Pit Bull Terrier cross'.

- In 1989 intense negative media reporting of dogs escalated following the death of an eleven-year-old who was attacked by two Rottweilers. This breed was frequently described by news media as the 'devil' or 'killer' dog.
- During 1991 there was a shift in media interest, perhaps for political reasons, from the Rottweiler to the American Pit Bull Terrier (APBT). In 1991 the words 'Pit Bull Terrier' appeared in 53% of headlines where the breed of dog was mentioned. The German shepherd appeared in 5.8% of cases, and the Rottweiler 11.8%. Increased media interest in the APBT in 1991 appears to have been stimulated by two attacks within a short period of each other, one involving a six year old girl. The APBT was typically reported by the print media as a breed used in the criminal underworld (*the hood*) for protection.

It would be unwise to underestimate the pernicious effect of mass media representations in perpetuating the view of the dog type/breeds identified in the DDA 1991, and similar legislation in other countries, as dangerous and behaviourally homogenous; a natural consequence of which would be increasing anxiety among the general public about the risk they pose. This increased perception of risk is not uncommon in relation to the reporting of a number of 'social problems' that receive salacious media coverage. Research suggests that the public's perception of issues such as immigration, benefit fraud and crime are widely out of kilter with the statistical evidence (Ipsos Mori (UK), August 2014).

The prototypical nature of many press reports about dog bite fatalities may be designed to ease comprehension – the 'availability heuristic'. This is a cognitive heuristic in which a person relies upon readily available knowledge rather than examining alternatives (Tversky and Kahneman, 1974). Therefore, material that is incongruent with past exemplars of aggressive and supposedly dangerous dog breeds/types is less likely to be employed. Closely allied to the 'availability heuristic' is the concept of confirmation bias – a tendency for people to favour information that confirms their preconceptions or hypotheses regardless of the accuracy of the information (Wason, 1968). Furthermore, within social psychology it is recognised that anxiety narrows the focus of attention, leading to the treatment of out-group members less as individuals and more as equivalent members of a category (Stephan and Stephan, 1984). Anxiety can also weaken the impact of stereotype-disconfirming information (Wilder and Shapiro, 1989; Wilder, 1993) and so affect public perception of risk.

The use of media headlines involving children offers editors the opportunity to draw on the contrast between 'good and evil', an integral feature of classic childhood fairy tales (Franz, 1974; Bettelheim, 2010). These narratives function at a deep psychological level, tapping into our primal fears (Figure 7.3). The disproportionate concern for child safety over recent decades (Piper et al., 2006; Sikes, 2008), coupled with a media feeding frenzy in the reporting of dog bite incidents involving children in the late 1980s, led policy makers to make a type of 'forced choice' (Lodge and Hood, 2002) to respond to the public's perceived threat from these 'devil dogs'.

In the exercise of power, it is important for governments to be seen to react to public concerns, and this was so for the British government of 1991. Possibly interested in presenting its traditionally punitive 'tough on crime' image, the Conservative government hastened

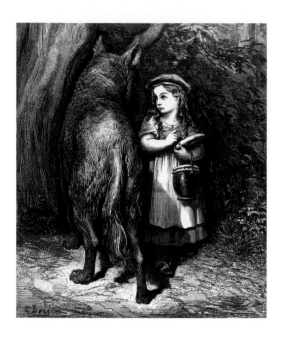

**Figure 7.3** *Red Riding Hood and The Wolf* by the artist Gustav Dore, 1883.

the passage of the DDA, 1991 through Parliament in a single day (Hansard, 1992). The professed objective of this *'panic policy making'* (Hunter and Brisbin, 2007) was to keep *'the public as secure as is conceivably possible'* (Radford, 2001). In addition to 'the Pit Bull Type', three 'fighting' breeds, were seemingly randomly identified in the DDA, 1991 – the Japanese Tosa, Dogo Argentino and Fila Brasileiro – as representing a risk to public safety.

Research suggests that the labelling of particular populations as 'dangerous' and/or 'deviant' serves an important function in satisfying society's need to effect some control over a perceived threat and powerfully affects public perception of the risk they pose (Durkheim, 1897; Cohen, 1972; 2002; Hall et al., 1978; Becker, 2008).

In Cohen's seminal study, *Folk Devils and Moral Panics*, he writes:

*'Societies appear to be subject, every now and then, to periods of moral panic. A condition, episode, person or group of persons emerges to become defined as a threat to societal values and interests; its nature is presented in a stylized and stereotypical fashion by the mass media.' 1972:9.*

## 7.4 The American Pit Bull Terrier – folk devil – brand aggression

During the late 1980s in the UK the American Pit Bull Terrier (APBT) emerged as a 'Folk Devil' – a breed portrayed in the media as the personification of the 'dangerous dog' and whose name became a metaphor for aggressiveness and tenacity. Myths began to circulate about this strange, new type of dog with 'locking jaws' and a propensity to bite, that persist today, despite a lack of evidence to support this (Collier, 2006).

Cohen's work (2002) on symbolisation can be usefully applied to our understanding of the public's perception of the APBT – satisfying the three requirements for the mass communication of a stereotype (See Box 7.1).

**Box 7.1  Three requirements for the mass communication of a stereotype**

**Word** – 'Pit Bull' becomes a metaphor for aggressiveness– media headlines commonly referring to this dog type as a *'Devil Dog'* of a particular threat to towards children, and having strong associations with public perceptions of working class delinquency (Jones, 2012). The latter, perhaps, responsible for the shift in media focus away from the Rottweiler.

**Objects** – Dogs of a particular morphological type come to symbolise the word (Figure 7.4). Breeds are principally identified from their appearance. Recent research suggests that the now iconic physical features of the Pit Bull strongly affect people's feelings of fear (Gazzano et al., 2013). Furthermore, the public's fear of these dogs has resulted in other dog types with similar physical features to experience what Goffman (1963) described as *courtesy stigma* (Twining et al,. 2000).

**Status** – The objects themselves become symbolic of a status (and the heightened emotions of moral outrage attached to that status). This symbolism powerfully fuels fear of the 'other' – racism (Hall, 1978) and breedism (Clarke, 2012; Clarke et al., 2013).

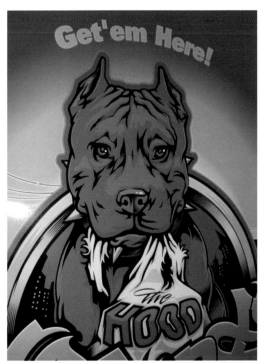

**Figure 7.4** Promotional poster for Hood Hounds collectible figures.

The media feature significantly in moral debates, often by setting the agenda – selecting those who might be deviant or socially problematic and transmitting claims (often through imagery) and manipulating the rhetoric for identifying deviant types (Hall et al., 1978; Cohen and Young, 1981; Cohen, 2002). It is in such media portrayals of dog types that we can see evidence of biased reporting bolstering the folk devil image of the Pit Bull type. Furthermore, lack of clarification of what is described in the Act as 'any dog of the *type* known as the Pit Bull Terrier' has resulted in confusion in interpretation (Hoffman et al., 2014) resulting in any dog of a stocky, muscular build being viewed with caution by members of the British public.

## 7.5  Recent media headlines – twenty-three years after the introduction of breed-specific legislation in the UK

More recently, in exploring the representation of 'aggressive dogs' in the British news media and the public perception of risk, Orritt and Harper (2014) highlight a number of key findings. Fatal dog bite stories score highly for 'newsworthiness' over the twelve news values identified by Ghavamnia and Dastjerdi (2013), particularly in relation to negativity and unambiguity:

*   Negativity – The tragedy of an event, 'emotional risk-based' media reporting of dog bite incidents typically included an emotional interview of close relatives describing the victim and events preceding their death.
*   Unambiguity – Media reporting of dog bite incidents typically involved succinct narratives relying on a clear angel/demon dichotomy, particularly incidents involving children. Dogs were frequently referred to as 'devil dogs' and victims typically portrayed as angelic and innocent. This is implicit in the following headline:

> *'Family of baby girl savaged to death by illegal American pit bull at her grandmother's house say they are "totally devastated" by loss of their "little princess"' (Daily Mail 10 October 2014)*

This was later followed by a reporting of the coroner's findings on 21 October 2014:

> *'This breed is classified under the dangerous dogs act for a reason – its dangerousness. The family in this case have paid the ultimate price for owning such a dog, the death of their six-month-old daughter.' (Daventry Express, UK, 21 October 2014)*

When breeds involved in dog bite fatalities do not fit the media narrative, there is a need to offer the public an explanation for this rather than challenging the crude ideological premise underpinning breed-specific legislation. Highlighting the dog as a *'stray'* or *'rescue'* assists in this as it suggests that, although breed is an important predictor or behaviour, this can occasionally be trumped by other factors (which may relate to antisocial behaviour tendencies that led to the previous rejection of the dog). Again, this type of reporting effectively labels the dog as culprit rather than victim, as illustrated by the following headlines: *'Dog that mauled Lexi, 4, to death was "park stray"'* (*Metro*, London, 7 November 2013), *'Newborn baby girl savaged to death by dog family rescued'* (*Daily Mail*, 19 February 2014).

## 7.6  Breed-related risk – the evidence

### 7.6.1  Dog bites and breeds

Data from the Department of Trade and Industry's home and leisure accident surveillance systems (Home Accident Surveillance System (HASS) and the Leisure Accident Surveillance System (LASS) for the period November 1987 to November 1988 record that in excess of 55,000 children were bitten during this period, but only three in 200 cases involved children being hospitalised for more than six days and no fatalities were recorded. Dog bites were

**Table 7.1** Breeds recorded in dog bites to children in the UK, November 1987 to November 1988 (Levene, 1991).

| HASS | | LASS | |
| --- | --- | --- | --- |
| Breed | Number | Breed | Number |
| Mongrel | 114 | Mongrel | 63 |
| German shepherd | 66 | German shepherd | 52 |
| Jack Russell | 49 | Jack Russell | 17 |
| Doberman | 22 | Doberman | 13 |
| Rottweiler | 13 | Rottweiler | 8 |
| | | Pit Bull Terrier | 1 |

common, but rarely serious (Levene, 1991). The breed of dog was recorded in 487 (36%) of HASS incidents and 237 (27%) of LASS incidents. Of the dog bite incidents where the breed of dog was named, only one recorded the APBT, with the vast majority involving mongrels (Table 7.1). This likely represents the breeds of dogs that were popular to own at the time, and the Pit Bull Terrier was rare. Looking at this data, to ban Pit Bulls and not German shepherds, Jack Russells, Dobermans and Rottweilers seems illogical.

More recently, a review of available data of registered dog bite fatalities from the ONS (UK) spanning 2005–13, cross-referenced with media reports portrays a similar picture concerning the risks posed by 'dangerous dogs' as since identified in the 1991 Act (Table 7.2), even when difficulties in identifying breed in such cases, as identified in previous chapters, are taken into consideration.

Despite media interest in reporting incidents involving 'Pit Bull types' or Bull Terriers, 88% of the dogs identified by breed in the British press (2005–13) involved in fatalities, were not 'dangerous' breeds as identified in the DDA, 1991 (Table 7.2). Furthermore, scientific evidence also reports no significant differences between Bull Terriers and Golden Retrievers in hypertrophy of aggressive behaviour towards humans (Ott et al., 2009). A dog bite fatality involving an unremarkable breed and adult is not nearly as newsworthy to the British press as an incident involving a Bull Terrier type and child. A similar phenomenon concerning the media representation of the Pit Bull has been found following research in the US (Delise, 2007).

## 7.6.2 *The impact of breed-specific legislation*

Breed-specific legislation engenders a misleading and false assumption that breeds that are not labelled as 'dangerous' are 'safe'. All types of dog have the potential to bite, and according to popular belief especially if the dog is not trained or socialised properly, or if it is isolated, neglected or encouraged to behave aggressively. Further, there is no evidence that breed alone is a useful predictor of a dog's propensity for aggressive behaviour towards humans (See Chapter 10; and also Duffy et al., 2008; Ott et al., 2009; BVA–BSAVA, 2010) or towards children (Levene, 1991; Watson, 2001; Kahn et al., 2003). Clearly, there needs to be a shift away from breed as a causal explanation for aggressive behaviour and towards a more open consideration of other more relevant factors to inform risk management of dog bite incidents (See Chapters 4, 29, 30 and 32).

**Table 7.2** Reported and registered dog bite fatalities in the United Kingdom, 2005–13.

| Year | Human Fatality | Age of Victim | Location | Media-reported breed | Canine Fatality |
|---|---|---|---|---|---|
| **2005** | Liam Eames (M) | 1 year | Family Home – Leeds | **American Bulldog (1)** | Dog Destroyed |
| | Anon (F) | 35–39 yrs | — | | |
| **2006** | Caydee-Lee Glaze (F) | 5 months | Grandparent's public house – Leicester | **Rottweilers (2)** | Dogs Destroyed |
| | Anon (M) | 30–34 yrs | — | | — |
| | Anon (M) | 60–64 yrs | — | | — |
| **2007** | Ellie Lawrenson (F) | 5 years | Grandmother's home – Merseyside | **Pit Bull Type (1)** | Dog Destroyed |
| | Archie-Lee Hirst (M) | 1 year | Grandparent's home – Yorkshire | **Rottweiler (1)** | Dog Destroyed |
| **2008** | Anon (M) | 1–4 yrs | — | | — |
| | Anon (M) | 65–69 yrs | — | | — |
| | Anon (F) | 75–79 yrs | — | | — |
| | Anon (F) | Under 1 year | | | — |
| **2009** | Jaden Mack (M) | 3 months | Grandmother's home – Wales | **Staff Bull Terrier (1) and Jack Russell Terrier (1)** | Dogs Destroyed |
| | Andrew Walker (M) | 21 years | Friend's home – Blackpool | **German shepherds (2)** | Dogs Destroyed |
| | John Paul Massey (M) | 4 years | Grandmother's home – Liverpool | **Pit Bull Type (1)** | Dog Destroyed |
| | Anon (M) | 55–59 yrs | — | | — |
| | Anon (M) | 75–79 yrs | — | | — |
| | Anon (M) | 80–84 yrs | — | | — |
| **2010** | Zumer Ahmed (F) | 18 mths | Family home – Sussex | **American Bulldog (1)** | Dog Destroyed |
| | Barbara Williams (F) | 52 yrs | Family home – Wallington Nr. Sutton | **Belgian Mastiff (1)** | Dog Destroyed |
| | Anon (F) | 80–84 yrs | — | | — |
| | Anon (F) | 85–89 yrs | — | | — |
| **2011** | Anon (M) | 35–39 yrs | — | | — |
| | Anon (M) | 50–54 yrs | — | | — |
| | Anon (M) | 70–74 yrs | — | | — |
| | Anon (M) | 75–79 yrs | — | | — |
| | Anon (M) | 85–89 yrs | — | | — |
| | Anon (F) | 75–79 yrs | — | | — |
| **2012** | Anon (M) | 55–59 yrs | — | | — |
| | Anon (F) | 50–54 yrs | — | | — |
| | Anon (F) | 50–54 yrs | — | | — |
| **2013** | Lexi Branson (F) | 4 years | Family Home – Leicestershire | **Bulldog type (1)** | Dog destroyed |
| | Jade Anderson (F) | 14 years | Friend's Home – Greater Manchester | **Bull Mastiff (1)** | Dogs destroyed |
| | Anon (M) | 60–64 yrs | — | **American Bulldog (1)** | — |
| | Anon (M) | 80–84 yrs | — | **Staff. Bull Terriers (2)** | — |
| | Anon (F) | 70–74 yrs | — | | |

Regrettably, stereotypical images of certain dog types undoubtedly have particularly powerful cultural capital and advertisers naturally seek to exploit the value placed on these by many young adults (Figures 7.5 and 7.6). Ownership of a 'dangerous' breed by individuals is a mode of expression (Overall and Love, 2001; Harding, 2014). Like brands, they offer the individual a particular social status and social cachet (Klein, 2009; Maher and Pierpoint, 2011), and this is likely to be especially so in the case of low-income families and alienated youth (Hayward and Yar, 2006; Hamilton, 2012; Rollins, 2014).

The demonisation of dog types, particularly those of the Pit Bull type, increased the social cachet of owning them among the most disenfranchised and often the most brand-savvy in UK society, who fear social exclusion by their peers – inner-city working class adolescents (see Chapter 6). Within the criminal sub-cultures in the UK these dog types are commonly traded as commodities (Harding, 2014; Rollins, 2014; Chapter 6) and used to instil fear in others (human and non-human animals).

Therefore, the increase in status or weapon dogs in the UK (League Against Cruel Sports, UK, 2014) used to attack other people or animals is perhaps an unsurprising consequence of breed-specific legislation. Therefore repealing breed-specific legislation presents a useful way to address the desirability and the cultural capital afforded by the ownership of these breeds/dog types. Indeed some regions have started to repeal such legislation (see Chapter 13) and the impact on human safety and youth culture towards dogs should be assessed.

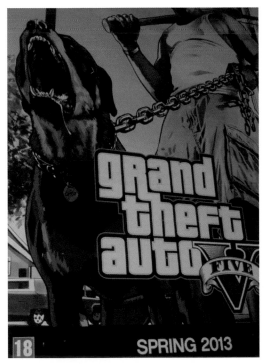

**Figure 7.5** Grand Theft Auto promotional poster, 2013.

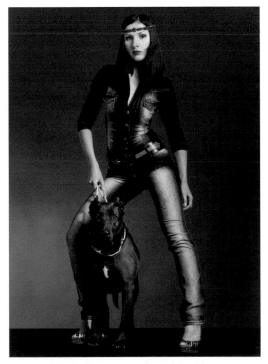

**Figure 7.6** Fashion shot of model with 'dangerous dog' type. (Photo: Adobe Stock)

## 7.7 Conclusion

Taking the UK as an exemplar, there appears to be a gap in how the public perceive the safety risk posed by dangerous dog breeds/types and the available evidence. This distorted reality may be explained by:

- The branding and symbolisation of particular breeds/types, perpetuated by the media, that left a legacy of stigmatisation from which it is difficult for members of these breeds/types and their owners to escape.
- The deviancy amplification spiral of particular dog types that ushered in breed-specific legislation, fuelled by fear and devoid of any scientific research. Seemingly, being tough on the issue of 'dangerous dogs' and reacting to populist perceptions of the risk they pose may have been seen as more important to those in power than engaging in any reasoned and informed debate.

What is often left out of this deviancy amplification spiral is the fear experienced by individual dogs that, because of labelling, stigmatisation and *spoiled identity* (Goffman, 1963) often find themselves poorly treated, and subject to destruction.

The dog needs to be recognised as a biological and cultural product – its behaviour cannot be characterised outside of a humans' and cultural and political context. To safeguard the public effectively and promote canine welfare it is important to combat the fundamentally crude and gross reductivist ideology perpetuated by the media and breed-specific legislation concerning 'dangerous' dogs and to develop a more nuanced understanding of this phenomena – the author suggests a useful first step would be to repeal breed-specific legislation.

## 7.8 References

*Air Bud* (1997). [Film] Directed by Charles Martin Smith, Walt Disney Pictures, Warner Brothers, UK.

Altheide, D. L. (2002). *Creating fear: News and the construction of crisis.* Transaction Publishers, New York, USA.

Appleby, D. L., Bradshaw, J. W., Casey, R. A. (2002). Relationship between aggressive and avoidance behaviour by dogs and their experience in the first six months of life. *The Veterinary Record,* 150(14), 434–438.

Barnes, J. E., Boats, B. W., Putnam, F. W., Dates, H. F., Mahlman, H. R. (2006). Ownership of high-risk ('vicious') dogs as a marker for deviant behaviours: implications for risk assessment. *Journal of Interpersonal Violence,* 21 1616–34.

Becker, H. S. (2008). *Outsiders.* Simon and Schuster. New York, USA.

Bettelheim, B. (2010). *The uses of enchantment: The meaning and importance of fairy tales.* Random House, New York, USA.

Borchelt, P. L. (1983). Aggressive behavior of dogs kept as companion animals: classification and influence of sex, reproductive status and breed. *Applied Animal Ethology,* 10, 45–61.

BVA-BSAVA (2010). Joint Response Dangerous Dogs Consultation (June 2010) www.bva.co.uk/uploadedFiles/Content/News-campaigns and policies/Policies/Companion animals (accessed 20 July 2014).

Clarke, T. (2012). Exploring Breed Diversity in Behaviour of the Domestic Dog (*Canis familiaris*) Acculturation – A Neglected Area of Study. PhD thesis. The University of Lincoln, UK.

Clarke, T, Cooper, J, Mills, D. (2013). Acculturation – Perceptions of breed differences in behavior of the dog (Canis familiaris) *Human-Animal Interaction Bulletin* 1 16–33.

Cohen, S. (1972). *Folk Devils and Moral Panics,* McGibbon and Kee Ltd, London, UK.

Cohen S. (2002). *Folk Devils and Moral Panics,* Third Edition, Routledge, Oxon, UK.

Cohen, S., Young, J. (eds) (1981). *The manufacture of news: Social problems, deviance and the mass media.* Constable, London, UK.

Collier, S. (2006). Breed-specific legislation and the pit bull terrier: Are the laws justified? *Journal of Veterinary Behavior: Clinical Applications and Research,* 1(1), 17–22.

*Daily Mail* headline – 10 November 2014 www.dailymail.co.uk/news/article-2787934/dog-savaged-six-month-old-baby-girl-death-grandmother-s-house-illegal-american-pit-bull-say-police.html#ixzz3IrVWABob (accessed 12 October 2014).

*Daily Mail* headline – 19 February 2014 www.dailymail.co.uk/home/sitemaparchive/day_20140219.html (accessed 10 March 2014).

*Dangerous Dogs Act, 1991* www.legislation.gov.uk/ukpga/1991/65/contents (accessed 10 July 2014).

*Daventry Express* www.daventryexpress.co.uk/news/local/family-paid-ultimate-price-for-owning-a-danger-dog-1-6369293 (accessed 20 October 2014).

Delise, K. (2007). *The Pit Bull Placebo. The Media, Myths and Politics of Canine Aggression.* National Canine Research Council, Anubis Publishing, Sofia, Bulgaria.

*Devil Dog, the Hound of Hell* (1978). [Film] Directed by Curtis Harrington, Wizan Productions, USA.

Dickens, C. (1838). *Oliver Twist*, Classic, 41, London, UK.

*Dogs of Hell; Rottweiler* (1982). [Film] Directed by Worth Keeler, USA.

Duffy, D. L., Hsu, Y., Serpell, J. A. (2008). Breed differences in canine aggression, *Applied Animal Behaviour Science,* 114 (3) 441–460.

Durkheim, É. (1897). Suicide. In Spaulding, J. and Simpson, G. (1951) *Suicide: A Study in Sociology.* The Free Press, New York, USA.

Ericson, R. V., Baranek, P. M., Chan, J. B. (1991). *Representing order: Crime, law, and justice in the news media.* Open University Press, Milton Keynes, UK.

*Fatal Attraction* (1987). [Film] Directed by Adrian Lyne, Paramount Pictures, USA.

Franz, M. L. V. (1974). *Shadow and evil in fairy tales.* Shambhala Publications Inc., Boston, USA.

Furedi, F. (2006). *Culture of fear revisited.* Continuum, London, UK.

Gazzano, A., Zilocchi, M., Massoni, E., Mariti, C. (2013). Dogs' features strongly affect people's feelings and behavior toward them. *Journal of Veterinary Behavior: Clinical Applications and Research,* 8, 213–220.

Ghavamnia, M., Dastjerdi, H. V. (2013). Evaluation in media discourse: contrasts among journalists in reporting an event. *Procedia-Social and Behavioral Sciences*, 70, 447–457.

Gladwell, M. (2006). Troublemakers: What pit bulls can teach us about profiling? *The New Yorker,* 81, 38–43.

Goffman, E. (1963). *Stigma: Notes on the Management of Spoiled Identity,* Prentice-Hall, New York, USA.

Goode, E., Ben-Yehuda, N. (2010). *Moral Panics: The Social Construction of Deviance.* Blackwell Publishers Ltd, Oxford, UK.

Hall, S., Critcher, C., Jefferson, T., Clarke, J., Roberts, B. (1978). *Policing the Crisis. Mugging, the State, and Law and Order.* The Macmillan Press Limited, London and Basingstoke, UK.

Hamilton, K. (2012). Low-income families and coping through brands: Inclusion or stigma? *Sociology,* 46, 74–90.

Hansard (House of Commons Debates) Sessions 1992–93. www.parliament.uk (accessed 20 August 2014).

Harding, S. (2014). *Unleashed: The Phenomena of Status Dogs and Weapon Dogs.* Policy Press, London, UK.

Hayward, K., Yar, M. (2006). The 'chav' phenomenon: Consumption, media and the construction of a new underclass. *Crime, Media, Culture,* 2, 9–28.

Herron, M. E., Shofer, F. S., Reisner, I. R. (2009). Survey of the use and outcome of confrontational and non-confrontational training methods in client-owned dogs showing undesired behaviors. *Applied Animal Behaviour Science,* 117, 47–54.

Hiby, E. F., Rooney, N. J., Bradshaw, J. W. S. (2004). Dog training methods: their use, effectiveness and interaction with behaviour and welfare. *Animal Welfare* 13, 63–69.

Hoffman, C. L., Harrison, N., Wolff, L., Westgarth, C. (2014). Is That Dog a Pit Bull? A Cross-Country Comparison of Perceptions of Shelter Workers Regarding Breed Identification. *Journal of Applied Animal Welfare Science,* 1–18.

Hunter, S., Brisbin, Jr., R. A. (2007). Panic Policy Making: Canine Breed Bans in Canada and the United States. Delivered at the 2007 Annual Meeting of the Western Political Science Association, Las Vegas, Nevada, 8–10 March.

IPSOS Mori (2014). Perceptions are not reality: Things the world gets wrong. Available at: https:www.ipsos.mori.com (accessed 1 November, 2014).

Johnson, S. (1751): Rambler (126) June 1 in Clark, J. C. D. (1994). Samuel Johnson: literature, religion and English cultural politics from the Restoration to Romanticism. Cambridge University Press. Cambridge, UK.

Jones, O. (2012). Chavs: The demonization of the working class. Verso Books, London, UK.

*Julia* (2008). Directed by Erick Zonca, Studio Canal, France.

Kahn, A., Bauche, P., Lamoureux, J. (2003). Child victims of dog bites treated in emergency departments: a prospective survey. *European journal of pediatrics,* 162, 254–258.

Klein, N. (2009*). No logo.* Fourth Estate, London, UK.

Lakestani, N. N., Waran, N., Verga, M., Phillips, C. (2005). Dog Bites in Children. *European Journal of Companion Animal Practice,* 15, 133–135.

League Against Cruel Sports (2014) Dog-fighting. Available at: www.league.org.uk/our-campaigns/dog-fighting (accessed 10 November, 2014).

Levene, S. (1991). Dog Bites to Children *British Medical Journal* 303: 466.

Lodge, M., Hood, C. (2002). Pavlovian Policy Responses to Media Feeding Frenzies? Dangerous Dogs Regulation in Comparative Perspective, *Journal of Contingencies and Crisis Management,* 10 1–13.

Maher, J., Pierpoint, H. (2011) Friends, status symbols and weapons: the use of dogs by youth groups and youth gangs. *Crime, law and social change,* 55, 405–420.

Meints, K., Racca, A., Hickey, N. (2010). Child–dog misunderstandings: children misinterpret dogs' facial expressions. In *Proceedings of the 2nd Canine Science Forum. Vienna,* Austria (Vol. 99).

*Metro* headline – 19 February 2014 http://metro.co.uk/2013/11/06/dog-that-mauled-lexi-branson-4-to-death-was-park-stray-4176967 (accessed 20 February 2014).

Morrongiello, B. A., House, K. (2004). Measuring parent attributes and supervision behaviors relevant to child injury risk: examining the usefulness of questionnaire measures. *Injury Prevention*, 10, 114–118.

*No Country for Old Men* (2007). [Film] Directed by Ethan Coen and Joel Coen, USA, Miramax Films.

ONS (2014) The 21st Century Mortality Files – Deaths Dataset, 2001–13 Available at: www.ons.gov.uk (accessed 10 October 2014).

Orritt, R., Harper, C. (2014). Similarities between the Representation of 'Aggressive Dogs' and 'Sex Offenders' in the British News Media. Available at: https://www.inter-disciplinary.net/probing-the-boundaries/wp-content/uploads/2014/05/orrittahpaper.pdf (accessed 10 October 2014).

Ott, S., Schalke, E., Hirschfeld, J., Hackbarth, H. (2009). Assessment of a Bullterrier bloodline in the temperament test of Lower Saxony – comparison with six dog breeds affected by breed specific legislation and a control group of Golden Retrievers. *DTW. Deutsche tierarztliche Wochenschrift*, 116, 132–137.

Overall, K. L, Love, M. (2001). Dog bites to humans – demography, epidemiology, injury, and risk. *Journal of the American Veterinary Medical Association*, 218 1923–34.

Pet Food Manufacturers Association, UK (2014). Available at: www.pfma.org.uk (accessed 1 October 2014).

Piper, H., Powell, J., Smith, H. (2006). Parents, Professionals, and Paranoia: the Touching of Children in a Culture of Fear. *Journal of Social Work*, 6, 151–167.

Podberscek, A. L. (1994). Dog on a tightrope: the position of the dog in British society as influenced by press reports on dog attacks (1988 to 1992). Anthrozoos: A Multidisciplinary *Journal of the Interactions of People & Animals*, 7, 232–241.

*Poltergeist* (1982). [Film] Directed by Tobe Hooper, SLM production Group, Metro Goldwyn Mayer, USA.

Radford, M. (2001). *Animal Welfare Law in Britain. Regulation and Responsibility*. Oxford University Press, Oxford, UK, 346–348.

Ragatz, L., Fremouw, W., Thomas, T., McCoy, K. (2009). Vicious dogs: the antisocial behaviours and psychological characteristics of owners. *Journal of Forensic Sciences*. 54 699–703.

Reisner, I. (1991). The pathophysiologic basis of behaviour problems. Veterinary Clinics of North America. *Small Animal Practice*, 21, 207–224.

Reisner, I. R., Shofer, F. S. (2008). Effects of gender and parental status on knowledge and attitudes of dog owners regarding dog aggression toward children. *Journal of the American Veterinary Medical Association*, 233, 1412–1419.

Rollins, J. (2014). *Status Dogs & Gangs*. CreateSpace Independent Publishing Platform, UK.

*Rottweiler* (2004). [Film] Directed by Brian Yuzna, Castelao Produccionas, Spain.

Shepherd, K. (2009). *BSAV Manual of Canine and Feline*, 2nd Edition, pages 13–16, Editors Horwitz, D.F and Mills, D.S.

Sikes, P. (2008). At the Eye of the Storm: An Academic('s) Experience of Moral Panic. *Qualitative Inquiry*, 14, 235–253.

Stephan, W. G., Stephan, C. W. (1984). The role of ignorance in intergroup relations. In Miller, N., Brewer, M. B (eds.) *Groups in contact: The psychology of desegregation*. Academic Press, Orlanda, Florida, USA.

Tami, G., Gallagher, A. (2009). Description of the behaviour of domestic dog (Canis familiaris) by experienced and inexperienced people. *Applied Animal Behaviour Science*, 120, 159–169.

*The Omen* (1976). [Film] Directed by Richard Donner, 20th Century Fox, UK.

2

Tversky, A. and Kahneman, D. (1974). Judgment under Uncertainty: Heuristics and Biases. *Science* 185, 1124–1131.

Twining, H., Arluke, A., Patronek, G. (2000). Managing the stigma of outlaw breeds: A case study of pit bull owners. *Society and Animals,* 8(1), 25–52.

*Tyrannosaur* (2011). [Film] Directed by Paddy Considine, Studio Canal, UK.

Valentine, G. (2004). *Public space and the culture of childhood.* Ashgate, Aldershot, UK.

Wason, P. C. (1968). Reasoning about a rule. *Quarterly Journal of Experimental Psychology* (Psychology Press) 20, 273–328.

Watson, L. (2001). Does breed specific legislation reduce dog aggression on humans and other animals? A review paper. Urban Animal Management Conference Proceedings 2003. www.ccac. net.au/files/Does-breed-specific-leg-reduce-UAM03Watson-0.pdf (accessed 20 November 2014).

Wilder, D. A. (1993). Freezing intergroup evaluations: Anxiety fosters resistance to counter stereo-typic information. In Hogg, M. A., Abrams, D. (eds.) 1993. *Group motivation: Social psychological perspectives.* Harvester Wheatsheaf, Hemel Hempstead, United Kingdom.

Wilder, D. A., Shapiro, P. N. (1989). Role of competition-induced anxiety in limiting the beneficial impact of positive behaviour by an out-group member, *Journal of Personality and Social Psychology,* 56, 60–69.

# Section 3
# Dog Bites and Risk

In Section 3, we consider the issue of dog bites and risk. As highlighted in the previous sections, the risk of a dog bite is commonly misunderstood or misrepresented. This includes both the absolute risk as well as the associated risk factors. In this section the issue of risk is considered from the perspective of a range of academic disciplines. In Chapter 8 Malgorzata Pilot and Fernanda Fadel consider the genetics of aggressive behaviour especially as it relates to dogs, but with a knowledge of what we can learn from the wider biological literature. A major theme identified throughout the text is the need for robust and biologically grounded definitions of aggression. To do this we need to appreciate the complexity of aggressive behaviour and understand the underlying mechanistic processes that regulate the likelihood of its expression, rather than consider it a simple entity that has simple genetic correlates. They conclude that there is still much to be done with the phenotyping (describing the key attributes) of aggressive behaviour. This point is developed further in the next chapter by Maya Braem Dubé, who examines the breadth of tests used to assess aggressive behaviour in dogs. The complexity of the task means that simple tests are often unreliable when examined in more detail. However, perhaps just as worrying is that for many forms of assessment, we have no idea at all as to the predictive value of these tests. This is true even for tests that are used within the legal system to determine the fate of a dog, before or after any aggressive incident.

The identification of simple associations between a variable (risk factor) and the outcome of a dog bite is commonplace, but in Chapter 10 Rob Christley and colleagues illustrate both the danger and fallacy of this practice. Drawing on the most comprehensive review of the risk factors for human-directed aggressive behaviour in dogs, undertaken by co-author Jenny Newman, they show how weak the evidence for many apparent associations really is. For even those associations where there is reasonable evidence, the causal nature of the relationship is unclear, and the reader would do well to refer back to Chapter 4 when considering this matter. Fatal attacks are rare but grab the headlines frequently because of their impact. Again there is a danger of simplistic assumptions being made about these cases, such as fatal attacks being the inevitable extreme form of response from dogs with a tendency to bite. Wim Van der Voorde and Dingeman Rijken, in Chapter 11, review dog bite-related fatalities in the scientific literature and highlight the error of this assumption, as well as how little we really know about these cases. These dogs are, understandably, often killed, but, perhaps less understandably, this often happens before an assessment is made of the dog to see what we can learn from the case. They emphasise the importance of a proper forensic investigation of the crime scene, so that no evidence is discarded, for example by destroying the dog or failing to examine it properly. This is a theme we return to in Section 4. Finally, Samantha Penrice and Marcello Ruta provide new data in Chapter 12 on how we might assess risk from a more detailed biomechanical consideration of jaw structure. It is often assumed that bite force is the primary risk factor to be considered in this regard, but this is shown to be a gross simplification, with different jaws equipped to deliver different types of bite and so posing different risks according to the circumstance.

In conclusion, this third section highlights the value of multi-disciplinary research into the risk of dog bites and the need not to make oversimplistic conclusions if we are genuinely interested in trying to manage the risk of dog bites effectively.

CHAPTER 8

# The Genetic Basis of Dog Aggression

## *Fernanda Fadel and Malgorzata Pilot*

## 8.1 Introduction

This chapter reviews current knowledge on the genetic basis of aggression and related behavioural traits (e.g. impulsivity, shyness–boldness) in the domestic dog. This is presented in the wider context of research on the genetics of aggression in other vertebrate species. Candidate genes that show correlation with aggressive tendencies in vertebrate model species are discussed, as well as the effect of these genes on neurobiological and physiological functions of the organism.

Dog aggression is discussed in its evolutionary context, considering the origin of the dog from the grey wolf and subsequent artificial selection. During the early stages of domestication, selection was likely to act against aggression towards known humans and conspecifics. During breed formation, selection could have led to diversification of aggression levels between breeds in certain contexts. We discuss studies on behavioural differences between breeds, and evaluate the concept of the 'aggressive breed' from a genetic perspective. Finally, we outline possible directions for further research on the genetic basis of aggressive behaviour in dogs.

## 8.2 Evolutionary context of aggression

Aggression is an aspect of behaviour that is of great interest for animal welfare and human safety. There is growing interest in understanding the genetics behind aggressive behaviour, especially in humans and dogs. However, one of the major obstacles is defining traits related to aggression and assigning dogs to such traits.

Being able to react aggressively in certain situations is beneficial from an evolutionary perspective, but not without risk (Ferguson and Beaver, 2009). Regardless of breed, all dogs are capable of showing aggression if they feel threatened. Some will react faster, some slower; some reactions will be just a warning signal, other reactions will be life threatening for the victim. The reaction threshold may vary with contexts and this might relate back to different key functions. As described by van den Berg et al. (2006):

*'There is individual variation in the tendency of dogs to display aggressive behaviour. This variation is the result of a complex system of interacting genes and environmental influences, which is poorly understood.'*

The domestication process probably selected animals for reduced fear-based aggression towards humans (Kukekova et al., 2012). Breed formation contributed to selection of different behaviours in different breed groups, mainly according to their working purpose (hunting, herding, pointing and retrieving). This behavioural selection also potentially secondarily selected for different levels of aggressive behaviour.

## 8.3  Assessing behaviour related to aggression

Identifying and classifying behavioural phenotypes is a major challenge in behavioural genetics (Overall et al., 2006). Behavioural traits are quantitative phenotypes, and different levels of a particular trait may be potentially adaptive in different contexts. An example is trait impulsivity: when foraging, there will be instances in which it is better to get a low value reward immediately than a higher value reward at a higher cost (of extended travelling time or waiting time), but in other instances the higher value reward might be a better choice (Mazur, 1994; Stevens and Stephens, 2010).

Behavioural phenotypes are influenced by genetic and environmental factors. Therefore, an important issue when understanding and categorising phenotypes is the influence of environmental factors on behaviour, and the extent of their contribution to a phenotype. This may be assessed by studying heritability. The main environmental factors that can affect a dog's behaviour are early life experiences, nutrition and social interactions both with humans and other dogs. It is believed that dogs are more prone to be affected by situations in an early period of their development (up to around six months) than later in life (Appleby et al., 2002). Individuals from non-domestic maternal environments and lacking urban experience in early life are more likely to show aggression towards unfamiliar humans and human avoidance behaviour, or aggression during veterinary visits (Appleby et al., 2002).

One of the biggest challenges when studying aggression is defining it in a way that can be measured (see Chapter 1). According to the Oxford Dictionary (2015), aggression is '(1) feelings of anger or antipathy in hostile or violent behaviour; readiness to attack or confront; (2) the action of attacking without provocation; (3) forcefulness'. In the field of animal behaviour, aggressivity is usually assessed in specific contexts that can be delimited and measured. There is a wide range of behavioural factors leading to aggression rather than one aggressive phenotype, and therefore classifying individuals into different categories related to aggression is a difficult task. Different experiments or assessments classify aggressive behaviour in different ways and there seems to be little consensus among researchers (van Rooy et al., 2014, see also Chapter 9). Labelling the individual as aggressive is not very precise when it comes to looking for the genetic basis of a phenotype. A more precise definition of different aspects of aggressive behaviour is currently needed, using appropriate qualifiers that may be contextual or related to other behavioural traits. Some examples of studies that define and delimit aggression to specific contexts are:

- The Canine Behavioural Assessment and Research Questionnaire (C-BARQ – Hsu and Serpell, 2003), which groups items into several behavioural traits, including at least three contexts of aggression: stranger-directed aggression, owner-directed aggression, and dog-directed aggression (van den Berg et al., 2006).
- Casey et al., (2014), who used their own questionnaire to examine human-directed aggression and divided it into three contexts: towards unfamiliar people on entering the house, towards unfamiliar people outside the house, and towards family members.
- The Dog Impulsivity Assessment Scale (DIAS – Wright et al., 2011), which measures one aspect of aggression related to impulsivity in response to novelty.

There is also a tendency to label breeds according to certain aggression stereotypes (Chapter 7), creating a 'breed profile', especially in the media (Chapter 5). Dog breeds are distinct genetic units that express specific phenotypic traits and vary in behaviour (Ostrander and Wayne, 2005) and if some behavioural traits are highly heritable, behavioural differences between breeds selected for different working purposes may be expected, but this does not mean all breed members conform to the stereotype. Nonetheless, some scientists suggest there are very specific behavioural characteristics to each breed (Svartberg, 2002). However, few studies have explored the differences in behavioural tendencies (e.g. DIAS – Wright et al., 2011) as opposed to specific behaviours as done in C-BARQ (Hsu and Serpell, 2003) that may be observed in different breed groups and which are considered to be remnants from past selection related to the original purpose of the breed (Mirkó et al., 2012). Further, few studies have explored individual differences in aggression. The majority of recent research points to the finding that the differences between individual dogs' behaviour within a breed often exceeds variation among breeds (Mehrkam and Wynne, 2014). Therefore, it is likely to be inaccurate to make a judgement on the behaviour of an individual dog solely based on its breed, and breed-level tendencies should not be generalised to make predictions about the individual (Clarke et al., 2013).

In addition, changes in dog breeding priorities, e.g. for appearance over behavioural function, over recent years are probably contributing to even greater behavioural variability within breeds than between breeds (Mirkó et al., 2012). Nowadays, dogs are bred for two main but quite different purposes:

1. Working dogs that perform a particular set of tasks useful for humans.
2. Show dogs that display a set of particular morphological traits.

Both may be used to produce individuals that are kept as pets, but the two lines may vary in their ability to adapt to this different function, and so the risk of aggressive behaviour. Many dog breeds have distinct working and show types that need to be taken into consideration when analysing behaviour since their selection is based on different behavioural characteristics that might influence results. Therefore, a behavioural trait can be analysed either in dogs as a whole, including as many breeds and mixed-breed dogs as possible; or focusing only on one breed or groups of breeds with the same working function, looking for differences within it.

There are several ways to assess behavioural traits in dogs (see Chapter 9), but in summary, some of the most established approaches include:

- *Behavioural experiments* which focus on the tendency of individuals to show a specific behaviour in a specific context at the time of testing, rather than the broader traits underlying behavioural expression (Gartstein and Rothbart, 2003). Conducting a wide range of behavioural tests over a range of contexts and at different times may be used to partly overcome this problem and infer underlying traits. These experiments are usually constrained by small sample sizes and large variability due to circumstances.
- *Psychometric questionnaires* which provide an alternative to the experimental approach, and address many of its constraints. Like those used in human psychology, they can be answered by the person who spends a significant amount of time with the subject (like parents reporting on their children, dog owners or professional dog handlers can report on their dogs). When it comes to questionnaires, research on human behaviour has been used as a basis for dog research, such as by adapting human psychometric scales for dogs (Gosling et al., 2003).
- *Clinical histories* that provide another approach to assess behavioural traits or classify individual dogs into different categories for aggressive behaviour. This may be combined with one of the previously mentioned approaches, and the methods are not exclusive. Some researchers include in the 'aggressive' category dogs that have been referred to a behaviour clinic for showing aggression towards the owner (mouthing, biting) and in the control category dogs that had not shown such behaviours (Amat et al., 2009; van den Berg et al., 2008). The problem with this approach is that some of the 'control' individuals may be subsequently moved to the 'aggressive' category and individuals may vary in their level of concern.

## 8.4　Methods for exploring behaviour genetics in dogs

There are currently four main approaches to studying behaviour genetics in dogs:

- The *candidate gene* approach targets a limited number of selected genes. They are selected a priori based on their suspected influence on a particular phenotypic trait. This can be followed by association studies of the genes identified. One of the disadvantages of this approach is the limited number of genes that are screened, potentially leaving out genes that might also be involved. The candidate gene approach can also be applied after GWAS (see below) as a follow-up study to verify its findings. It is an effective approach when candidate gene positions and functions are already known (e.g. Våge et al., 2010b).
- *Linkage studies* are conducted using related individuals, some of which show the modified phenotype (mainly diseases and disorders in humans) in order to identify its genetic basis. The segregation of genetic markers is compared within families that show a high frequency of the disease in order to identify the genes or genomic regions that are playing a role in the disease (Teare and Barrett, 2005). Several individuals from the same family both showing and not showing the phenotype have to be sampled for this approach.
- *Genome-wide association studies (GWAS)* are based on screening genome-wide variability

among individuals in order to identify genetic variants associated with a certain phenotypic trait by comparing groups of individuals differing in the level of this trait. This method is a good starting point to look for candidate genes (i.e. genes which are likely to be associated with the trait in question). Inbreeding in dogs led to large linkage disequilibrium (combinations of linked genes in a non-random way). Because of this large number of strong associations between alleles, considerably less loci need to be genotyped in dogs to detect associations using GWAS when compared to humans (Sutter et al., 2004; Lindblad-Toh et al., 2005; Boyko, 2011; Hall and Wynne, 2012). This is a great advantage of carrying out GWAS with dogs. On the down side, a large sample is usually still required for this approach (Eichler et al., 2010). Alleles that occur with very high frequency in the population may be undetectable by GWAS (Karlsson et al., 2013; Park et al., 2011; Tang et al., 2014). This is the case when some risk alleles are almost fixed in the population studied, and therefore even controls may carry them in a heterozygous state. However, this is more likely to be a problem when GWAS is focused on one dog breed only. GWAS has been used successfully in dogs to identify candidate genes for obsessive compulsive disorder in Doberman pinschers (Tang et al., 2014).

- *Heritability* analysis is based on comparison of behavioural traits between closely related individuals in order to infer how much phenotypic variation in an individual is due to genetic factors v non-genetic factors (i.e. environment or chance). This method gives an estimate of the extent to which a trait is inherited genetically, but does not indicate which genes are influencing the trait. This method is useful for selecting behaviour in breeding programmes, but not for identifying genetic determinants.

## 8.5  The genetics of canine aggressive behaviour

### 8.5.1  Heritability studies

There has not been much research focused directly on the genetic basis of aggression in dogs. A few studies show the heritability of behavioural traits in dogs, especially concerning boldness, fear, reactivity (Ariyomo et al., 2013; Branson and Rogers, 2006), but it is important to look carefully at how these traits have been defined when interpreting them, as different traits may be defined under the same name. Some of these studies suggest that these behavioural traits might be correlated with other heritable traits such as coat colour (Pérez-Guisado et al., 2006) and paw preference or lateralisation (Branson and Rogers, 2006).

So far, there have been two heritability studies in dogs published that focused on aspects of aggression. One of them looked into the heritability of 'dominance aggression' (defined by the authors as aggressive behaviour within the context of territory, food, objects, or persons) in English cocker spaniels (ECS) (Pérez-Guisado et al., 2006). This study examined fixed (i.e. sex and coat colour) and genetic factors in 51 ECS aged seven weeks using the Campbell Test. In this test a puppy is placed in a new place without distractions and with a person that the puppy has not encountered before. The test is divided into five parts: social attraction, following, restraint, social dominance and elevation dominance. Each part is scored depending on the puppy's reaction (Campbell, 1972). The results showed that each coat colour was associated with a significantly different response. Golden coat was related to greater 'dominance' behaviour while particolour coats corresponded to less 'dominant' behaviour, with black coat in the middle. Similar results regarding coat colour and aggression were also reported by Podberscek and Serpell (1997). Regardless of colour, males scored higher for 'dominance aggression' than females. 'Dominance' behaviour was shown to be heritable, with a heritability value of 0.20 (meaning that additive genetic variance constitutes 20% of phenotypic variance in the population studied). There was also a maternal factor, with estimated heritability from dams being more than twice than that from sires (Pérez-Guisado et al., 2006), but this study did not control for early maternal-puppy interaction effects, which may skew the results in favour of an apparent dam effect.

The second study compared aggressive behaviour in Golden Retrievers using some of the factors relating to aggressive behaviour from the C-BARQ questionnaire (Hsu and Serpell, 2003; van den Berg et al., 2006). The highest heritability estimates were for human-directed aggression (0.77) and dog-directed aggression (0.81), and the correlation between the two factors was very low (Liinamo et al., 2007).

### 8.5.2  Behavioural traits correlated with aggressive behaviour

There are other behavioural traits that correlate with aggressive behaviour, e.g. fearfulness, impulsivity, shyness–boldness, and their assessment may allow for a more specific definition of phenotype (for a review see Rayment et al., 2014):

- Impulsivity: this can be described as the inability to inhibit behaviour in the presence of salient cues. This wider conceptualisation of the term impulsivity as a trait can be psychometrically profiled by dog carers (Wright et al., 2011). Impulsivity is a widely studied trait in humans (Seo et al., 2009) and is precisely defined in dogs (Wright et al., 2012). The Dog Impulsivity Assessment Scale (DIAS), is a validated psychometric questionnaire used to score elements of impulsivity in dogs – i.e. general tendency underpinning behavioural expression in general (Wright et al., 2011). Besides the Overall Questionnaire Score (OQS), the DIAS consists of three independent behavioural factors derived from principal components analysis of scores (Wright et al., 2011). These have been termed: behavioural regulation, aggression threshold and response to novelty, and responsiveness. The scores for all factors vary greatly among individuals (Wright et al., 2011), showing the potential of DIAS to phenotype impulsivity.
- Shyness–boldness: Boldness is the propensity of an individual to take risks (Wilson et al., 1994). This dimension is well established in ecology (Wilson et al., 1994) and often includes aspects of fearfulness and impulsivity, which can relate to aggressive behaviour. In zebrafish (*Danio rerio*), heritability of boldness has been found to account for 76% of phenotypic variance, while aggressiveness accounted for 36% (Ariyomo et al., 2013). Researchers have been using personality tests to score boldness in dogs for work selection (Svartberg, 2002).
- Fearfulness: this is the general capacity to react to a variety of potentially threatening situations (Boissy, 1995). Fearful responses are often associated with the expression of aggressive behaviour in dogs and several behavioural questionnaires and tests include subscales related to this dimension of behaviour (Duffy et al., 2008; Svobodová et al., 2008). In puppies, consistency of estimates of fearfulness seem to be weak, but stronger

and predictable in adults, meaning that this personality dimension does not have a good predictive validity from puppyhood to adulthood (Fratkin et al., 2013).

### 8.5.3 *Biological candidates and physiological correlates to aggressive behaviour*

Several studies have been trying to identify underlying causes of aggression in several animal species. Most of the findings so far are in the area of physiology, which can also be a starting point for genetics. The majority of studies on the genetic basis of aggression have focused on humans or rats (*Rattus norvergicus*), but can potentially be relevant to dogs due to similarities in mammalian physiology. Genes that regulate or are involved in the pathways of certain neurotransmitters are good candidates for studying certain aspects of the genetics of aggressive behaviour.

Research on the genetics of human aggression often focuses on 'violent behaviour'; defined as 'the intentional use of physical force, threatened or actual, against oneself, another person, or against a group or community, that either results in or has a high likelihood of resulting in injury, death, psychological harm' (World Health Organisation, 2002). Cohorts of humans with a record of violent behaviour at several levels have been compared to the normal population, taking into account childhood trauma, economic background or other common environmental factors that might influence the expression of violent behaviour in the population (Seo et al., 2009). Similarly, individual dogs can potentially be classified according to different levels or forms of aggressive behaviour, and environmental factors can be accounted for, such as early life environment and history (breeder, rescue, pet shop, etc.), diet, and socialisation with humans and dogs.

Most research results point to a significant influence of serotonin and dopamine on aggressive behaviour. Some of the biological and physiological correlates that have been identified or studied in relation to aggressive behaviour are considered below:

*   Serotonin and dopamine: These are two key neurotransmitters involved in the regulation of emotional behaviour. Serotonin has excitatory and inhibitory function in the brain, regulating several emotional responses. Impulsive aggression in humans and animals has been associated with low levels of serotonin (5-HT) in several studies (e.g. Davidson et al., 2000; Daw et al., 2002; Everitt and Robbins, 2000; Seo et al., 2009; Wright et al., 2012). Dopamine is involved in behavioural activation, motivated behaviour and reward processing. Studies on rats and squirrel monkeys (*Saimiri sciureus*) also show that hyperactivation of the dopamine system leads to increased impulsive aggression, suggesting that there is substantial influence of dopamine in modulation of aggressive behaviour (Everitt and Robbins, 2000; Seo et al., 2009). Wright et al. (2012) showed that dogs that scored high for impulsivity using the DIAS had low levels of serotonin metabolites and high ratio of serotonin-dopamine metabolites in urine measurements.

    There is a strong indication that the serotonin and dopamine systems interact at the neurophysiological level, meaning that impairment of the serotonergic system can influence the regulation of the dopaminergic system specifically in the context of emotional responses (Daw et al., 2002). The interaction between the two systems is widely believed to be reciprocal in regulating emotional behaviour (Daw et al., 2002). For example, appetitive behaviours (instinctive physical needs) are encouraged by dopamine and discouraged by serotonin (Daw et al., 2002; Ikemoto and Panksepp, 1999). Therefore, considering that serotonin regulates dopamine in the limbic reward-ing system, it is possible that low levels of serotonin lead to high levels of dopamine, resulting in impulsive behaviour. It is also possible that both serotonin hypoactivity and dopamine hyperactivity occur in individuals with a high tendency towards impul-sive aggression (Seo et al., 2009). In summary, dopaminergic hyperactivity may exert an additive effect on proneness to aggressive behaviour secondary to serotonergic dysfunction (Seo et al., 2009). In clinical neuroscience, high levels of serotonin have been frequently correlated with impulsive aggression in humans, but more studies are needed to examine the interaction between serotonin and dopamine in impulsive individuals (Seo et al., 2009).

Amat et al. (2013) compared serotonin serum concentration from blood samples between nineteen aggressive English cocker spaniels (ECS) and twenty aggressive dogs of other breeds (Amat et al., 2013). The dogs were presented at an animal behav-iour clinic reporting aggression towards family members, strangers and other dogs. The concentration levels of serum serotonin were significantly lower in aggressive ECS ($p<0.05$) than other breeds. The authors speculate that this difference could be explained by genetic factors, epigenetic differences (lack of mother care in ECS, early nutritional issues), and inconsistent and/or punishment training methods. The authors conclude that serotonin levels are very likely to influence aggressive behav-iour. Silver foxes have also been studied extensively regarding behavioural genetics. Through the 'Farm Fox Experiment', two breeding lines were selected: one 'tame' and one 'aggressive/control'. Tame foxes showed higher levels of serotonin and tryptophan hydroxylase in the midbrain and hypothalamus compared to the control foxes (Kukekova et al., 2012).

There is a general consensus that serotonin and dopamine are related to the expres-sion of impulsivity, but the exact mechanisms through which this occurs and how these variations relate back to trait impulsivity are still unclear (Rayment et al., 2014).

• *Serotonin receptor genes*: The serotonin receptors (5-hydroxytryptamine receptors or 5-HT receptors) are proteins that mediate excitatory and inhibitory neurotransmission, and are activated by serotonin.

In the silver fox, tame foxes have lower density of 5-HT1A serotonin receptors in the hypothalamus (Kukekova et al., 2012). A stop codon in HTR2B (serotonin receptor 2B) identified exclusively in the Finnish population was associated with substance abuse and risk of displaying impulsive behaviour in humans; and knockout of the same gene in mice led to increase in impulsive behaviours (Bevilacqua et al., 2010).

Three studies focused on specific breeds of dogs analysed the role of serotonin receptors in association with aggressive behaviour, with mixed findings. An association study of English cocker spaniels examined single-nucleotide polymorphisms (SNPs) occurring in or in the close vicinity of sixteen neurotransmitter-related genes and found HTR1D and HTR2C to be significantly associated with the 'aggressive phenotype' (ECS referred to a behaviour clinic due to human-directed aggression) (Våge et al., 2010a). In golden retrievers, there was no association between serotonin receptors 1A, 1B, and 2A, and the serotonin transporter with the 'aggressive phenotype' after performing mutation screens, linkage analysis, an association study, and a quantitative genetic analysis (van den Berg et al., 2008). The golden retrievers included in the 'aggressive phenotype' were dogs referred to a behavioural clinic because of their aggressive behaviour. In Shiba Inus, the analysis of relationships between behavioural traits, defined through a psychometric questionnaire, and genotype of fifteen polymorphisms in eight neuro-transmitter-related genes showed no association between HTR1A and HTR1B and the 'aggressive phenotype' (Takeuchi et al., 2009). The variation in these results reflects the complexity of the phenotype in question and the fact that each study is measuring aggression in different contexts (clinical history from ECS and golden retrievers, and questionnaires from Shiba Inus).

• *Dopamine transporter gene*: Dopamine transporters regulate signals in dopaminergic synapses and remove dopamine from extracellular space (Mortensen and Amara, 2003). Most breeds of dogs are homozygous for a two-tandem repeat allele of the dopamine trans-porter gene, while in the Belgian Malinois breed sampled in the USA the one-tandem repeat allele is overrepresented in either heterozygous or homozygous state. Preliminary findings showed an association of the one-tandem copy in the Malinois with owner-reported seizures, loss of responsiveness to environmental stimuli, episodic aggression, and hyper-vigilance (Lit et al., 2013).

• *Dopamine D4 receptor gene and tyrosine hydroxylase (TH) gene*: These are dopaminergic genes involved in encoding the D4 subtype dopaminergic receptor and enzyme tyrosine hydroxylase, respectively. Police working German shepherd dogs with one specific allele of DRD4 scored significantly higher in the activity-impulsivity dimension of the Dog-Attention Hyperactivity Disorder Rating Scale (Hejjas et al., 2007). German shepherd dogs that had at least one short allele of the TH gene were more active-impulsive com-pared to dogs carrying two copies of the long allele. The instruments used for measuring activity-impulsivity were Dog-Attention Hyperactivity Disorder Rating Scale and an Activity-Impulsivity Behavioural Scale (Kubinyi et al., 2012). Association of the DRD4 and TH gene alleles and activity-impulsivity was later found in Siberian huskies, with short alleles of both genes correlated with high scores for activity-impulsivity (Wan et al., 2013).

• *Monoamine oxidase A (MAO-A) gene.* This is an enzyme that removes amine groups from (deaminates) serotonin, dopamine, norepinephrine and epinephrine, and is coded for by the MAO-A gene (Hotamisligil and Breakefield, 1991). According to genetic studies in humans, variation in this gene may be associated with aggression and also with depression (Brunner et al., 1993; Haberstick et al., 2005; Tiihonen et al., 2014). This gene is located in the chromosome X both in dogs (Klukowska et al., 2004) and in humans (Meyer-Lindenberg et al., 2006). Several studies have shown an association between the MAO-A gene and aspects of aggressive behaviour in humans and in dogs (e.g. Houpt, 2007; Meyer-Lindenberg et al., 2006; Persson, 2013).

In humans, research points to a significant gene-environment interaction between low-activity MAO-A genotype and rearing environment on adult antisocial behav-iour (Byrd and Manuck, 2014). GWAS and candidate gene approach indicate that the low-activity genotype of the MAO-A gene on predisposition to violence (Haberstick et al., 2005). The low-activity MAO-A genotype contributes to a low dopamine turnover rate. The MAO-A gene has also been found to be associated with impulsivity and aggressivity in a Dutch family where a rare mutation caused a complete deficiency of the MAO-A enzyme (Brunner et al., 1993).

One of the studies to target monoamine oxidase genes (both MAO-A and MAO-B) in dogs, focused on gene expression in brain tissues of English cocker spaniels and found no association between these two genes and human-directed aggressive behaviour (Våge et al., 2010b). Kwon et al. (2013) relate the variation in MAO-A and MAO-B genes with personality in working dogs using several approaches.

- *CDH genes*: The CDH gene codes neuronal cadherin, which belongs to a family of proteins responsible for neuronal membrane adhesion. Its low activity leads to neuronal membrane dysfunction.

In the Finnish human population, it has been shown that low activity genotypes of the CDH13 gene and the MAO-A gene are highly associated with extreme violent behaviour (Tiihonen et al., 2014).

## 8.5.4  Gene expression in brain tissues

A number of studies have looked into gene-specific differences in expression between brain parts and different phenotypes. Saetre et al. (2004) compared gene expression in the frontal lobe, the amygdala and the hypothalamus (regions involved in cognition and/or emotion) between dogs and wolves. They found differences in mRNA expression mainly in the hypothalamus, which could be the result of strong selection for domesticated behaviour in dogs and suggest that assessing gene expression in this region of the brain could potentially shed light on differences in other behavioural phenotypes among dogs. A more recent study shows brain-biased expression for genes related to complex cognitive behaviours in outbred Chinese indigenous dogs and German shepherds when compared to grey wolves (Li et al., 2013). This suggests rapid changes in gene expression in the brain following domestication (Li et al., 2013). The tame and control foxes from the Farm Fox Experiment have also been compared based on gene expression in brain tissues. The main finding was a difference in mRNA levels in hemoprotein related genes between the two lines, indicating that these genes might modulate tameness (Lindberg et al., 2007).

Differential gene expression in brain tissues has been found between nine aggressive dogs and eleven non-aggressive dogs (Våge et al., 2010a). The phenotyping was done using questionnaires based on aggressive behaviours towards humans; the control group did not show these behaviours. Increased expression of genes UBE2V2 and ZNF227 were significantly associated with increased Odds Ratio (OR) for aggressive behaviour. Zinc finger protein 227 (ZNF227) is predicted to be a transcriptional regulator in humans, which is possibly associated with behavioural change (Våge et al., 2010a), although no particular mechanism was proposed in that study. The UBE2V2 participates in several cell functions and is likely involved in pathways associated with aggressive behaviour. These results should be interpreted with caution because of the small sample size, but this preliminary data on differential gene expression in the canine brain provides useful information for future work (Våge et al., 2010a).

## 8.6 Future research

One of the major problems in genetic studies of aggression is phenotype classification, and so more research needs to be directed towards addressing this challenge. The creation of phenotyping protocols to be followed based on well-established research would help to guide future genetics studies and allow for a direct comparison between studies via meta-analysis.

The evidence of the interaction between serotonin hypofunction and dopamine hyperfunction, suggests that future studies should focus on investigating these in individuals displaying impulsive and/or aggressive behaviour as well as the genes involved in regulating these systems (Seo et al., 2009).

As more reliable ways of quantifying behavioural traits become available, i.e. using validated questionnaires, screening the dog genome for different behavioural phenotypes will become more accessible. However, even in human studies, the sensitivity and specificity of studies on the genetic basis of aggression is still too low for screening, for example with a view to preventing crime (Tiihonen et al., 2014). Even when candidate genes are identified with high likelihood, we still have to take into consideration that environmental factors will play a major role in behavioural expression (e.g. substance abuse in humans (Tiihonen et al., 2014), and early life environment in dogs). Therefore, when genes related to impulsivity and aggressive behaviour are identified, they are only an additional tool to be used for screening dogs, which may be combined with other behavioural assessments.

Better understanding of the genetic background of aggressive behaviour will help plan breeding programmes according to the use of the dogs. This knowledge could be used to inform the development of laws (Våge et al., 2010a) based on individual risk rather than using the behavioural stereotypes of breed to assess risk. Knowledge of the genetic basis of aggressive behaviour may also aid decisions concerning appropriate medication for animals with undesirable behaviours (Våge et al., 2010a).

## 8.7 References

Amat, M. et al. (2009). Aggressive behavior in the English cocker spaniel. *Journal of Veterinary Behavior: Clinical Applications and Research*, 4(3), pp.111–117.

Amat, M. et al. (2013). Differences in serotonin serum concentration between aggressive English cocker spaniels and aggressive dogs of other breeds. *Journal of Veterinary Behavior: Clinical Applications and Research*, 8(1), pp.19–25.

Appleby, D. L., Bradshaw, J. W. S., Casey, R. A. (2002). Relationship between aggressive and avoidance behaviour by dogs and their experience in the first six months of life. *The Veterinary Recor,* 150, pp.434–438.

Ariyomo, T. O., Carter, M., Watt, P. J. (2013). Heritability of boldness and aggressiveness in the zebrafish. *Behavior Genetics*, 43, pp.161–167.

van den Berg, L. et al. (2008). Evaluation of the serotonergic genes htr1A, htr1B, htr2A, and slc6A4 in aggressive behavior of Golden Retriever dogs. *Behavior Genetics*, 38(1), pp.55–66.

van den Berg, L. et al. (2006). Phenotyping of aggressive behavior in Golden Retriever dogs with a questionnaire. *Behavior Genetics*, 36(6), pp.882–902.

Bevilacqua, L. et al. (2010). A population-specific HTR2B stop codon predisposes to severe impulsivity. *Nature*, 468(7327), pp.1061–6.

Boissy, A. (1995). Fear and fearfulness in animals. *Quarterly Review of Biology*, 70(2), pp.165–191.

Boyko, A. R. (2011). The domestic dog: man's best friend in the genomic era. *Genome Biology*, 12(2), p.216.

Branson, N. J., Rogers, L. J. (2006). Relationship between paw preference strength and noise phobia in *Canis familiaris*. *Journal of Comparative Psychology*, 120(3), pp.176–83.

Brunner, H. G. et al. (1993). Abnormal behavior associated with a point mutation in the structural gene for a monoamine oxidase A. *Science*, 262, pp.578–580.

Byrd, A. L., Manuck, S. B. (2014). MAOA, childhood maltreatment, and antisocial behavior: Meta-analysis of a gene-environment interaction. *Biological Psychiatry*, 75(1), pp.9–17.

Campbell, W. E. (1972). A behavior test for puppy selection. *Modern Veterinary Practice*, 5, pp.29–33.

Casey, R. A. et al. (2014). Human directed aggression in domestic dogs (*Canis familiaris*): Occurrence in different contexts and risk factors. *Applied Animal Behaviour Science*, 152, pp.52–63.

Clarke, T., Cooper, J., Mills, D. (2013). Acculturation – Perceptions of breed differences in behavior of the dog (*Canis familiaris*). *Human-Animal Interaction Bouletin*, 2(1), pp.16–33.

Davidson, R. J., Putnam, K. M., Larson, C. L. (2000). Dysfunction in the neural circuitry of emotion regulation — A possible prelude to violence. *Science*, 289(July), pp.591–595.

Daw, N. D., Kakade, S., Dayan, P. (2002). Opponent interactions between serotonin and dopamine. *Neural Networks*, 15, pp.603–616.

Duffy, D. L., Hsu, Y., Serpell, J. A. (2008). Breed differences in canine aggression. *Applied Animal Behaviour Science*, 114(3-4), pp.441–460.

Eichler, E. E. et al. (2010). Missing heritability and strategies for finding the underlying causes of complex disease. *Nature Reviews. Genetics*, 11(2008), pp.446–450.

Everitt, B. J., Robbins, T. W. (2000). Second-order schedules of drug reinforcement in rats and monkeys: measurement of reinforcing efficacy and drug-seeking behaviour. *Psychopharmacology*, 153(1), pp.17–30.

Ferguson, C. J., Beaver, K. M. (2009). Natural born killers: The genetic origins of extreme violence. *Aggression and Violent Behavior*, 14(5), pp.286–294.

Fratkin, J. L., Sinn, D. L., Patall, E. A., Gosling, S. D. (2013). Personality consistency in dogs: a meta-analysis. *PLoS One*, 8(1), e54907.

Gartstein, M. A., Rothbart, M. K. (2003). Studying infant temperament via the Revised Infant Behavior Questionnaire. *Infant Behavior and Development*, 26(1), pp.64–86.

Gosling, S.D., Kwan, V. S. Y. and John, O. P. (2003). A dog's got personality: a cross-species comparative approach to personality judgments in dogs and humans. *Journal of Personality and Social Psychology*, 85(6), pp.1161–9.

Haberstick, B.C. et al. (2005). Monoamine oxidase A (MAOA) and antisocial behaviors in the presence of childhood and adolescent maltreatment. *American Journal of Medical Genetics - Neuropsychiatric Genetics*, 135 B, pp.59–64.

Hall, N. J., Wynne, C. D. L. (2012). The canid genome: Behavioral geneticists' best friend? *Genes, Brain and Behavior*, 11, pp.889–902.

Hejjas, K. et al. (2007). Association of polymorphisms in the dopamine D4 receptor gene and the activity-impulsivity endophenotype in dogs. *Animal genetics*, 38(6), 629–633.

Hotamisligil, G. S., Breakefield, X. (1991). Human monoamine oxidase A gene determines levels of enzyme activity. *American Journal of Human Genetics*, pp.383–392.

Houpt, K. A. (2007). Genetics of canine behavior. *Acta Veterinaria Brno*, 76(3), pp.431–444.

Hsu, Y., Serpell, J. A. (2003). Development and validation of a questionnaire for measuring behavior and temperament traits in pet dogs. *Journal of the American Veterinary Medical Association*, 223(9), pp.1293–300.

Ikemoto, S., Panksepp, J. (1999). The role of nucleus accumbens dopamine in motivated behavior: a unifying interpretation with special reference to reward-seeking. *Brain Research Reviews*, pp.6–41.

Karlsson, E. K. et al. (2013). Genome-wide analyses implicate 33 loci in heritable dog osteosarcoma, including regulatory variants near CDKN2A/B. *Genome Biology*, 14, p.R132.

Klukowska, J. et al. (2004). Identification of two polymorphic microsatellites in a canine BAC clone harbouring a putative canine MAOA gene. *Animal Genetics*, 35, pp.75–76.

Kubinyi, E. et al. (2012). Polymorphism in the tyrosine hydroxylase (TH) gene is associated with activity-impulsivity in German shepherd Dogs. *PloS one*, 7(1), e30271.

Kukekova, A. V. et al. (2012). Genetics of behavior in the silver fox. *Mammalian genome: official journal of the International Mammalian Genome Society*, 23(1–2), pp.164–77.

Kwon, Y. et al. (2013). Bioinformatic analysis of the canine genes related to phenotypes for the working dogs. *Journal of Life Science*, 23(11), pp.1325–1335.

Li, Y. et al. (2013). Artificial selection on brain-expressed genes during the domestication of dog. *Molecular Biology and Evolution*, 30(8), pp.1867–1876.

Liinamo, A. E. et al. (2007). Genetic variation in aggression-related traits in Golden Retriever dogs. *Applied Animal Behaviour Science*, 104(1–2), pp.95–106.

Lindberg, J. et al. (2007). Selection for tameness modulates the expression of heme related genes in silver foxes. *Behavioral and Brain Functions*, 3, p.18.

Lindblad-Toh, K. et al. (2005). Genome sequence, comparative analysis and haplotype structure of the domestic dog. *Nature*, 438(7069), pp.803–19.

Lit, L. et al. (2013). Characterization of a dopamine transporter polymorphism and behavior in Belgian malinois. *BMC Genetics*, 14(1), p.45.

Mazur, J. E. (1994). Effects of intertrial reinforcers on self-control choice. *Journal of the Experimental Analysis of Behavior*, 61(1), pp.83–96.

Mehrkam, L. R., Wynne, C. D. L. (2014). Behavioral differences among breeds of domestic dogs (*Canis lupus familiaris*): Current status of the science. *Applied Animal Behaviour Science*, 155, pp.12–27.

Meyer-Lindenberg, A. et al. (2006). Neural mechanisms of genetic risk for impulsivity and violence in humans. *Proceedings of the National Academy of Sciences of the United States of America*, 103(16), pp.6269–74.

Mirkó, E. et al. (2012). Preliminary analysis of an adjective-based dog personality questionnaire developed to measure some aspects of personality in the domestic dog (*Canis familiaris*). *Applied Animal Behaviour Science*, 138(1–2), pp.88–98.

Mortensen, O. V. and Amara, S. G. (2003). Dynamic regulation of the dopamine transporter. *European Journal of Pharmacology*, 479, pp.159–170.

Ostrander, E. A., Wayne, R. K. (2005). The canine genome. *Genome Research*, 15(12), pp.1706–16.

Overall, K. L., Hamilton, S. P., Chang, M. L. (2006). Understanding the genetic basis of canine anxiety: phenotyping dogs for behavioral, neurochemical, and genetic assessment. *Journal of Veterinary Behavior: Clinical Applications and Research*, 1(3), pp.124–141.

Oxford Dictionaries (2015). Oxford University Press. Available at: www.oxforddictionaries.com (Accessed May 2015)

Park, J. H. et al. (2011). Distribution of allele frequencies and effect sizes and their interrelationships for common genetic susceptibility variants. *Proceedings of the National Academy of Sciences*, 108(44), pp.18026–18031.

Pérez-Guisado, J., Lopez-Rodríguez, R. and Muñoz-Serrano, A. (2006). Heritability of dominant–aggressive behaviour in English cocker spaniels. *Applied Animal Behaviour Science*, 100(3–4), pp.219–227.

Persson, M. (2013). Behaviour genetics in the domestic dog: Introduction essay. *Genewell – Avian Behavioural Genomics and Physiology Group*.

Podberscek, A., Serpell, J. A. (1997). Environmental influences on the expression of aggressive behaviour in English cocker spaniels. *Applied Animal Behaviour Science*, 52, pp.215–227.

Rayment, D. J. et al. (2014). Applied personality assessment in domestic dogs: Limitations and caveats. *Applied Animal Behaviour Science*, 163, pp.1–18.

van Rooy, D. et al. (2014). Holding back the genes: Limitations of research into canine behavioural genetics. *Canine Genetics and Epidemiology*, 1(1), p.7.

Saetre, P. et al. (2004). From wild wolf to domestic dog: Gene expression changes in the brain. *Molecular Brain Research*, 126, pp.198–206.

Seo, D., Patrick, C. J., Kennealy, P. J. (2009). Role of serotonin and dopamine system interactions in the neurobiology of impulsive aggression and its comorbidity with other clinical disorders. *Aggressive Violent Behaviour*, 13(5), pp.612–625.

Stevens, J. R., Stephens, D. W. (2010). The adaptive nature of impulsivity. *Faculty Publications, Department of Psychology, University of Nebraska – Lincoln*. Paper 519.

Sutter, N. B. et al. (2004). Extensive and breed-specific linkage disequilibrium in *Canis familiaris*. *Genome Research*, 14, pp.2388–2396.

Svartberg, K. (2002). Shyness–boldness predicts performance in working dogs. *Applied Animal Behaviour Science*, 79(2), pp.157–174.

Svobodová, I. et al. (2008). Testing German shepherd puppies to assess their chances of certification. *Applied Animal Behaviour Science*, 113(1–3), pp.139–149.

Takeuchi, Y. et al. (2009) Association analysis between canine behavioural traits and genetic polymorphisms in the shiba inu breed. *Animal Genetics*, 40, pp.616–622.

Tang, R. et al. (2014). Candidate genes and functional noncoding variants identified in a canine model of obsessive-compulsive disorder. *Genome Biology*, 15(3), p.R25.

Teare, M. D., Barrett, J. H. (2005). Genetic linkage studies. *Lancet*, 366, pp.1036–44.

Tiihonen, J. et al. (2014). Genetic background of extreme violent behavior. *Molecular Psychiatry*, pp.1–7.

Våge, J. et al. (2010a). Differential gene expression in brain tissues of aggressive and non-aggressive dogs. *BMC Veterinary Research*, 6, pp.34.

Våge, J. et al. (2010b). Association of dopamine- and serotonin-related genes with canine aggression. *Genes, Brain, and Behavior*, 9(4), pp.372–8.

Wan, M. et al. (2013). DRD4 and TH gene polymorphisms are associated with activity, impulsivity and inattention in Siberian husky dogs. *Animal genetics*, 44(6), 717–727.

Wilson, D. S. et al. (1994) Shyness and boldness in humans and other animals *Trends in Ecology and Evolution*, 9(11), pp.442–446.

World Health Organisation (2002). *World report on violence and health*.

Wright, H. F., Mills, D. S., Pollux, P. M. J. (2012). Behavioural and physiological correlates of impulsivity in the domestic dog (*Canis familiaris*). *Physiology and Behavior*, 105(3), pp.676–82.

Wright, H. F., Mills, D. S., Pollux, P. M. J. (2011). Development and Validation of a Psychometric Tool for Assessing Impulsivity in the Domestic Dog (*Canis familiaris*). *International Journal of Comparative Psychology*, 24, pp.210–225.

# CHAPTER 9

# Tests for Aggression and Prediction of Aggression

*Maya Braem Dubé*

## 9.1 Introduction

Affective aggression is a complex of behaviours, with diverse behavioural motivations, based on an individually experienced stress (negative emotion). This stress response is in response to internal and/or external factors. Understanding that aggression is often the result of the interplay of multiple internal and external factors is important when developing an evaluation method, as well as when deciding what answers an evaluation method should give, which method to choose in which situation and how to interpret the behaviour shown.

This chapter aims to give an insight into how aggression can be evaluated, why tests might be necessary for this, what needs to be taken into consideration and what is appropriate for which contexts.

## 9.2 Influences on aggression

The various internal and external influences on aggression need to be appreciated in order to understand not only how it needs to be assessed (i.e. what factors need to be controlled for), but also the limitations of a given test (i.e. its generalisability).

Internally influencing factors include:

- The physical (Beaver et al., 2003) and psychological well-being (Overall, 2007; Reisner et al., 2005; Shihab et al., 2011) of the individual. This includes the emotional state of the individual (Mills et al., 2012; Panksepp, 2004; Panksepp, 2005); which itself will be influenced by proximate factors such as:
    - Level of stress tolerance
    - Sensitivity to arousal.
- Behavioural styles (active versus passive response tendencies) for coping with stress (Benus et al., 1991; Horváth et al., 2007; Koolhaas et al., 1999; Riemer et al., 2013); which is obviously dependent upon ultimate factors such as:

- Learning experiences (Appleby et al., 2002; Veenema, 2009).
- Genetic predisposition (Saetre et al., 2006). This includes a range of specific factors related to inherited traits (Liinamo et al., 2007; Strandberg et al., 2005; Van der Berg, 2003, 2006), including personality (Goodloe and Borchelt, 1998; Gosling et al., 2003; Maejima et al., 2007; and breed-related associations (Bradshaw and Goodwin, 1999; Duffy et al., 2008; Hart and Hart, 1985; Scott and Fuller, 1965; Starling et al., 2013), both of which may reflect molecular variation in neuro-transmitter systems (Carrillo et al., 2009; Eisenberger et al., 2007; Rosado et al., 2010; Våge et al., 2010).

As aggression is shown in specific contexts, external circumstances also impact the likelihood of exhibiting an aggressive response. The following external factors are thought to play a role in aggressive behaviour:

3

- Social relationships: with the owner (Serpell, 1996; Topál et al., 1998) or other individuals of the same or other species.
- The owner's choice and clarity of communication method (Hiby and Rooney, 2004; Horváth et al., 2008; Jagoe and Serpell, 1996) and the degree of reciprocity of communication between dog and owner.
- The owner's personality and current emotional state (O'Farrell, 1997; Udell and Wynne, 2008)
- The quality and suitability of the animal's previous environment, especially its initial developmental and current physical surroundings particularly within the context of how these will affect current perceptions (Beerda et al., 1999; Podberscek and Serpell, 1997; Foyer et al., 2013; Reisner et al., 2005).

## 9.3 How can we assess aggressive behaviour?

There are two basic ways of getting information about a pet animal's behaviour: indi-rectly by asking a person close to the animal to describe his or her pet's reactions in certain situations, or directly by observing the dog's behaviour in more or less stand-ardised contexts.

**Indirect evaluation:** In a literature review of studies evaluating temperament of dogs, Jones & Gosling (2005) found 18% of described methods were ratings by questionnaire and/or interview. Although these can be subjective and subject to rater bias, this is not necessarily the case and questionnaires have the potential to be a reliable means of evaluating behaviour (Jones and Gosling, 2005).

**Direct evaluation:** According to Jones and Gosling (2005), direct evaluation in the form of tests that evaluate a dog's reaction to specific stimuli in controlled and standard-ised situations accounts for 33% of methods described, while direct observation of dogs in non-controlled environments, exposing them to more 'natural' stimuli, (for example, in behaviour consultations) represent 16% of described methods. Some advantages and disadvantages of the two types of evaluation described above are summarised below (Table 9.1).

**Table 9.1** Potential advantages and disadvantages of indirect and direct evaluation methods.

| | Indirect evaluation<br>Questionnaires and interviews | Direct evaluation<br>Tests and observation |
|---|---|---|
| **Potential Advantages** | • No additional stress for the dogs<br>• Inclusion of a variety of situations possible<br>• Easier to look for behaviour tendencies and personality traits<br>• No infrastructure necessary | • Direct observation rather than through views of a third party<br>• May increase objectivity especially if following strict interpretation protocol<br>• Standardisation possible<br>• Direct comparison of different dogs and same dogs over time possible |
| **Potential Disadvantages** | • Reliant on subjective view of third party observer<br>• Dishonesty<br>• Communication misunderstandings<br>• Lack of knowledge and skills to correctly evaluate behaviour | • Stressful for dogs and owner<br>• Limited number of situations possible<br>• Momentary picture, i.e. unable to extrapolate to everyday life if single test unless shown to be very reliable<br>• Infrastructure necessary |

## 9.4  Are we testing what we want to be testing?

In recent years, there has been increased realisation of the need for scientific evidence regarding the evaluation of behaviour traits and personality, whether by behaviour test or questionnaire (Bennett et al., 2012; Diederich and Giffroy, 2006; Hsu and Serpell, 2003; Ley et al., 2009; Mornement, 2009; Paroz et al., 2008; Svartberg, 2005; Taylor and Mills, 2006; Valsecchi et al., 2011; Van der Berg et al., 2003; Van der Berg et al., 2010; Van der Borg et al., 2010). Despite this there are significant gaps in the quality metrics of available tests, and it is not always clear if the basic requirements for a scientifically sound process have been followed. When developing any means of evaluating a behaviour, the following factors should be explicit (Taylor and Mills, 2006):

• **Objective**: It must be defined clearly what exactly is being evaluated, e.g. aggression in specific situations, aggressive tendency, only aggression or aggression as part of a wider assessment of temperament/personality, etc.
• **Aim**: The aim of the evaluation must be clear: is it about predicting future behaviour or suitability, e.g. for working dogs? Is it about evaluating current or future dangerousness/risk, e.g. in legal situations? Is it part of a behaviour consultation with a view to managing the problem? Is it a fundamental study that might be examining risk factors that might influence aggression?
• **Standardisation**: The test situations ideally should be standardised, especially if the aim is to be able to compare outcomes between several dogs, e.g. when testing suitability for a certain task or consistency of behaviour over time. This means the situations should always be the same with regard to location, timing, presented stimuli, length of time the animal is exposed to a stimulus, sequence of stimuli, scoring system and recorded behaviours. In real life, things are not perfect, as it is impossible to control for all influencing factors, especially the internal ones. However, attempts can be made to get as close to this kind of standardisation as possible. Standardisation can, however,

also have its disadvantages, as these test situations often do not reflect everyday situations and cannot cover all possible contexts. Hence extrapolation from the test results to everyday life may not be possible with a standardised test.

Standardisation not only applies to the actual test situations, but also to the scoring system, which, ideally, should be objective, based on discrete observable behaviours rather than interpretations, which can be subjective. However, as Wilsson and Sundgren (1997a) point out, the subjective evaluation by an experienced person allows the interpretation of an entire complex of behaviours (such as aggressive tendencies) rather than just evaluating the specific reaction to an isolated test situation; this may actually be a more powerful way of discriminating between individuals or conditions (Mills et al., 2006). Hence, the scoring system depends on what is being evaluated and why.

- **Reliability**: The test must be demonstrably reliable:
  - The same observer should evaluate the same dog in the same situation the same way in repeated observations (intra–observer reliability).
  - Two different observers should evaluate the same dog in the same situation the same way (inter-observer reliability).
  - The same dog should show the same behaviours in the same situation when retested (test–retest reliability). Test–retest reliability (Taylor et al., 2006) or temporal reliability (Epstein, 1983) is important when something supposedly consistent, such as temperament is being evaluated (Mornement, 2009).
  - There must be a correlation between items that make up a single factor, e.g. one might have several situations that contribute to the overall assessment of 'interspecific aggression', such as a situation where a person passes by the dog and a situation of a person handling a dog. These measures should correlate if they are measuring a single construct (internal consistency).
- **Validity**: The test must be valid, i.e. it is really measuring what we intend it to measure. Epstein (1983) emphasises that when 'measuring' a complex construct, such as personality or a behaviour trait, which would include aggressivity, this must consist of an aggregation of evaluations over several situations, because the tendency varies with the situation. There are several types of validity. For example, two separate situations assessing interspecific aggression, such as 'a person walking past the dog' and 'a person handling the dog', may both be measuring aggressive behaviour and so have content validity, but might be measuring the tendency in different circumstances, so will not necessarily agree. The trait is composed of the response across a wide range of circumstances. If several traits or behaviours are evaluated, it can happen that factors expected to evaluate one trait may correlate with other factors. The extent of this correlation makes up the 'construct validity'. Construct validity again can be subdivided into 'convergent' and 'discriminant validity'. The former relates to the situation when two constructs that we expect to relate to each other are shown to actually relate to each other. The latter describes the opposite, i.e. we have two constructs we expect not to be related and this is also found in the test situation. If separate methods are used to evaluate the same dog's behaviour, e.g. a test and a questionnaire, this can be used to establish 'concurrent validity'. If the assessment of an animal's behaviour correlates with its behaviour in a similar situation in the future, 'predictive validity' is established.

- **Feasibility**: The test must be feasible and realistic for those needing to use it. A test that is used to evaluate many dogs in a short period of time cannot be too long, whereas it might be acceptable to have a longer test that is evaluating the potential dangerousness of a dog for the courts (see Chapter 18). A test for puppies cannot be as long or complex as a test for adult dogs, and, from a practical point of view certain individuals (human and canine) might not be as suitable as others for testing.

## 9.5  The issue of predictability

**Predictability and the consequences of false predictions:** In the case of aggression, the ultimate purpose of an assessment is usually to predict the future likelihood of this behaviour being shown, whether this be for breeding and selecting working dogs, or public safety and legal issues. The question arises whether aggression *per se*, which has such a multifactorial basis, can actually be predicted with much accuracy. It might be argued that evaluation does not make sense in isolation from context or other traits. In order to predict a response, a certain degree of consistency must be assumed within the individual, over time, and over circumstances (Fratkin et al., 2013, Taylor and Mills, 2006). However, animals are subject to learning, and hence, even if the external aspect of the evaluation is standardised, there is no way to standardise the 'internal' state of the individual. Hence, an 'absolute prediction' is impossible and unrealistic (Epstein, 1983; Taylor and Mills, 2006). The complexity of the trait will inevitably result in lower predictability than might be hoped or assumed by some.

Whether a method has 'good predictability' depends not only on the behavioural variable of interest e.g. aggression, and the characteristics of the individual, but also on the choice of the most suitable method to answer the question. Even though some studies have found some predictability from puppy tests (Slabbert and Odendaal, 1999), the point in time when the first assessment is done is of importance. Behaviours evaluated in puppies tend to have a low predictive value for adult behaviours (Fratkin et al., 2013; Riemer et al., 2014; Wilsson and Sundgren, 1997b), and this includes aggression. The time lapse between two evaluations is likely to correlate with predictability, with it being higher for shorter intervals (Fratkin et al., 2013). The less time an animal is exposed to factors, the less likely it is that these factors will influence the outcome. The practical importance of the scientific integrity of the evaluation methods can be appreciated from the potential consequences of incorrect conclusions. Apart from the financial consequences of a false prediction (e.g. an unsuitable working dog continuing with training), the consequences could be a matter of life or death. Individuals falsely evaluated to be aggressive (false positives) might be euthanised despite there being no justifiable reason, while individuals who slip through the net and are not correctly identified as a significant risk (false negatives) may destroy the lives of others (Bräm et al., 2008). Hence, there are ethical, legal and welfare implications to the decision to test, how to test and also not to test, which should be recognised and discussed, in advance.

## 9.6  The scientific quality of behavioural tests

As already mentioned, we must have a clear idea of the questions we wish to ask: Do we want to focus on one particular aspect of aggressive behaviour, or are we looking at aggressive behaviour as part of a larger concept, such as a dog's personality or suitability for a certain task?

Very few published evaluation methods focus solely on aggression as an independent entity or a specific aspect of this, perhaps because aggression is multifactorial and must be considered in context (Epstein, 1983). However, one of the few circumstances in which the focus is mainly on aggressive behaviour is in the legal context when evaluating the potential dangerousness of a dog. Nonetheless, aggressive tendency is only one part of this evaluation with other factors, such as the physical attributes of the dog, at risk individuals, the local context and the behaviour of the handler needing to be considered as well (Chapter 18, Horisberger et al., 2004; Hussain, 2005; Guy et al., 2001). Following reports of many fatal incidents involving dog attacks worldwide, several countries have implemented laws that supposedly aim to reduce the risk of injuries caused by dog bites. Some of these laws, controversially focus on specific breeds, while others focus on other factors, such as those mentioned above, e.g. the dog's behaviour independent of breed or the owner's handling of the dog in situations. Many of these laws require tests to assess the dog's aggressive behaviour as a means of assessing potential dangerousness, e.g in Germany or certain cantons of Switzerland. However, there is no consensus as to how these tests are to be structured or implemented (Bräm et al., 2008; Diederich and Giffroy, 2006; Mornement, 2009).

Possibly the most widely known test for aggression from the scientific literature was developed by Netto and Planta in 1997 (revised in 2002). The original aim was to identify and exclude from breeding excessively aggressive individuals belonging to three 'potentially aggressive breeds' in the Netherlands. The final version of the test consists of forty-three subtests in which the dogs are presented with various stimuli in a controlled environment. The dogs' biting/attack behaviour in the test situations has shown convergent and discriminant validity with information on the biting history collected through questionnaires. The dogs were categorised into three categories based on their biting history as given by their owners: non-biters, dog-biters, and human-biters. The authors found a significant difference in their aggressive behaviours during the test situations between the non-biters and dog-biters (p = 0.05) and the human-biters (p = 0.003), respectively. A high test-retest reliability was found for total attack (r = 0.78, p < 0.0001) and biting/attack behaviour (r = 0.68, p < 0.0001). This test has been used as a basis for many other tests to evaluate aggressive behaviour in dogs.

However, due to the number of subtests involved, this test is quite demanding both for the dog and owner. In an attempt to address this issue, Klausz and colleagues (2013) developed a short, four-minute test focusing on human-directed aggression. They compared fear-related and aggressive behaviours shown in five test situations (friendly greeting, taking a bone away, threatening approach, tug-of-war, rolling over) by a set of dogs that, based on owner information a) had never bitten, b) had bitten once and c) had bitten more than once. Individuals that had bitten once showed significantly more signs of fear during the test than dogs in the other two groups. The authors conclude that *'fear-related aggression problems are most typical in the case of dogs that have no tendency to bite, but in rare cases, failing all else, they will bite'* (p.184). This concurs with the proposal that there is a high correlation between fear and aggression (Appleby et al., 2002; Haverbeke et al., 2009) to an extent, but it also underlines that aggression, and perhaps multiple bite episode, can be the result of other emotional states and associated behavioural motivations.

This study exemplifies the problem of tests that focus on only one aspect of behaviour, as a lot of other important information relating to behavioural tendencies underlying the risk may be missed. A more comprehensive picture is gained when direct and indirect information sources are combined (Bennett et al., 2012).

Aside from the tests that have gone through some form of scientific validation process, many independently developed tests are being used worldwide that have little or no scientific evidence to support their value. A comparison of the scores of 'intra-specific behaviour' (i.e. interdog responses) and 'inter-specific behaviour' (i.e. human directed responses) achieved in three tests that claim to include the evaluation of aggression showed inconsistent results within and between them (Bräm et al., 2008) and raises questions about their validity.

## 9.7  The scientific quality of indirect evaluations of aggression

The Canine Behavioural Assessment and Research Questionnaire (C-BARQ) (Hsu and Serpell, 2003) is probably the most widely used indirect canine behaviour evaluation tool (http://vetapps.vet.upenn.edu/cbarq/about.cfm). The current version consists of 100 questions describing the different ways in which dogs typically respond to common events, situations, and stimuli in their environment. The C-BARQ is simple to use and can be completed by anyone who is reasonably familiar with a dog's typical, day-to-day behaviour. On average, it takes ten to fifteen minutes to complete and is available for use by owners, professionals, and researchers. Van der Berg et al. (2010) have reported that C-BARQ is reliable for assessing stranger-directed aggression in German shepherd dogs, golden retrievers and Labrador Retrievers and could be used to identify '*the best and worst performing dogs regardless of sex, neutering or breed*' (p. 141). However, its reliability in a wider context in relation to the evaluation of aggressive behaviour remains unknown, and it is limited in the range of mechanistic explanations offered for the behaviour (fear aggression).

## 9.8  The practical use of behavioural test information

### 9.8.1  Breeding dog selection

Many kennel clubs throughout the world require animals to pass some form of behaviour evaluation in order to be accepted for breeding (Bräm et al., 2008; Fuchs et al., 2005; Paroz et al., 2008; Ruefenacht et al., 2002; Svartberg, 2002, 2005; Svartberg and Forkman, 2002). These tests typically include an evaluation of at least an element of aggression, which, if shown, is taken note of, but it is not the only focus of interest for assessing suitability. Some breeds are perceived to require a certain degree of aggressive behaviour, e.g. German shepherd dogs (Fuchs et al., 2005; Haverbeke, 2009; Ruefenacht et al., 2002), whereas others do not wish to have any aggression shown in their tests, e.g. American Staffordshire Terriers (Braem et al., 2008).

In an international survey of behaviour testing by kennel clubs, it was found that of the twenty-four national respondents, only three (Switzerland, Poland and Thailand) required a behaviour test for all registered breeds in order to receive breeding approval; another seven countries required an obligatory behaviour test for some breeds, of which three countries required behaviour tests for working breeds. However, up to now, there are no specific guidelines as to what these assessments should include, and their implications may be unclear. For example, the most frequently reported reasons in Swiss kennel clubs for not passing the behaviour part of the tests are fearfulness and aggression, however, in only 8% of the cases did this lead to exclusion from breeding (Scherrer, 2007). Quite apart from any quality specific issues, this questions whether the theoretical importance of including aggressive behaviour in breeding evaluation is actually put into practice.

The issue of canine aggressivity being viewed differently in different circumstances also applies to the context of the type of work the dog may be wanted for e.g. guiding the blind versus police work (Ennik et al., 2006). Thus even within a breed, there may be a desire for different tendencies in this regard.

### 9.8.2 Working dog selection

Certain breeds are typically used for specific working dog tasks, with German shepherds and Belgian shepherds (as military and police dogs), golden retrievers and Labrador Retrievers (as assistance dogs) being the most frequently described for assessment in the literature.

Training a working dog involves considerable investment in time, energy and money (Serpell and Hsu, 2001). Hence there is a demand for tools that might help the selection of animals at an early age that are more suitable for certain tasks as adults. It might therefore be expected that greater investment would be made to establish the quality of the tests, and there is more published in the scientific literature on these tests, but key quality metrics are still missing (Table 9.2). Studies with this particular focus tend to test young dogs (usually under the age of twelve months, sometimes as early as eight weeks) and look at the predictive validity of measures for future suitability for or success in work.

### 9.8.3 Shelter dog evaluation

When adopting a dog, both the new owner as well as the person rehoming the dog should want to make sure that the dog and the new home are as compatible as possible. In the ideal situation, information can be gathered from the original owner giving up the animal, the animal's behaviour during its stay at the shelter and the new owner adopting the animal to help inform this process. However, the history of the dog may not be known or only partially known, or there may be uncertainty about the honesty of the information gained. In order to evaluate this problem, Segurson et al. (2005) gave questionnaires to owners relinquishing dogs to animal shelters, and told them either the information was confidential or not. The people in the confidential group reported a significantly higher frequency of owner-directed aggression (p = 0.001) and fear of strangers (p = 0.025) than did the other group. No significant differences between the two groups were found for the remaining five factors (stranger-directed aggression, dog-directed aggression or fear, non-social fear, separation-related problems, attachment or attention-seeking behaviour).

A plethora of tests are being used worldwide, and there is a scarcity of quality metrics to support the use of any of these tests (Mornement et al., 2010; Sigrist, 2007). Of particular importance in this situation is a recognition that the new home may differ considerably

**Table 9.2** Examples of studies looking into evaluating behaviour of (future) working dogs, their evaluation type and the behaviours evaluated.

| Author | Aim | Population characteristics | Assessment age | Behaviour dimensions assessed and/or their structure | Validity and reliability | Results |
|---|---|---|---|---|---|---|
| Wilsson et al., 1997a and 1997b | To investigate whether the behaviour test can be used to select dogs for different kinds of work and for breeding | N = 2107 German shepherd, Labrador Retriever Service dogs (police dog, guide dog) | 450–600 days | 10 behaviour characteristics assessed Factor analysis revealed 4 factors: Mental stability, cooperation or willingness to please, affability, ardour | Predictive validity not referred to as such, but tested by comparison with dogs being accepted to training or not. The importance of reliability is mentioned, but not investigated. | Similarities in behaviour traits between categories of service dogs compared with dogs not suitable for service. Breed differences, e.g. GSD higher in sharpness and defence drive, Labradors higher in nerve stability, lower in reaction to gunfire, higher in cooperation. Subjective evaluation of complex behaviour parameters can be used to select suitability of different types of service dogs belonging to different breeds as service dogs. Primary information received from the test should be regarding the individual. |
| Slabbert and Odendaal, 1999 | To predict suitability for police dog work through a behaviour test | N = 167 German shepherd Police dogs | 8 weeks (obstacle, retrieval) 12 weeks (retrieval, startle, gunshot) 16 weeks (startle) 6 months (aggression) 9 months (aggression) | Behaviour evaluated in relation to a number of contexts they would be likely to encounter in a working context | Inter-rater reliability given as comparison of evaluation by 4 independent evaluators. Predictive validity: Retrieve (8 weeks), aggression (6 and 9 months) combined predicted 81.7% of unsuccessful dogs and 91.7% of successful police dogs. | Decision on suitability made at 18–24 months. Retrieval at 8 weeks and aggression at 9 months were found to be suitable selective criteria. 82% of dogs with low aggression scores (at 9 months) did not become police dogs, 55% with high aggression scores did become police dogs. |

**Table 9.2** (continued).

| Author | Aim | Population characteristics | Assessment age | Behaviour dimensions assessed and/or their structure | Validity and reliability | Results |
|---|---|---|---|---|---|---|
| Sinn et al., 2010 (building on Wilsson et al., described above) | To investigate the predictive relationship between behavioural traits and important working outcomes | N = 977 Belgian shepherd, German shepherd Military working dogs | Test 1 – before purchasing Test 2 – at off-vendor site, n = 65 Test 3 – prior to training, n = 477 | Factor analysis revealed: Object focus, Sharpness, Human focus, Search focus | Predictive validity for working outcome studied. Inter-rater reliability for all 15 items good (0.77) Test-retest good for most short intervals (>0.50), decreased with longer intervals (<0.40) | Good inter-rater reliability, good short-term, but not long-term test-retest reliability. No prediction of work outcome by age, sex or early test behaviour Aggregation of item scores to estimate personality more powerful than using single item behaviours alone. |
| Svartberg, 2002 | To investigate the relationship between the shyness-boldness trait and working dog performance (low, middle, high) | N = 2655 German shepherd, Tervueren Working dogs | Test between 12–18 months of age | Factor analysis revealed: Playfulness, Curiosity/Fearfulness, Chase-proneness, Sociability, Aggressiveness | Predictive validity of behaviour traits for work success. | A relationship between boldness and work success was found. |
| Svartberg et al., 2005 | To test the validity of behaviour traits for predicting typical behaviour in everyday life | N = 697 16 breeds Working dogs | Retrospective comparison with test done 1–2 years prior to questionnaire (dog age at test 12–24 months) | Factor analysis revealed: Playfulness, chase-proneness, curiosity/fearfulness, sociability, aggressiveness, distance-playfulness | Convergent validity for playfulness, curiosity/fearfulness, sociability, and distance-playfulness Chase-proneness related to human-directed play interest and non-social fear. Aggressiveness low association with all behavioural factors of the questionnaire. | Behavioural problems based on social and non-social fear were predicted, but not other behavioural problems. |

3

**Table 9.2** Examples of studies looking into evaluating behaviour of (future) working dogs, their evaluation type and the behaviours evaluated.

| Author | Aim | Population characteristics | Assessment age | Behaviour dimensions assessed and/or their structure | Validity and reliability | Results |
|---|---|---|---|---|---|---|
| Wilsson & Sinn, 2012 | To test the predictive validity of subjective and behavioural ratings in working dogs. Physical engagement ($z = 2.69$, $p < 0.001$ in test, $z = 3.35$, $p < 0.001$ in subjective rating) and confidence ($z = 2.51$, $p < 0.05$ in subjective rating) strongest predictors of training completion | $N \sim 496$ German shepherd Military working dogs | 15–18 months | 25 behaviour ratings 13 subjective ratings 5 behavioural ratings: Confidence, physical engagement, social engagement, aggression, environmental sureness 3 subjective ratings: engagement, confidence, aggression | Predictive validity of behaviour ratings on working outcome. Only minor differences in predictive validity between the two methods (1.7–6.6%) | Both ratings correctly predicted 70.3–78.3% of dogs that did or did not complete training. |
| Rocznik et al., 2015 | To examine the content validity of the Transportation Security Administration detection-dog puppy test | $N = 34$ German shepherd, Labrador Retriever, Malinois, Chesapeak Bay retriever, Tervueren | 3, 6, 9, and 12 months | 15 traits in the test 8 behaviour categories in the questionnaire | Content validity established at face value by comparison of traits deemed important by handlers in the field and traits tested in the test. | 13 of the 15 behaviour traits rated in the test were deemed important by the handlers. Test does not measure all the traits important for handlers. |
| Serpell & Hsu, 2001 | To develop and validate a questionnaire for assessment of behaviour and temperament in 1-year-old guide dogs | $N = 1097$ Labrador Retriever, Golden Retriever, Labrador x Golden Retriever cross Guide dogs | 1 year | Factor analysis revealed 8 factors: Stranger-directed fear/aggression, non-social fear, energy level, owner-directed aggression, chasing, trainability, attachment, dog-directed fear/aggression | Convergent validity: 14 of the 16 expected associations between rejection reason and behaviour factor were statistically significant. Discriminant validity: only 3 of the 56 predicted non-associations were statistically significant. | Good construct for the evaluation of the behaviour of the studied population. |

from that to which the dog had adapted previously, and this may alter the risk of aggression that may not have been apparent previously (Appleby et al., 2002; Haverbeke et al., 2009). For example:

- A dog that has been living isolated as a breeding bitch for most of its life might start showing aggressive behaviours when placed in a home in a busy city because it is exposed to chronic stress in the form of excessive sensory load from all the people, sounds, smells, etc., encountered.
- By contrast, a dog might show aggressive tendencies in the stressful shelter setting, but not when adopted into a calmer environment.

There are two ways to verify information obtained through a behaviour test: prospectively by comparing the test results with future behaviour (e.g. by retesting after a certain time period or contacting the new owners) or retrospectively, by comparing them to the dog's history. In a retrospective study, Christensen and colleagues (2007) looked at the aggressive behaviour of sixty-seven dogs that had passed a temperament test and had been adopted from shelters and found that certain types of aggressive tendencies were not reliably predicted by the temperament tests. In another retrospective study of 2,017 dogs in shelters, Bollen and colleagues (2008) found the most significant retrospective predictor of aggression was failure of the behavioural evaluation test conducted at the time of entry into the shelter (OR 11.83, p < 0.0005). There was a significant association between dogs that were evaluated to be 'unsocial' in the behaviour test and the absence of aggressive behaviours according to the six-month follow-up (p = 0.005). Dogs estimated as being 'borderline' were more likely to be returned to the shelter for problems with aggression (p = 0.028). Eighty-six per cent of the dogs that failed the behaviour evaluation did so in several of the subtests, which might indicate that these dogs have a general tendency to choose aggression in a range of stressful situations. During the two-year study period 1,033 dogs were adopted; when compared to the numbers of the previous year (1,002 adoptions and 190 returned), using the behaviour evaluation over a two-year period reduced the total return of dogs to the shelter from 19% (190 of 1,002 dogs) to 14% (142 of 1,033 dogs) (p = 0.001) and the return of dogs based on aggression problems was reduced from 5 to 3.5%. Additionally, the frequency of dogs returned based on serious aggression was reduced during the study years. However, it remains unknown if this decrease is within the realms of normal fluctuation, and repeat follow up over subsequent years would be useful.

## 9.9 Conclusion

Aggression is part of the normal behavioural repertoire of dogs. At best, simple tests will most likely identify animals with the most extreme tendencies, and if more is expected than this, then the demands of what is being asked need to be appreciated.

As it is impossible in real-life situations to control for all the influencing factors that might affect a dog's behaviour after the time when the animal was assessed (by a questionnaire or a test), predicting aggression as an isolated behaviour very rarely makes sense. It perhaps is more realistic to attempt to get a grasp of the larger picture of the animal's personality and behavioural tendencies when under certain types of potentially stressful circumstances, ideally based on information collected from its past in combination with some kind of observational method, covering as many potential triggers as possible.

## 9.10 References

Appleby, D. L., Bradshaw, J. W. S., Casey, R. A. (2002). Relationship between aggressive and avoidance behaviour by dogs and their experience in the first six months of life, *Veterinary Record*, 150, 434–438.

Beaver, B., Haug, L. I. (2003). Canine behaviors associated with hypothyroidism, *Journal of the American Animal Hospital Association*, 39, 431–434.

Beerda, B., Schilder, M., Van Hooff, J., DeVries, H. W., Mol, J. A. (1999). Chronic stress in dogs subjected to social and spatial restriction. 1. Behavioral responses, *Physiology & Behavior*, 66, 233–242.

Bennett, S. L., Litster, A., Weng, H., Walker, S. L., Luescher, A. U. (2012). Investigating behavior assessment instruments to predict aggression in dogs, *Applied Animal Behaviour Science*, 141, 139–148.

Benus, R. F., Bohus, B., Koolhaas, J. M., Vanoortmerssen, G. A. (1991). Heritable Variation for Aggression as a Reflection of Individual Coping Strategies, *Experientia*, 47, 1008–1019.

Bollen, K. S., Horowitz, J. (2008). Behavioral evaluation and demographic information in the assessment of aggressiveness in shelter dogs, *Applied Animal Behaviour Science*, 112, 120–135.

Bradshaw, J. W. S., Goodwin, D. (1999). Determination of behavioural traits of pure-bred dogs using factor analysis and cluster analysis; a comparison of studies in the USA and UK, *Research in Veterinary Science*, 66, 73–76.

Braem, M., Doherr, M. G., Lehmann, D., Mills, D., Steiger, A. (2008). Evaluating aggressive behavior in dogs: a comparison of 3 tests, *Journal of Veterinary Behavior: Clinical Applications and Research*, 3, 152–160.

Carrillo, M., Ricci, L. A., Coppersmith, G. A., Melloni, R. H. (2009). The effect of increased serotonergic neurotransmission on aggression: a critical meta–analytical review of preclinical studies, *Psychopharmacology*, 205, 349–368.

Christensen, E., Scarlett, J., Campagna, M., Houpt, K.A. (2007). Aggressive behavior in adopted dogs that passed a temperament test, *Applied Animal Behaviour Science*, 106, 85–95.

Diederich, C., Giffroy, J. (2006). Behavioural testing in dogs: A review of methodology in search for standardisation, *Applied Animal Behaviour Science*, 97, 51–72.

Duffy, D. L., Hsu, Y., Serpell, J. A. (2008). Breed differences in canine aggression, *Applied Animal Behaviour Science*, 114, 441–460.

Eisenberger, N. I., Way, B. M., Taylor, S. E., Welch, W. T., Lieberman, M. D. (2007). Understanding genetic risk for aggression: clues from the brain's response to social exclusion, *Biological Psychiatry*, 61, 1100–1108.

Ennik, I., Liinamo, A. E., Leighton, E., van Arendonk, J. (2006). Suitability for field service in 4 breeds of guide dogs, *Journal of Veterinary Behavior: Clinical Applications and Research*, 1, 67–74.

Epstein, S. (1983). Aggregation and beyond. Some basic issues on the prediction of behavior, *Journal of Personality*, 3, 360–392.

Foyer, P., Wilsson, E., Wright, D., Jensen, P. (2013). Early experiences modulate stress coping in a population of German shepherd dogs, *Applied Animal Behaviour Science*, 146, 79–87.

Fratkin, J. L., Sinn, D. L., Patall, E. A., Gosling, S. D. (2013). Personality consistency in dogs: a meta-analysis, *PLoS ONE*, 1–19.

Fuchs, T., Gaillard, C., Gebhardt-Henrich, S., Ruefenacht, S., Steiger, A. (2005). External factors and reproducibility of the behaviour test in German shepherd dogs in Switzerland, *Applied Animal Behaviour Science*, 94, 287–301.

Goodloe, L. P., Borchelt, P. L. (1998). Companion dog temperament traits, *Journal of Applied Animal Welfare Science*, 1, 303–338.

Gosling, S. D., Kwa, V. S. Y., John, O.P. (2003). A dog's got personality: a cross-species comparative approach to personality judgments in dogs and humans, *Journal of Personality and Social Psychology*, 1161–1169.

Guy, N. C., Luescher, U. A., Doohoo, S. E., Miller, J. B., Doohoo, I. R., Spangler, E., Bate, L. A. (2001). A case series of biting dogs: characteristics of the dogs, their behaviour, and their victims, *Applied Animal Behaviour Science*, 74, 43–57.

Hart, B. L., Hart, L. A. (1985). Selecting pet dogs on the basis of cluster analysis of breed behavior profiles and gender, *Journal of the American Veterinary Medical Association*, 186, 1181–1185.

Haverbeke, A., De Smet, A., Depiereux, E., Giffroy, J. M., Diederich, C. (2009) Assessing undesired aggression in military working dogs, *Applied Animal Behaviour Science*, 117, 55–62.

Hiby, E., Rooney, N. (2004). Dog training methods: their use, effectiveness and interaction with behaviour and welfare, *Animal Welfare*, 13, 63–69.

Horisberger, U., Stärk, K. D. C., Rüfenacht, J., Pillonel, C., Steiger, A. (2004). The epidemiology of dog bite injuries in Switzerland characteristics of victims, biting dogs and circumstances, *Anthrozoös*, 17, 320–339.

Horváth, Z., Botond-Zoltán, I., Magyar, A., Miklósi, A. (2007). Three different coping styles in police dogs exposed to a short-term challenge, *Hormones and Behavior*, 52, 621–630.

Horváth, Z., Dóka, A., Miklósi, A. (2008). Affiliative and disciplinary behavior of human handlers during play with their dog affects cortisol concentrations in opposite directions, *Hormones and Behavior*, 54, 107–114.

Hsu, Y., Serpell, J. A. (2003) Development and validation of a questionnaire for measuring behavior and temperament traits in pet dogs, *Journal of the American Veterinary Medical Association*, 223, 1293–1300.

Hussain, S. G. (2005) Attacking the Dog-Bite Epidemic: Why Breed-Specfic Legislation Won't Solve the Dangerous-Dog Dilemma, *Fordham Law Review*, 74, 28–47.

Jagoe, A., Serpell, J. (1996). Owner characteristics and interactions and the prevalence of canine behaviour problems, *Applied Animal Behaviour Science*, 47, 31–42.

Jones, A. C., Gosling, S. D. (2005). Temperament and personality in dogs (canis familiaris): A review and evaluation of past research, *Applied Animal Behaviour Science*, 95, 1–53.

King, T., Martson, L. C., Bennett, P. C. (2012). Breeding dogs for beauty and behaviour: Why scientists need to do more to develop valid and reliable behaviour assessments for dogs kept as companions, *Applied Animal Behaviour Science*, 137, 1–12.

Klaassen, B., Buckley, J. R., Esmail, A. (1996). Does the dangerous dogs act protect against animal attacks: a prospective study of mammalian bites in the accident and emergency department, *Injury*, 27, 89 91.

Klausz, B., Kis, A., Persa, E., Miklósi, A., Gácsi, M. (2013). A quick assessment tool for human-directed aggression in pet dogs, *Aggressive Behavior*, 40, 178–188.

3

Koolhaas, J. M., Korte, S. M., de Boer, S. F., Van der Vegt, B. J., Van Reenen, C. G., Hopster, H., De Jong, I. C., Ruis, M. A., Blokhuis, H. J. (1999). Coping styles in animals: current status in behavior and stress–physiology, Neuroscience & *Biobehavioural Reviews*, 23, 925–935

Ley, J. M., McGreevy, P., Bennett, P. B. (2009). Inter-rater and test-retest reliability of the Monash Canine Personality Questionnaire–Revised (MCPQ–R), *Applied Animal Behaviour Science*, 119, 85–90.

Liinamo, A. E., van der Berg, L., Leegwater, P. A. J., Schilder, M. B. H., von Arendonk, J. A. M., van Oost, B. A. (2007). Genetic variation in aggression-related traits in Golden Retriever dogs, *Applied Animal Behaviour Science*, 104, 95–106.

Maejima, M., Inoue-Murayama, M., Tonosaki, K., Matsuura, N., Kato, S., Saito, Y., Weiss, A., Murayama, Y., Ito, S. (2007). Traits and genotypes may predict the successful training of drug detection dogs, *Applied Animal Behaviour Science*, 107, 287–298.

Mills, D. S., Ramos, D., Estelles, M. G., Hargrave, C. (2006). A triple blind placebo-controlled investigation into the assessment of the effect of Dog Appeasing Pheromone (DAP) on anxiety related behaviour of problem dogs in the veterinary clinic. *Applied Animal Behaviour Science*, 98(1), 114–126.

Mills, D., Braem Dube, M., Zulch, H. (2012). *Stress and Pheromonatherapy in Small Animal Clinical Behaviour*, 1st edition, Wiley-Blackwell.

Mornement, K. M. (2009), Reliability, validity, and feasibility of existing tests of canine behaviour, *Proceedings of the AIAM Annual Conference on Urban Animal Management*.

Mornement, K. M., Coleman, G. J., Toukhsati, S., Bennett, P. C. (2010). A Review of Behavioral Assessment Protocols Used by Australian Animal Shelters to Determine the Adoption Suitability of Dogs, *Journal of Applied Animal Welfare Science*, 13, 314–329.

Netto, W. J., Planta, D. J. U. (1997). Behavioural testing for aggression in the domestic dog, *Applied Animal Behaviour Science*, 42, 243–263.

O'Farrell, V. (1997). Owner attitudes and dog behaviour problems, *Applied Animal Behaviour Science*, 52, 205–213.

Overall, K. (2007). Working bitches and the neutering myth: sticking to the science, *The Veterinary Journal*, 173, 9–11.

Panksepp, J. (2004). *Affective Neuroscience: the Foundation of Human and Animal Emotions,* 1st edition, Oxford University Press.

Panksepp, J. (2005). Affective consciousness: core emotional feelings in animals and humans, *Consciousness and Cognition*, 14, 30–80.

Paroz, C., Gebhardt-Henrich, S., Steiger, A. (2008). Reliability and validity of behaviour tests in Hovawart dogs, *Applied Animal Behaviour Science*, 115, 67–81.

Podberscek, A. L., Serpell, J. A. (1997). Environmental influences on the expression of aggressive behaviour in English Cocker Spaniels, *Applied Animal Behaviour Science,* 52, 215–227.

Reisner, I. R., Houpt, K. A., Shofer, F. S. (2005). National survey of owner-directed aggression in English Springer Spaniels, *Journal of the American Veterinary Medical Association*, 227, 1594–1603.

Riemer, S., Müller, C., Vir´qnyi, Z., Huber, L., Range, F. (2013). Choice of conflict resolution strategy is linked to sociability in dog puppies, *Applied Animal Behaviour Science*, 149, 36–44.

Riemer, S., Müller, C., Virányi, Z., Huber, L., Range, F. (2014). The Predictive Value of Early Behavioural Assessments in Pet Dogs – A Longitudinal Study from Neonates to Adults, *PLoS ONE*, 9.

Rocznik, D., Sinn, D. L., Thomas, S., Gosling, S. D. (2015). Criterion analysis and content validity for standardized behavioral tests in a detector-dog breeding program, *Journal of Forensic Sciences*, 60, 10.1111/1556-4029.12626.

Rosado, B., García-Belenguer, S., León, M., Palacio, J. (2007). Spanish dangerous animals act: Effect on the epidemiology of dog bites, *Journal of Veterinary Behavior: Clinical Applications and Research*, 2, 166–174.

Rosado, B., García-Belenguer, S., Palacio, J., Chacón, G., Villegas, A., Alcalde, A. I. (2010). Serotonin transporter activity in platelets and canine aggression, *The Veterinary Journal*, 136, 104–105.

Ruefenacht, S., Gebhardt-Hendrich, S., Miyake, T., Gaillard, C. (2002). A behaviour test on German shepherd dogs: heritability of seven different traits, *Applied Animal Behaviour Science*, 79, 113–132.

Saetre, P., Strandberg, E., Sundgren, P. E., Pettersson, U., Jazin, E., Bergström, T. F. (2006). The genetic contribution to canine personality, *Genes, Brain and Behavior*, 5, 240–248.

Scherrer, C. (2007). Wesensprüfungen bei Rassehundeclubs in der Schweiz – Ergebnisse eine Befragung, Doctoral Dissertation, University of Berne, Switzerland.

Scott, J. P., Fuller, J. L. (1965). *Genetics and the Social Behavior of the Dog: the classic study*. The University of Chicago Press, Chicago, USA.

Segurson, S. A., Serpell, J. A., Hart, B. L. (2005). Evaluation of a behavioral assessment questionnaire for use in the characterization of behavioral problems of dogs relinquished to animal shelters, *Journal of the American Veterinary Medical Association*, 227, 1755–1761.

Serpell, J. A. (1996). Evidence for an association between pet behavior and owner attachment levels, *Applied Animal Behaviour Science*, 47, 49–60.

Serpell, J. A., Hsu, Y. (2001). Development and validation of a novel method for evaluating behavior and temperament in guide dogs, *Applied Animal Behaviour Science*, 72, 347–364.

Shihab, N., Bowen, J., Volk, H. A. (2011). Behavioral changes in dogs associated with the development of idiopathic epilepsy, *Epilepsy & Behavior*, 21, 160–167.

Sigrist, C. (2007). Die Beurteilung der Persönlichkeit von Tierheimhunden anhand eines einfachen Tests oder einer kombinierten Testmethode, Doctoral Dissertation, University of Berne, Switzerland.

Sinn, D. L., Gosling, S. D., Hilliard, S. (2010). Personality and performance in military working dogs: Reliability and predictive validity of behavioral tests, *Applied Animal Behaviour Science*, 127, 51–65.

Slabbert, J. M., Odendaal, J. S. J. (1999). Early prediction of adult police dog efficiency – a longitudinal study, *Applied Animal Behaviour Science*, 64, 269–288.

Starling, M. J., Branson, N., Thomson, P. C., McGreevy, P. D. (2013). 'Boldness' in the domestic dog differs among breeds and breed groups, *Behavioural Processes*, 97, 53–62.

Stoll, H. F. (2010). Wesensprüfungen als Teil der Zuchtzulassng von Rassehunden, Doctoral Dissertation, University of Bern, Switzerland.

Strandberg, E., Jacobsson, J., Saetre, P. (2005). Direct genetic, maternal and litter effects on behaviour in German shepherd dogs in Sweden, *Livestock Production Science*, 93, 33–42.

Svartberg, K. (2002). Shyness-boldness predicts performance in working dogs, *Applied Animal Behaviour Science*, 79, 157–174.

Svartberg, K. (2005). A comparison of behaviour in test and in everyday life: evidence of three consistent boldness-related personality traits in dogs, *Applied Animal Behaviour Science*, 91, 103–128.

Svartberg, K., Tapper, I., Temrin, H., Radesäter, T., Thorman, S. (2005). Consistency of personality traits in dogs, *Animal Behaviour*, 69, 283–291.

Taylor, K. D., Mills, D. S. (2006). The development and assessment of temperament tests for adult companion dogs, *Journal of Veterinary Behavior: Clinical Applications and Research*, 1, 94–108.

Topál, J., Miklósi, A., Csányi, V., Dóka, A. (1998). Attachment behavior in dogs (Canis familiaris): A new application of Ainsworth 's (1969) Strange Situation Test, *Journal of Comparative Psychology*, 112, 219–229.

Udell, M. A. R., Wynne, C. D. L. (2008). A Review of Domestic Dogs' (Canis Familiaris) Human-Like Behaviors: Or Why Behavior Analysts Should Stop Worrying and Love Their Dogs, *Journal of the Experimental Analysis of Behavior*, 89, 247–261.

Våge, J., Wade, C., Biagi, T., Fatjó, J., Amat, M., Lindblad-Toh, K., Lingaas, F. (2010). Association of dopamine- and serotonin-related genes with canine aggression, *Genes, Brain and Behavior*, 9, 372–378.

Valsecchi, P., Barnad, S., Stefanini, C., Normando, S. (2011). Temperament test for re–homed dogs validated through direct behavioral observation in shelter and home environment, *Journal of Veterinary Behavior*, 6, 161–177.

Van der Berg, L., Schilder, M. B. H., Knol, B. W. (2003). Behavior genetics of canine aggression: behavioral phenotyping of Golden Retrievers by means of an aggression test, *Behavior Genetics*, 33, 469–483.

Van der Berg, L., Schilder, M. B. H., DeVries, H., Leegwater, P. A. J., van Oost, B. A. (2006). Phenotyping of Aggressive Behavior in Golden Retriever Dogs with a Questionnaire, Behavior Genetics, 36, 882–902.

Van der Berg, S. M., Heuven, H. C. M., van den Berg, L., Duffy, D. L., Serpell, J. A. (2010). Evaluation of the C-BARQ as a measure of stranger–directed aggression in three common dog breeds, *Applied Animal Behaviour Science*, 124, 136–141.

Van der Borg, J. A. M., Beerda, B., Ooms, M., Silveira de Souza, A., van Hagen, M., Kemp, B. (2010). Evaluation of behaviour testing for human directed aggression in dogs, *Applied Animal Behaviour Science*, 128, 78–90.

Veenema, A. H. (2009). Early life stress, the development of aggression and neuroendocrine and neurobiological correlates: What can we learn from animal models? *Frontiers in Neurendocrinology*, 30, 497–518.

Wilsson, E., Sinn, D. L. (2012). Are there differences between behavioral measurement methods? A comparison of the predictive validity of two ratings methods in a working dog program, *Applied Animal Behaviour Science*, 158–172.

Wilsson, E., Sundgren, P. E. (1997a). The use of a behaviour test for the selection of dogs for service and breeding. 1. Method of testing and evaluating test results in the adult dog, demands on different kinds of service dogs, sex and breed differences, *Applied Animal Behaviour Science*, 53, 279–295.

Wilsson, E., Sundgren, P. E. (1997b). The use of a behaviour test for selection of dogs for service and breeding. 2. Heritability for tested parameters and effect of selection based on service dog characteristics, *Applied Animal Behaviour Science*, 54, 235–241.

# CHAPTER 10

# Risk Factors for Dog Bites – An Epidemiological Perspective

*Jenny Newman,  *Robert Christley, Carri Westgarth, Kenton Morgan

★*Co-lead authors*

## 10.1 Introduction

Epidemiology is the study of health-related events in populations, rather than in individual animals. Traditionally, epidemiological methods have been applied to the study of diseases, but they are readily applied to issues relevant to dog aggression, including injuries and behaviours. Typically, epidemiologists use the term 'outcome' to refer to the disease or other health-related event being investigated. Epidemiological methods are used to explore how frequently outcomes occur, how common they are in a population, their distribution within and across populations, and to identify factors affecting the likelihood of the occurrence of these outcomes. Hence, these approaches can be applied in order to identify factors that make dogs more likely to exhibit aggressive behaviour, or to bite. This knowledge can aid development of interventions and other measures likely to reduce the public health and animal welfare burden of dog aggression, and epidemiology has an important role in assessing the efficacy of such interventions.

Hence, the aim of epidemiology is to identify patterns of occurrence of an outcome, whether that pattern is changing over time or geographically, and whether the pattern varies between individuals with different characteristics. For example, is it more or less common in older than younger animals?

However, as epidemiology addresses risk on a population level it is not able to determine whether a specific individual will develop a given outcome. Rather, epidemiology seeks to provide an understanding of the probability of possible outcomes and identify factors that may alter that probability, based on evidence *from the population within which an individual belongs*. For example, Wake, Stafford and Minot (2006) reported that 38% of veterinary science and veterinary nursing students enrolled in one university reported having been bitten by a dog, and that a greater proportion of male students reported being bitten; the findings of such a study cannot be used to accurately identify specific individuals that will be bitten in the future, and while the results apply to those students studied, findings from the same university in other years, from similar students at different universities, or from entirely different types of groups, may differ by a greater or lesser extent. Epidemiology explores associations between potential risk factors and outcomes. However, as epidemiological studies are designed to identify associations, rather than to establish causal relationships directly, it should always be remembered that **'association is not the same as causation'**, and that associations may arise for a number of reasons (see below). Furthermore, the conclusions of a particular epidemiological study apply most directly to the population on which the study was conducted and extrapolation to other populations, such as in a different place or time, or with different characteristics should only be done with caution. The ability to draw valid conclusions from a study to other populations is referred to as **external validity** or **generalisability**. Even when applying the results of an epidemiological study directly to the population in which the study was conducted, the (*internal*) validity of the findings are reliant on robust design and conduct of each step of the study; problems at any stage can render the conclusions unreliable and possibly misleading.

Numerous studies have adopted epidemiological approaches to investigate issues related to dog bites, and findings have been summarised in review studies (For example, see Overall and Love, 2001). In this chapter we will:

- Present an overview of epidemiological design principles and how they must be used to evaluate the level of evidence that can be provided by epidemiological studies;
- Critical analysis of dog aggression research indicates that evidence regarding specific risk factors is weak.
- Present findings from a systematic review of evidence for risk factors for human-directed dog aggression.
- Explore how epidemiological methods may be optimised in future studies.

---

**Text box 10.1  Epidemiological terms for describing how common is an event**

**How common is an outcome?** (see Porta, 2008, for more information)

**Prevalence**: the number of individuals with the outcome (e.g. people with dog bite injuries) in a given population (e.g. the people in a particular town or suburb), usually presented as a proportion or percentage.

Usually prevalence refers to a specified point in time, and can be more precisely called the *point prevalence*.

**Incidence**: the number of individuals that develop the outcome (i.e. <u>new</u> events, such as a dog bite) within a stated period as a proportion of the individuals at risk, usually presented as a proportion or percentage, and must refer to the time period.

## Text box 10.2 Epidemiological terminology relating to risk

**Is the risk of an outcome associated with another factor?** (see Porta, 2008, for more information)

**Risk factor**: any variable that influences the frequency or occurrence of an outcome. Hence a risk factor is something that makes the outcome more or less likely to occur (e.g. smoking is a risk factor for lung cancer, as it makes lung cancer more likely to occur). The term *potential* risk factor is often used where it is (as yet) uncertain whether the factor alters the risk of the outcome.

**Relative risk (RR)**: a measure of how many times greater (or lower) the risk is in one group compared to another, where group membership is defined by the presence or absence of a particular (potential) risk factor. For example, are males (i.e. the potential risk factor) at greater risk of being bitten by a dog (the event or outcome) compared to females?

Relative risks can take any positive value. A relative risk of 1 indicates the risk in both groups is the same; a relative risk greater than 1 indicates the risk factor increases the risk of the outcome, whereas a relative risk between zero and one indicates the risk factor reduced the risk (i.e. is protective).

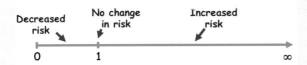

**Odds ratio (OR):** another method of assessing whether a risk factor is associated with the occurrence of an outcome (i.e. similar to relative risk). Odds ratios can be calculated in situations where the risk in the exposed and unexposed groups cannot be estimated (such as in case-control studies; see below). Odds ratios are also generated by some common statistical analyses, such as logistic regression. When the outcome is rare, an odds ratio will be approximately equal to the relative risk.

**Attributable Risk (AR)**: the additional risk in individuals *exposed* to (i.e. with) a risk factor that can be attributed to exposure to that factor. In other words, this is the number of cases above the background level that can be attributed on the factor being examined and is an indication of the number of cases of the outcome that could be prevented if the exposure to risk factor could be prevented entirely.

Hence, if the incidence of bites in a year by intact male dogs is 55.1 per 1,000 dogs compared to 7.7 per 1,000 for neutered male dogs (data from Shuler et al., 2008) then the attributable risk = 55.1–7.7 = 47.8, implying that for every 1,000 male dogs that are neutered 47.8 bite incidents are avoided per year.

## 10.2  Types of common epidemiological study designs

In order for the results of epidemiological studies to be of high validity, essential steps need to be followed during the design and implementation of the investigation. Numerous types of epidemiological study designs have been described, each with its own strengths and weaknesses, and each able to address somewhat different questions. Here we outline several common designs (Figure 10.1). It is vital that appropriate study designs be used when undertaking an epidemiological investigation. It is worth noting that it is not always possible to undertake the 'best' type of study; for example, it would be unethical to conduct a randomised controlled trial to assess whether dogs severely mistreated at a young age were more likely to subsequently display aggressive behaviours, if to do so would require deliberate mistreatment of animals. Hence, we often need to utilise data from studies that may be considered somewhat less robust than the 'gold standard', but when doing so we should always pay careful attention to all potential study limitations.

Furthermore, although careful conduct of recognised epidemiological study designs can maximise the validity of the results, there always remains a risk of 'incorrect' findings due to bias, confounding or just chance.

**Case studies and case series** provide descriptions of individual cases or groups of cases, respectively. These can be very useful, particularly when providing new information or highlighting previously unrecognised potential risk factors. However, as there is no comparison (control) group, these types of studies do not provide evidence of causation and should only be used to generate hypotheses to be tested in more robust studies. For example, Shetty et al. (2005) report on 250 cases of animal bites presenting to a hospital clinic. Although they find that males account for approximately twice as many cases as females, they are unable to determine the reason for this. Nevertheless, the findings suggest that the gender of the victims should be considered in further studies. Similarly, a review of another 250 dog bite incidents in Guelph, Canada, (Szpakowski, et al., 1989) reported that around 60% of incidents occurred within the dogs' home territory and also identified variation in the number of incidents per month. Such findings could be investigated in future investigations.

**Before-and-after** studies examine the frequency of the outcome of interest at one or more time points either side of a change of interest. For example, a study may examine the frequency of dog bites in a community before and after initiation of an educational campaign. A weakness of these studies is that it can be difficult to be sure that other things, which may also affect the frequency of the outcome, have simultaneously not changed over time. For example, the occurrence of a widely reported serious dog attack may directly change people's behaviour, or change their receptiveness to the educational initiative. Before-and-after studies can be improved by including 'control' populations and/or by staggering the introduction of the intervention over time. For example, Rosado et al., 2007 investigated the annual number of reported dog bite incidents in Aragón, Spain, from 1995 to 2004. By comparing the data from before and after introduction of breed-specific legislation in 2000, the authors suggest that the legislation was not successful in reducing the number of people injured by dog bites. However, they also point out a number of factors (such as changes to the dog population and to the tendency to report dog bites), which may have occurred over the study period and that may have affected their results. These issues highlight one of the major shortcomings of this type of study; that, in addition to the intervention of the event of interest, there may be a great many things that could affect the outcome of interest that could also change over time. Even if these can be identified, it often can be difficult or impossible to tease out the influence of the intervention of interest from that of the other factors.

**Ecological studies** measure and compare entire populations or groups, rather than the individuals within groups. For example, the frequency of serious dog bites might be compared between two or more regions with different dog control legislation. Although making use of data that may be readily available, these studies have several weaknesses. It is often difficult, if not impossible, to identify other things that may vary between the regions. For example, differences in dog bites may be related to subtle cultural variation, rather than to the legal frameworks in place. In addition, ecological studies of potential risk factors and outcomes that apply to individuals still measure these factors at the population level and this may result in the *ecological fallacy*. This occurs when the associations evident between populations are different to those at the individual level. For example, an ecological study comparing dog bite frequency among regions of England found that hospital admissions for dog bites were between two and three times greater for the most economically deprived compared to the least deprived areas (Winter, 2015). While this association is worthy of further investigation, of itself it does not prove that social deprivation is a risk factor for dog bites. First, there may be other factors, such as rates of dog ownership, that may vary with deprivation indices and which may affect dog bite rates. Secondly, the study does not provide evidence that, within any particular area, people in the more deprived parts of that area are at greatest risk. This somewhat surprising fact arises because an association observed at an aggregated level (i.e. at the level of regions) may not hold true for individuals within these populations (the *ecological fallacy*).

**Cross-sectional studies** investigate a particular population at a specific time, taking a 'snapshot' of the outcomes or diseases present and, sometimes, concurrently measuring the presence of a range of potential risk factors within the population. Hence, cross-sectional studies may be used to answer questions such as 'how common is this event in this population?' (*descriptive cross-sectional studies*) or 'is this event more common in animals with certain characteristics?' (*analytic cross-sectional studies*). For example, Gilchrist et al. (2008) surveyed almost 10,000 households using a cross-sectional study design. Although they included some descriptive results (e.g. that 16.6 adults and 13.1 children per 1,000 reported incurring a dog bite in the previous twelve months), they also undertook analyses to compare the rate between different sub-groups (e.g. the risk varied with the number of dogs in the household, with households without a dog being at lowest risk).

As it may be impossible to measure the characteristics of an entire population, it is more common that measurements are made on a subset of the population, i.e. a sample of the entire population is taken. It is paramount that this sample is a representative selection of the intended population, such that every member of the population is equally likely to be selected, independent of their characteristics. The study by Gilchrist et al. (2008) used a random digit dialling telephone survey approach to contact people in all 50 states in the USA. While this method can provide good coverage of a population, recent reduction in the number of houses with a landline phone, the increase in use of mobile phones and socio-economic variation in phone ownership means some bias may be expected using this approach. A convenience sample does not meet this criterion and is likely to be biased. There are many examples of convenience samples among scientific studies of dog bites. For example, Blackwell et al., 2008 investigated the relationship between training methods and the occurrence of behaviour problems using a convenience sample by recruiting owners during dog walks or when visiting a veterinary hospital.

It is also worth noting that, as analytic cross-sectional studies measure the outcome and the potential risk factors at the same time, often they cannot identify whether the risk factor or event occurred first, except under specific circumstances, such as where the risk factor is something the animal was born with, for example its sex.

**Case-control studies** examine a group that have had the outcome under study, for example dogs that have bitten, and compare them to those that have not. Hence, in a case-control study, individuals with the outcome of interest are identified and enrolled in the study (the *cases*). In addition a sample of other individuals that have not had the outcome are also enrolled, as a comparator, or *control*, group. A key feature of case-control studies is that eligibility for inclusion in the study is determined by an individual's status with respect to the outcome under study. Once the case and control groups are identified, the characteristics of each group can be measured and compared, and the likelihood of specific characteristics occurring in each group calculated.

A key issue with case-control studies is to ensure that an appropriate control sample is selected. This is often surprisingly difficult. One test of the appropriateness of the control group is whether an animal within it, if it were to develop the outcome of interest, could have been included within the case group; if not, it is not an appropriate control.

Gershman et al., (2015) used a case-control study design to investigate dog-related risk factors for bites to non-household members. They recruited cases from dogs reported to a centre in Denver, USA, for a first bite episode to a non-household member in which the victim required medical attention. Controls were neighbour-matched dogs with no history of biting a non-household member. The controls were selected by random digit telephone dialling, using the first five digits of the owner's phone number (as these numbers referred to specific geographic areas). A clear assumption using this sampling method is that control dogs identified through the random dialling process would have been recruited as cases had they bitten a non-household member; for the reader, it is difficult to judge the extent to which this is true.

One common issue with case control studies is recall bias. This arises when information recalled by cases (or their owners) is systemically different to that recalled by the controls. For example, it is possible that the experience of their dog having bitten someone may affect case dog owners' recall or reporting of past events, such as previous nips, bites or growls (perhaps as part of their explanation for the bite event) and this differential recall, compared with that by owners of control dogs, could influence the apparent effect of these factors on the risk of biting.

**Cohort studies** follow a group of individuals over a period of time, measuring the presence of risk factors and diseases, or other outcomes, at the beginning of, and at time points throughout, the study. Like most epidemiological studies, cohort studies are usually undertaken on a subset of the population of interest. A key benefit of cohort studies is that they enable determination of whether or not exposure to a potential risk factor occurred prior to the occurrence of the outcome. An additional benefit is that well-designed cohort studies can assess the effect of multiple potential risk factors on any one of multiple outcomes. *Prospective* cohort studies may not be suited to the investigation of rare outcomes or those that take a very long time to develop, as they would need to include very many individuals or follow them for a long period of time, respectively, in order to be sure to observe sufficient outcomes. An alternate approach is to conduct the study *retrospectively*. Although this approach may be cheaper and quicker compared to prospective cohort studies, the reliance on existent data may constrain the range and quality of the data available for analysis. For example, Martin (2001) retrospectively compared a cohort of dogs that attended puppy socialisation classes with a cohort of littermates that had not attended such classes. Similarly, Howe et al. (2001) contacted owners of dogs that had had early (<24 weeks of age) or late (≥24 weeks of age) gonadectomy (i.e. de-sexing) in order to compare the occurrence of a range of behavioural and other outcomes between these groups.

**Randomised controlled trials** (RCT) are often said to be the gold standard for demonstrating causal relationships between risk factors and outcomes. In many ways they are similar to cohort studies, in that they follow a group of individuals, some of whom are exposed, and others not exposed, to the potential risk factor of interest. The key difference is that whereas the cohort study uses natural exposures, randomised trials intervene to allocate the exposure to some individuals and not to others. For example, Chapman et al. (2000) randomly allocated a bite-prevention educational intervention to children in some schools and not to children in other (control) schools, prior to assessment of the frequency with which the children in each group interacted with a dog that was unknown to them. As the children (or, more correctly, their schools) had been allocated randomly to the intervention or control group, it is likely that the groups were, on average, similar to each other in all respects, except for the intervention itself. This represents the key advantage of the RCT design, in that this process of randomisation of the intervention can prevent the effects of confounding (see below) that may otherwise cause bias in the results.

RCT studies require an intervention, so it may not be possible, or ethical, to use them to investigate the effects of some potential risk factors. For example, Guy et al. (2001) investigated the risk factors for dog bites to owners using a cross-sectional study design. Many of the factors associated with a history of biting behaviour, such as the presence of teenage children in the household and a history of skin disease, could not have been incorporated as interventions into a RCT.

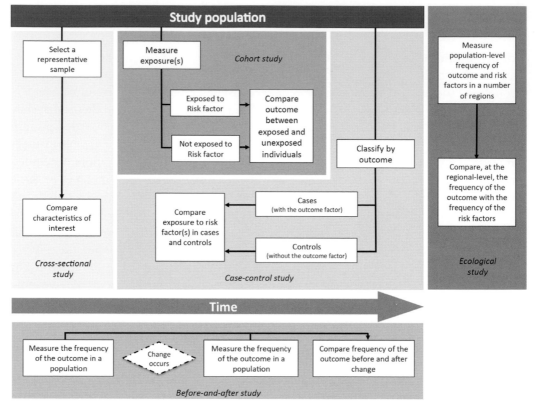

**Figure 10.1** Selected epidemiological study designs and their relationship to time.

## 10.3 'Accuracy' in epidemiological studies

A major problem with epidemiological studies examining dog bites relates to the quality of many of these studies. For a study to generate accurate results it must have both high **precision** and high **validity**, where precision is a measure of the amount of random error and validity is a measure of the amount of systematic error (bias) (see Text box 10.3). Studies should be designed to minimise both these types of error. As it is not possible to remove the effects of these errors entirely, it is important to evaluate the extent to which a particular study's results may be influenced by random and systematic error and to consider the potential impact on a study. Some examples of issues within the dog aggression literature are provided below, in the section 'Common limitations in epidemiological investigations of risk factors for aggression by dogs'.

## 10.4 Systematic reviews and meta-analyses

A **systematic review** entails synthesis of existing study results using a highly methodical, pre-specified series of steps. These steps determine how studies should be identified, appraised,

## Text box 10.3 Types of error and bias

**Random error** occurs due to chance and can be thought of as the 'background noise' against which the study is conducted. Random error often arises because epidemiological studies select a sample of a larger population, rather than the entire population, but it can arise at other stages as well. Increasing the size of the study sample will reduce random error. That is, a study would get a more precise estimate of the proportion of dogs in a rescue centre that are female if it randomly selected twenty-five animals, rather than five.

**Bias** occurs when errors vary systematically within the study. Some of the major types of bias are selection bias, information bias and confounding.

**Selection bias** arises when the subjects included in a study or, more specifically, in the data analysed, are systematically different to those not included and/or the criteria for selection of the study subgroups varies systematically within the study. For example, in one of the cross-sectional studies mentioned above, Blackwell et al. (2008) investigated the relationship between training methods and the occurrence of behaviour problems using a convenience sample of dog owners recruited during dog walks or when visiting a veterinary hospital. It is unlikely that the participants recruited in such a way will be representative of the underlying, but unobserved, populations in those locations due to the many factors related to the dog and the owner that may systematically influence the frequency and duration of dog walking and of attendance at veterinary hospitals. Hence, caution is needed when extrapolating from observations made on these participants to the population at large.

Selection bias may occur at almost all stages of an epidemiological study, and hence many types have been described (Sackett, 1979). Selection bias is best minimised through careful design and conduct of a study.

**Information bias** occurs when errors in measurement vary systematically between study subjects. Information bias can be further defined as misclassification bias or measurement error. **Misclassification bias** occurs when there is error in the categorisation of an exposure or outcome variable. For example, a nip from a small dog may be more likely to be classified as 'play', whereas if a large dog was involved in a similar situation it may tend to be classified as a bite. It is easy to see how such biases may arise, and that they may induce misleading conclusions.

The term **measurement bias** is applied to errors in continuous measurements, where the amount of error varies in a systematic way. If two different assays were used to measure cortisol, and one was used to assay dogs deemed to be 'aggressive' and the other used for dogs said to be 'non-aggressive', apparent differences between the aggressive and non-aggressive dogs could be simply due to systematic differences in the amount of error of each assay.

Some forms of information biases may be minimised through careful planning, for example use of only a single assay for all dogs or, if this is not possible, random allocation of dogs to each of the assays (irrespective of their status as 'aggressive' or 'non-aggressive'. In some cases it may be possible to correct for information biases following data collection, but it is usually preferable to prevent these biases in the first place.

3

## Text box 10.4  Confounding

**Confounding** occurs when there is a 'confusion of effects' in which the true association between the risk factor and outcome of interest is influenced by the effect of a third variable, the confounding variable. For example, a study may be designed to investigate whether dogs that lie on the sofa are more likely to bite. However, other variables, such as size, may change the risk that a dog will bite and also the probability it will be allowed to lie on the sofa. If these associations with size exist, the estimate of the effect of lying on the sofa on the risk of a dog biting will lack validity. For a variable to confound the association between a risk factor and an outcome it should fulfill the following criteria:

- It should be a risk factor for the outcome
- It should be associated with the risk factor
- It should not be on the causal pathway between the risk factor and the outcome.

The first two criteria were evident in the example: lying on the sofa is associated with size and, in this example, we are assuming that size is a risk factor for a biting. To meet the third criterion any effect of lying on the sofa on the risk of biting should not occur through an effect on size: clearly lying on the sofa does not cause an animal to be bigger or smaller, so this criterion is met. In contrast, if the risk factor of interest was, in fact, size, part of the effect of size on the risk of biting may be mediated through lying on the sofa, so the latter may not meet the third criterion. Hence, size may be a confounding variable of the relationship between lying on the sofa and biting, but lying on the sofa will not confound the relationship between size and biting.

Confounding can be controlled either at the design stage of a study or during analysis. During the design stage, researchers may control confounding by:

(a) *Restricting* the study population (e.g. in our example, only including small dogs);
(b) *Matching* during selection (e.g. for each dog that lies on the sofa enrolled in the study, a dog of similar size that does not lie on the sofa is enrolled), or;
(c) *Randomisation* of an intervention. This may be possible in the example study, as we could randomly allocate dogs be allowed, or not, to lie on the sofa.

During the analysis stage, confounding can be controlled through:

(a) *Stratificated* analysis where the data are analysed within strata of the confounder, (e.g. 'small' and 'large' dogs are analysed separately);
(b) *Multivariable regression* methods: these are statistical procedures that can account for the effect of one variable, the confounder, while examining the effect of the risk factor of interest.

In addition, if it is found that there is no association between the potential confounder and the risk factor of interest, then confounding will not occur as in this eventuality the second criterion is not met.

selected and their results synthesised. The aim is to only include studies that address the question of interest directly and that are of sufficiently high quality to be considered reliable. Sometimes, **meta-analyses** may be undertaken to statistically combine the results of a number of high quality studies.

A systematic review, completed in 2011, aimed to identify and synthesise all available robust evidence of risk factors for human-directed dog aggression (Newman, 2012). The review identified and examined studies undertaken between 1 January 1960 and 31 December 2010. In total, 27,565 publications were screened and 164 relevant studies underwent detailed appraisal of methodological quality. Despite this highly inclusive design, no robust high quality evidence for any risk factor for human-directed dog aggression was identified; most studies only provided low quality evidence.

From this systematic review, just eight studies were deemed to meet the inclusion criteria, and these were judged to provide moderate quality evidence (Table 10.1); in the main these studies offer hypotheses for future work, rather than robust evidence of causal effects. Among the conflicting evidence identified in the systematic review (Table 10.2) one factor stood out with consistent findings across three studies (which included three breeds of dog) – that aggression may be, at least in part, heritable. Hence, despite considerable conjecture in both lay and professional publications regarding risk factors for dog aggression, no high quality, robust evidence was identified in this systematic review.

It must be noted that this absence of evidence does not suggest that there are no factors that alter the risk of human-directed dog aggression, but simply that current research (at least up to 2010) does not provide robust evidence of the effect of these factors. To this end, the findings of this systematic review establish a baseline on which future research can build. Focus should perhaps turn to those factors most amenable to modification. Due to the likely influence of heritability, breeding practices selecting non-aggressive dams and sires have much potential. Furthermore, the complex web of cultural, socio-demographic and experiential factors that influence dog husbandry and management practices provides multiple potential opportunities for intervention and reduction of risk; limited and conflicting evidence for an effect of husbandry on the risk of aggression and biting was identified and this area requires more research. However, it is imperative that any future investigations of human-directed dog aggression are of sufficiently high methodological standard that the evidence provided is able to inform development of preventive strategies and legislation.

## Summary of moderate quality evidence identified by systematic review

### 10.4.1 Dog-related factors

#### Breed, sex and age of dog

Among the moderate quality evidence identified in the systematic review (categorised as 2+)[1] there are limited and conflicting findings for an effect of breed, sex and age of a dog (signalment) on risk.

---

1   See Table 10.3 for an explanation of the grading system used in the systematic review.

Three observational studies examined the effect of age on risk; none found an association (Gershman, et al., 1994; Guy, et al., 2001; Reisner, et al., 2005). The same three studies also examined the effect of the dog's sex on risk, with conflicting findings. In the survey of owner-directed aggression in English Springer Spaniels, male dogs were significantly more likely than females to exhibit aggression towards a household member (OR 1.7; CI 1.2–2.3; Reisner, et al., 2005). In their study of Canadian vet-visiting dogs, Guy, et al. (2001) identified that there was an interaction between the weight of a dog, its sex, and risk of biting a household member, with females being increasingly likely to bite with decreasing weight. Gershman, et al., (1994) found that male dogs were at greater risk of having been reported for biting a non-household member (OR 6.2; CI 2.5–15.1).

Two of these studies were of aggression or bites to household members (Guy, et al., 2001; Reisner, et al., 2005) and one to non-household members (Gershman, et al., 1994); this may partly explain the conflicting evidence identified. Furthermore, Guy, et al., (2001) considered regular visitors to the home to be household members, while they could have been classed as non-household members by Gershman, et al., (1994). Thus there is heterogeneity across the target groups of these studies.

The effect of breed on risk of human-directed dog aggression was examined in two studies (Gershman, et al., 1994; Guy, et al., 2001); no evidence reaching the inclusion standard was identified. Breed was controlled for in five studies by either restricting the study to specific breeds (Reisner, et al., 2005; Saetre, et al., 2006; Strandberg, et al., 2005) or using internal controls (DeNapoli, et al., 2000; Dodman, et al., 1996) and was not reported in a further study (Chen, et al., 2000). Gershman, et al., (1994) identified that dogs considered to be predominantly German shepherd or Chow breeds were at increased risk of biting a non-household member, but this was considered low quality evidence (2-) as a result of issues associated with breed identification, the method of analysis for breed and the low numbers of other breeds within the study population. In their case-control study of risk factors for dog bites to household members, Guy et al. (2001) found no association between breed and dogs having bitten. In this study, as the authors acknowledge, there were sixty-two different breeds represented among the 202 purebred dogs, rendering the number of dogs belonging to each breed very small. Thus power to detect differences is likely to have been insufficient.

## Neutering

Three studies examined the effect of neutering on risk of human-directed dog aggression, with conflicting findings (Gershman, et al., 1994; Guy, et al., 2001; Reisner, et al., 2005). The case control study of Guy, et al. (2001) identified no significant effect of neutering on risk of biting a household member (OR 0.8; CI 0.4–1.9). The majority of dogs (87.5%) in this study were neutered, reducing the study's ability to detect an effect. Reisner, et al. (2005) found that, overall, neutered dogs were more likely to be reported to be aggressive towards household members (OR 1.7; CI 1.3–2.4). When male and female dogs were analysed independently the association with neutering only persisted in the female dogs, with neutered females having an odds ratio of 1.9 (CI 1.3–2.8) compared to intact females; the odds ratio for neutered male dogs was not available in the paper. In contrast, Gershman et al. (1994) found that sexually intact dogs were at greater risk of biting (OR 2.6; CI 1.1–6.3). Subgroup analysis of those victims below twelve years of age found this relationship was no longer statistically significant (OR 2.3; CI 0.7– 7.3). Thus, while evidence of moderate quality (2+) was identified that neutering may affect risk, no conclusion can be drawn from the conflicting findings without further robust research. Prospective longitudinal research into the effects of neutering would be required in order to elicit the causal direction of any association with risk of human-directed aggression, as some dogs are neutered because they are aggressive towards other dogs or people (Reisner, et al., 2005).

### Behavioural History

There is limited evidence that various aspects of a dog's current or past behaviour are associated with their future propensity to exhibit aggression and bite (Guy et al., 2001; Reisner et al., 2005); in particular, there is moderate quality evidence (2+) that a history indicating past aggressive acts increases the risk of future aggressive acts. This requires further high quality investigation.

In their study of risk factors for bites to a household member, Guy et al. (2001) found that dogs that were reported to have exhibited aggression over food in the first two months of ownership were more likely to have bitten (OR 3.1; CI 1.1–9.0), compared to those that had not exhibited aggression over food. Those that had scored highly for excitability during the same period were also more likely to have bitten (OR 1.1; CI 1.0–1.3). These aspects of behavioural history were only examined in those dogs acquired prior to six months of age. More recent behavioural history was recorded in this study, but not included in multivariable models due to the high number of interactions and difficulty in establishing the causal direction of any relationship identified.

Reisner et al. (2005) reported that English Springer Spaniels exhibiting owner-directed aggression were more likely to have a history of aggression towards familiar non-household members; with odds ratios of 18.3 (CI 2.1–138.8) and 4.0 (CI 1.5–10.9) for those with a history of aggression towards a familiar child and adult, respectively. There was also an association between a dog having a history of aggression towards unfamiliar children within the dog's own territory and exhibiting aggression towards a household member (OR 2.6; CI 1.1–6.1). In addition, this study found an association between having exhibited aggression towards other dogs and risk of aggression towards household members (OR 1.9; CI 1.3–2.7).

In contrast to the two studies examining bites to household members or regular visitors to the home, Gershman et al. (1994) did not identify any association between factors in the behavioural history, including previous bites to household members, and biting a non-household member.

### Medical History

It is well recognised that ill-health can influence behaviour (Dantzer, 2001; Graham et al., 2006; Overall, 2003; Reisner, 1991). It is also suggested that the converse may be true (Black, 2002; Graham et al., 2006). Illness in an animal is often first recognised by deviation from their usual behaviour pattern (Overall, 2003). While there is some evidence for an association between pruritic or malodorous skin conditions and biting a household member (OR 1.9; CI 1.0–3.4; Guy et al., 2001), the association of aggression and health requires more extensive study, ideally with a longitudinal design across the general dog population and not restricted to vet-visiting dogs.

3

*Heritability*

The only consistent finding of moderate quality evidence (grade 2+) was that a degree of the variation in tendency to human-directed dog aggression is heritable; this was identified across three studies (Reisner et al., 2005; Saetre et al., 2006; Strandberg et al., 2005) and three breeds of dog (English Springer Spaniel, Rottweiler and German shepherd).

Saetre et al. (2006) and Strandberg et al. (2005) performed pedigree analyses on the findings of the Swedish Working Dog Association Dog Mentality Assessment (DMA) between 1989 and 2001 in 5,694 German shepherd dogs and 4,589 Rottweiler dogs. This work investigated the heritability of a range of behavioural traits within the cohort using a standardised behavioural test. It was determined that only aggression appeared to be inherited independent of other traits, with other behaviours falling along a broad spectrum of canine personality previously denoted as the 'shyness–boldness dimension' (Svartberg, 2002). Within the study population, in both breeds, 10% of the aggression shown towards a person who appeared suddenly was controlled by additive genetics and the remainder could be attributed to non-genetic factors (Saetre et al., 2006; Strandberg et al., 2005). When studying the maternal heritability of behaviour among the German shepherd dogs in this population Strandberg et al. (2005) did not find an influence from maternal pedigree. This aspect of their study suggested that the environmental effect on the litter had a larger influence on behaviour displayed during the standardised test.

In their cross-sectional survey of owner-directed aggression in English Springer Spaniels, Reisner et al. (2005) found that, of 1,053 adult dogs, the 48.4% reported by their owners to have a history of owner-directed aggression were significantly more likely to have one particular breeding kennel within their four generation pedigree (OR 1.6; CI 1.1–2.3). This kennel was specifically studied because of its noted frequent presence in the pedigrees of dogs being referred to the authors for management of aggression. The kennel was present in 34% of the pedigrees in the study. Reisner et al. (2005) acknowledge that this finding may reflect non-genetic factors associated with the kennel under study.

While, as with any pedigree analysis, the findings of each of these studies can only be applied to the study population, these works highlight a risk factor potentially modifiable over generations and thus requiring future robust research.

## 10.4.2 Target-related factors

No robust evidence was identified for an association between risk of being bitten and factors related to the person being bitten. This area was little studied in the research meeting the quality threshold of the systematic review.

Chen et al. (2000) examined bites to postal workers in Taiwan. Those working in rural areas were significantly more likely to be bitten, with an incidence of 1.0 dog bites for each person-working year in rural areas, compared to an incidence of 0.5 bites per person for each working year in urban districts (OR 2.7; CI 1.4–5.3). It is difficult to extrapolate these findings to the general population or even postal workers in other countries; however, with growing concern over the impact of dog aggression on the welfare of postal workers (Langley, 2012) this study does highlight an area requiring further study. No association between degree of urbanisation and the risk of a dog biting a household member or regular visitor to the home was identified amongst Canadian vet-visiting dogs (Guy et al., 2001).

### 10.4.3 Owner-related factors

An association was identified between one or more children below ten years of age sharing the home with the dog and risk of biting non-household members (OR 3.5; CI 1.6–7.5; Gershman et al., 1994). Where the recipient of the bite was below the age of twelve years the odds ratio increased to 6.9 (CI 1.8–26.1). This may have resulted from increased opportunities for interaction with non-household members, especially children, in households with children of their own. Guy et al. (2001) found no association between children living within the dog's household and risk of biting a household member. However, this study did find an association between the risk of a dog biting and the number of teenagers in the dog's home. The risk of biting increased with each additional teenager (OR 2.1; CI 1.3–3.4).

#### Early life

The pedigree analysis of Strandberg et al. (2005) examined the magnitude of the effect of litter and maternal environment in German shepherd dogs and found that the effect of the litter environment was greatest. The nature of this study did not permit further investigation as to which factors of the litter environment this related. Guy et al. (2001) did not identify an association between the early experiences of a dog and its subsequent risk of owner-directed aggression.

There is limited evidence, from the study of owner-directed aggression in English Springer Spaniels, for an effect of the source of acquisition on risk of aggression (Reisner et al., 2005), however there are a multitude of uncontrolled potential confounders of this effect. Neither Gershman et al. (1994) nor Guy et al. (2001) were able to identify an effect of the source of acquisition on risk in their studies of bites to non household members and household members respectively.

Guy et al. (2001) found that allowing a dog to sleep on the bed during the first two months of ownership was independently associated with risk of the dog subsequently having bitten a household member (OR 1.9; CI 1.1–3.5). In contrast, Reisner et al. (2005) found no independent association between a range of aspects of husbandry and risk of owner-directed aggression. This included no evidence of an association with allowing the dog to sleep on the owner's bed.

No evidence was identified for an effect of training (Gershman, et al., 1994; Guy, et al., 2001; Reisner, et al., 2005), owner socio-demographics (Reisner, et al., 2005), purpose for ownership (Gershman, et al., 1994; Guy, et al., 2001; Reisner, et al., 2005), or experience and knowledge of dogs and their behaviour (Guy, et al., 2001).

#### Diet

There is some limited evidence for an effect of dietary protein and tryptophan content on the level of aggression expressed towards either owners or visitors from two randomised trials with internal cross-over design (evidence quality 1+; DeNapoli, et al., 2000; Dodman, et al., 1996). The presentation of the results in these papers prevented extraction of appropriate summary statistics. Hence, the following summary of these results is largely qualitative, and we caution against over-interpretation of the presented p-values.

Dodman et al. (1996) found that dietary protein content made no significant difference to the primary problem behaviour of dogs exhibiting owner-directed aggression (p = 0.5) or hyperactivity (p = 0.13), nor their control dogs. However, in the group of twelve dogs whose main reported behavioural issue was aggression towards visitors to their home, low or medium dietary protein content was associated with a reduction in the reported intensity of the aggression (p = 0.04) as compared to high dietary protein content. On further evaluating this group, the effect was present in those seven dogs that scored highly for fearfulness (p <0.0001) but failed narrowly to reach statistical significance in the remainder of the group (p = 0.054); this requires further investigation. DeNapoli et al. (2000) undertook a similar trial, examining the effect of high and low protein diets with and without tryptophan supplementation on the level of aggression in a population of thirty-eight privately owned dogs. This study found that overall the lowest visitor-directed aggression scores were recorded while being fed a low protein, tryptophan-supplemented diet and that the high protein unsupplemented diet was associated with the highest owner-directed aggression scores.

These studies were small in both numbers and duration, and while similar in design they analysed their data differently. Dodman et al. (1996) only found an effect within individual groups and DeNapoli et al. (2000) only when the study population was analysed as a whole. This inconsistency, in addition to the very small population size and the use of subgroup analyses, raises concerns as to the validity of the findings. The effect of dietary protein content on the risk of aggression requires further investigation. It is also not possible to be confident that the effect can be generalised to protein level, as implied by the authors, or specific dietary formulations.

In conclusion, this systematic review found that currently a robust evidence base for risk factors of human-directed dog aggression was lacking. In order to examine thoroughly the evidence base, capturing evidence across the spectrum of circumstances, interactions, severity and targets, it was necessary to maintain a broad focus. This permitted studies of all potential risk factors, including any as yet unidentified by the study team, to be included in the review if they met the required methodological standard. In recognition of the diverse range of study designs and the abundance of observational studies undertaken in this field, all studies (whether observational or interventional in design) had the potential to be included if they were found to provide at least moderate quality evidence. Given this broad focus, low evidential threshold and the multiple methodological reasons for exclusion of the majority of the studies failing to reach this threshold, this review provides a pragmatic and practical assimilation of the current evidence base. The review identified no high quality evidence and very limited evidence of moderate quality. It is vital that future research in this area is of a high methodological standard in order for it to be able to add to the currently sparse evidence base.

## 10.5 Common limitations in epidemiological investigations of risk factors for aggression by dogs

From the systematic review of risk factors for human-directed dog aggression described above a number of common limitations in the methodology and interpretation were found and we discuss these below.

**Table 10.1** Studies of the effect of specific factors reaching the standard for inclusion in narrative systematic review.

| Study | Study type | Level | Study population size | Population characteristics | Outcome measures | Main factors studied | Potential risk factors identified |
|---|---|---|---|---|---|---|---|
| DeNapoli et al., 2000 | Randomised crossover trial | 1+ | 38 (33 analysed) dogs. | Privately owned dogs | Change in aggression score | Protein and tryptophan content of diet | High protein associated with highest dominance aggression. Low protein, tryptophan supplemented, associated with lowest territorial aggression. |
| Dodman, Reisner et al., 1996 | Randomised crossover trial | 1+ | 50 dogs. | Privately owned dogs | Change in aggression score | Protein content in diet | No overall effect. Reduced protein content reduced only fear related territorial aggression. |
| Saetre, Strandberg et al., 2006 | Cross-sectional | 2+ | 5,694 German shepherd dogs, 4,589 Rottweiler dogs. | Dogs that underwent the Dog Mentality Assessment by the Swedish Working | Finding of aggressive traits during the Swedish DMA. | Heritability of an aggressive behaviour trait. | Evidence of heritability. |
| Strandberg, Jacobsson et al., 2005 | Cross-sectional | 2+ | 5,959 German shepherd dogs (5 excluded). | Dog Association between 1989 & 2001. | | Heritability of an aggressive behaviour trait. Maternal and litter environment. | Evidence of heritability. Greater environmental effect than genetic. |
| Chen, Tang et al., 2000 | Cross-sectional | 2+ | 192 postal workers. | Postal workers. | Bite during course of work. | Socio demographics. Experience. Location. | Working in rural area. |
| Gershman, Sacks et al., 1994 | Case-control | 2+ | 178 geographically matched pairs of dogs. | Registered dogs reported for biting a non-household member and geographically matched controls. | Bite to non-household member requiring hospital attendance. | Signalment. Size. Acquisition. Husbandry. Behaviour history. Discipline. | Male dog, entire, living with children, chained in yard. |
| Guy, Luescher et al., 2001 | Case-control | 2+ | 353 dogs; 227 cases, 126 controls. | General veterinary caseload in Canada. | Bite to household member. | Signalment, Weight. Home environment. Medical history. Behaviour history. Husbandry. | Interaction between weight and sex - small female dogs at greatest risk. Teenage children in home. History of skin disorder. Behaviour history. |
| Reisner, Houpt et al., 2005 | Cross-sectional | 2+ | 1,053 dogs. | Adult, American Kennel Club registered, English Springer Spaniels | Owner-directed aggression and bite | Signalment. Breeding. Acquisition. Behaviour history. | Male dogs. Neutered females. Specific kennel in pedigree. Source of acquisition. Aggression towards other targets. |

3

**Table 10.2** Risk factors investigated by studies reaching evidential threshold.

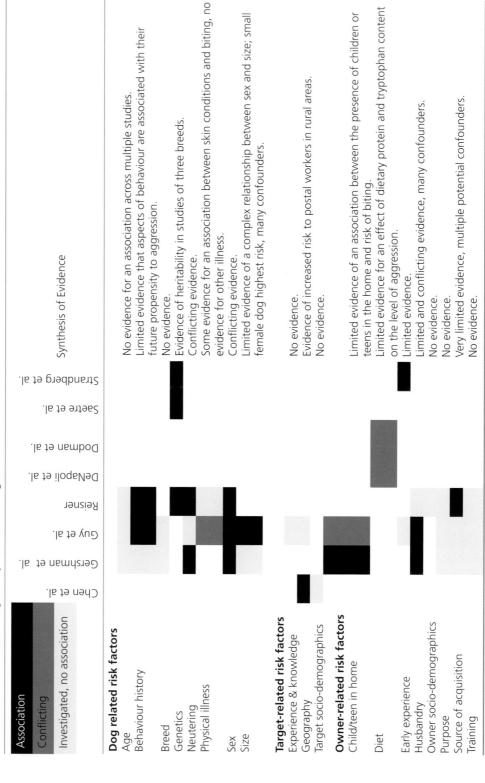

Legend:
- ■ Association
- ■ Conflicting
- ☐ Investigated, no association

Studies (columns): Chen et al., Gershman et al., Guy et al., Reisner, DeNapoli et al., Dodman et al., Saetre et al., Strandberg et al.

| Risk factor | Synthesis of Evidence |
|---|---|
| **Dog related risk factors** | |
| Age | No evidence for an association across multiple studies. |
| Behaviour history | Limited evidence that aspects of behaviour are associated with their future propensity to aggression. |
| Breed | No evidence. |
| Genetics | Evidence of heritability in studies of three breeds. |
| Neutering | Conflicting evidence. |
| Physical illness | Some evidence for an association between skin conditions and biting, no evidence for other illness. |
| Sex | Conflicting evidence. |
| Size | Limited evidence of a complex relationship between sex and size; small female dog highest risk, many confounders. |
| **Target-related risk factors** | |
| Experience & knowledge | No evidence. |
| Geography | Evidence of increased risk to postal workers in rural areas. |
| Target socio-demographics | No evidence. |
| **Owner-related risk factors** | |
| Child/teen in home | Limited evidence of an association between the presence of children or teens in the home and risk of biting. |
| Diet | Limited evidence for an effect of dietary protein and tryptophan content on the level of aggression. |
| Early experience | Limited evidence. |
| Husbandry | Limited and conflicting evidence, many confounders. |
| Owner socio-demographics | No evidence. |
| Purpose | No evidence. |
| Source of acquisition | Very limited evidence, multiple potential confounders. |
| Training | No evidence. |

**Table 10.3** The hierarchy of evidence utilised in the systematic review, adapted from SIGN (n.d.).

| Level | Description of studies meeting this level |
| --- | --- |
| 1++ | High quality meta-analyses, systematic reviews of RCTs, or RCTs with a very low risk of bias |
| 1+ | Well-conducted meta-analyses, systematic reviews, or RCTs with a low risk of bias meta-analyses, systematic reviews, or RCTs with a high risk of bias |
| 1- | Meta-analyses, systematic reviews, or RCTs with a high risk of bias |
| 2++ | High quality systematic reviews of case control, cohort or analytical cross-sectional studies. High quality case control, cohort and cross-sectional studies with a very low risk of confounding or bias and a high probability that the relationship is causal |
| 2+ | Well-conducted case control, cohort or analytical cross-sectional studies with a low risk of confounding or bias and a moderate probability that the relationship is causal |
| 2- | Case control, cohort or analytical cross-sectional studies with a high risk of confounding or bias and a significant risk that the relationship is not causal |
| 3 | Non-analytic studies, e.g. case reports, case series, descriptive cross-sectional studies |
| 4 | Expert opinion |

## 10.5.1 Defining outcome, what is a bite?

Many studies of risk factors for dog bites do not actually make it clear what is meant by a 'dog bite' (see also Chapter 1). Even among those studies that do provide an explicit definition, a range of definitions have been used.

Guy et al. (2001) defined a bite as 'the upper or lower teeth making contact with the victim's skin with sufficient pressure to cause a visible injury such as an indentation, welt, scrape or bruise, puncture or tear in the skin. A dog mouthing a person's skin without applying sudden pressure is not considered a bite'. This definition does not, however, implicitly identify the act as aggressive. A puppy in play, for example, may perform an act that would meet these criteria for a bite, without any aggressive intent. Hence, a study based on the definition of a bite used by Guy et al. (2001) would include bites that had occurred within a variety of contexts.

In contrast, Messam et al. (2008) sought to identify non-play bites and, to this end, asked three questions:

1.  Not during play, in the last two years, did the dog ever hold on to or catch a part of any person's body with its teeth and cause a wound?
2.  Not during play, in the last two years, did the dog ever hold on to or catch a part of any person's body or clothes with its teeth but not cause a wound?
3.  During play, in the last two years, did the dog ever hold on to or catch a part of any person's body with its teeth and cause a wound?

Responding in the affirmative to either of questions 1 and 2 resulted in the dog being classed as a biting dog in this study.

As can be seen from these two definitions the same dog could readily be classified as a biting dog in one study but not the other. As the choice of definition should be determined by the particular research question being investigated, these definitions (or others) could be suitable for some studies, but not others. However, such variation in the definition of dog bites means that it may be difficult, or even impossible, to compare directly findings of different studies.

Frequently studies use an outcome of bites requiring medical attention, reported to authorities or, on some occasions, both. While this provides a clear definition, identification of bite cases will be influenced by a host of factors, including those that determine whether an individual chooses to attend for medical treatment. For example, if a child and adult each suffered a bite wound of similar severity, it is possible that the child would be more likely to be taken for medical attention than the adult. It will also include both play and non-play bites, as both are able to cause injury.

## 10.5.2 Sample size

The systematic review described above did not identify any robust evidence that breed has an effect on the risk of a dog biting. This may be because breed is not, in itself, a risk factor. However, even where studies have been of robust design they have lacked the 'statistical power' to establish whether breed is a risk factor for dogs biting. The case control study of Guy et al. (2001) suffered in this respect; of the 353 dogs recruited, 202 were purebred representing sixty-two different breeds; consequently there were just a handful of dogs representing most breeds. Gershman, et al. (1994) recruited similar numbers of dogs to their case control study, with most breeds being represented by fewer than ten individuals. Despite this lack of evidence, in many jurisdictions legislation intended to reduce the risk of severe dog bite incidents pays particular attention to the breed of a dog. The findings of this systematic review indicate that breed-specific legislation has no firm evidence base, either for or against.

## 10.5.3 Sample selection

Many dog bite risk factor studies utilise populations selected by convenience, with a high risk of introducing bias. All types of convenience sampling in observational studies carries the likelihood that those who are convenient, or more likely to be sampled, are not representative of the overall population under study, by virtue of the factors increasing their likelihood of being sampled.

## 10.5.4 Comparator group

Studies designed to establish risk factors require a control or comparator group. As a result of their lack of a comparator group, case series and case studies do not provide robust evidence for the effect of potential risk factors, but can provide useful information for generating hypotheses to be tested in larger studies. Therefore, attempts to draw solid conclusions about risk from these studies should be strongly avoided.

Registry-based populations are often used as a comparator group in risk factor analysis. Within these populations only a limited amount of information is known about the individuals and, perhaps more critically, information concerning those not captured within the register is lacking. Without knowledge of the population not represented, it is impossible to gauge the effect of a factor on risk. This is problematic as factors affecting the likelihood of an owner to register or license a dog may confound the relationship with risk of a dog biting.

## Text box 10.5  Why convenience sampling is problematic

**Recruitment via advertisements placed in dog-related magazines** (Baranyiová et al., 2005; McGreevy and Masters, 2008) where bias may be introduced due to the characteristics of the readership of such magazines, in addition to those who choose to participate having read the advertisement.

**Internet-based surveys** (Duffy et al., 2008; Cornelissen and Hopster, 2010) have a similar propensity to introduce volunteer bias, in addition to bias resulting from the factors making an owner more likely to access internet-based information. However, there is evidence from some fields of research that this method of recruitment may produce populations with characteristics comparable to more traditional methods.

**Recruitment of dogs being walked in public places.** (Hiby et al., 2004; Perez–Guisado and Munoz–Serrano, 2009) Studies that recruit in this manner are at risk of not being representative of the general dog population. Dogs most likely to be recruited would be those that were walked (a) more frequently and/or for longer periods of time (b) during the working day in (c) public areas. These three factors (and probably more) are likely to be related to a host of potential confounders interwoven with the behaviour of dog and owner.

**Registries of bite incidents.** Multiple factors influence an individual's decision to report a bite incident to authorities, even where it is compulsory to do so. The study described by Shuler et al. (2008), for example, reported that, although multiple parties are required to report dog bites in the county where the study was conducted, the reported bite rate was 40% below the national estimated rate of bites attending emergency departments. This, in turn, is thought to represent only a fifth of all dog bites (Cornelissen and Hopster, 2010). The characteristics of the dogs, owners and recipients involved in unreported bite incidents are not captured if only those reported are examined. Similar issues relate to studies using medically attended bites as an inclusion criteria.

### 10.5.5 Confounding

Without appropriate accounting for all confounding variables, false conclusions may be drawn. Many studies fail to adequately account or control for confounding in both designing their study and analysing the data. In part, this results from the lack of identification of potential confounders before the study commences. Without this, controlling for confounders is impossible. Some studies, such as that of Messam et al. (2008) recognised the presence of confounding, but not its importance to their findings. Figure 10.2 depicts the inter-relationships identified by Messam et al. (2008) between factors potentially associated with non-play bites. Diagrams of this nature should form an essential component of the planning stages of all studies in order to identify and subsequently control for potential confounders.

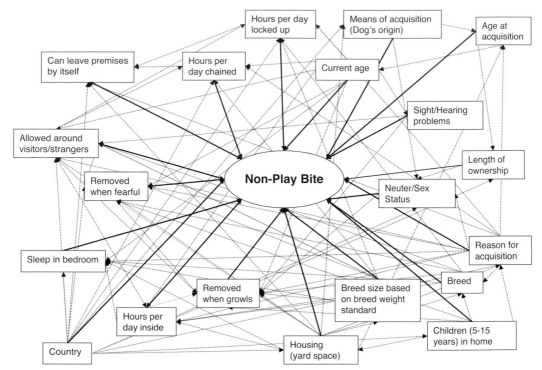

**Figure 10.2** The directed acyclic diagram used by Messam et al. to visualise a hypothesised causal web of dog bites, and thus identify potentially confounded relationships. Bold lines represent causal relationships between exposures and non-play bites. Dotted lines represent causal relationships between exposures. Reprinted from Messam et al. (2008) The human–canine environment: A risk factor for non-play bites? *The Veterinary Journal*, 177; 205–215, Copyright (2008), with permission from Elsevier.

## 10.5.6 *Measurement*

Measurement methods, of both the outcome and exposure to study factors, are often not reproducible or validated. A poor outcome definition frequently compounds this problem. A number of studies investigating the epidemiology of aggression have used the opinion of owners, veterinarians, other animal care workers as measures of the outcome and/or the study factors. For example, Fatjó et al. (2006) explored the epidemiology of a number of behavioural problems through a survey of veterinarians' opinions, while Bradshaw et al. (1996) used rankings by veterinarians and dog care professionals to assess the behavioural characteristics (including aggression) of a range of dog breeds. Such evidence cannot provide robust evidence of causation, and such information, even when expressed by an experienced and knowledgeable body of people, is low level, potentially biased, evidence. Indeed, such studies are investigating beliefs about, for example, breed preponderance to aggression, rather than actual differences between the breeds (see Chapter 7).

Breed determination by the target of aggression, where the breed is not subsequently verified, is further problematic as a result of the effect of cognitive biases. For example, those being bitten by an unknown dog may subconsciously misidentify the dog as of a breed that they perceive to be aggressive. Measurement of breed is especially problematic where the breed of cases was identified by the victim and the breed of controls by the owner. A robust method of measuring outcome or exposure would be objective, validated, reproducible and unbiased, with cases and controls assessed in an identical manner.

Whether a study is observational or interventional, blinding reduces the risk of introducing measurement or observer bias. Bias is potentially introduced by prior knowledge of outcome by the person measuring exposure to a study factor, or conversely of exposure to a potential risk factor when measuring outcome. If, for example, an interviewer knows that a dog has been reported to have bitten they may interpret the owner's responses differentially to when they know the dog has not bitten, making measurement of exposure to risk factors unreliable.

## 10.5.7 Analysis

Analysis of epidemiological studies may often require relatively complex statistical approaches; these are often outside the experience of people undertaking the research and hence simpler, but less robust, methods are often used. However, another problem may arise because modern statistical software enables conduct of complex statistical analyses without requiring knowledge of their correct and appropriate applications.

Multivariable analysis is commonly applied in epidemiology to determine the effects of individual factors by controlling for the confounding effect of other measured factors within an analytical model and presenting findings for the effect of a variable after adjustment for confounders. However, many studies report only univariable findings (i.e. simple associations). In such circumstances (and as described in the section on confounding, above), incorrect conclusions may be drawn from data as the estimate of the effect on the outcome of the risk factor of interest may be influenced by one or more other, confounding, variables.

## 10.6 Design priorities in future research

- It is vital that any future work exploring the risk factors for bites from dogs be undertaken to a high methodological standard.
- **Longitudinal studies** are likely to provide the most robust evidence with the ability to better determine the direction of causal relationships.
- Study populations should be recruited at **random** with all members of a population having the same likelihood of being approached. Randomisation is fundamental to reducing the risk of introducing selection bias.
- A priori development, examination and critique of putative **causal webs**, as illustrated in Figure 10.2, should be undertaken, permitting identification, measurement and control of **potential confounders**.
- **Sample size and power calculations** should be undertaken in order that populations of sufficient size can be recruited to reduce the risk of failing to identify an effect that is present (type II error).
- **Outcome and risk factors must be defined clearly and objectively.**
- Comparator populations must be derived from **the same population as the cases.**

- **Measurement** of both outcome and exposure to risk factors must be reliable and reproducible. **Blinding** reduces the risk of introducing measurement or observer bias.
- **Analysis** should permit identification of the effect of individual factors on risk. For observational studies this is likely to require multivariable analysis so that the effect of confounders can be controlled.

## 10.7 References

Baranyiová, E., Holub, A., Tyrlík, M., Janáčková, B., Ernstová, M. (2005). 'The influence of urbanization on the behaviour of dogs in the Czech Republic.' Acta Veterinaria Brno 74(3): 401–409.

Black, P. H. (2002). Stress and the inflammatory response: A review of neurogenic inflammation. *Brain, Behavior, and Immunity* 16, 622–653.

Blackwell, E. J., Twells, C., Seawright, A., Casey, R. A. (2008). 'The Relationship between Training Methods and the Occurrence of Behavior Problems, as Reported by Owners, in a Population of Domestic Dogs.' *Journal of Veterinary Behavior: Clinical Applications and Research* 3(5): 207–17. http://linkinghub.elsevier.com/retrieve/pii/S1558787807002766 (11 September 2014).

Bradshaw, J. W. S., Goodwin, D., Lea, A. M., Whitehead, S. L. (1996). A survey of the behavioural characteristics of pure-bred dogs in the United Kingdom. Veterinary Records, 138: 465–168.

Chapman, S., Cornwall, J., Righetti, J., Sung, L. (2000). 'Preventing Dog Bites in Children: Randomised Controlled Trial of an Educational Intervention.' *BMJ (Clinical research ed.)* 320(7248): 1512–13.

Chen, S. C. et al. (2000). An epidemiologic study of dog bites among postmen in central Taiwan. *Chang Gung Med J* 23, 277–283.

Cornelissen, J. M., Hopster, H. (2010). 'Dog bites in The Netherlands: a study of victims, injuries, circumstances and aggressors to support evaluation of breed specific legislation.' Vet J 186(3): 292–298.

Dantzer, R. (2001). Cytokine-Induced Sickness Behavior: Mechanisms and Implications. *Annals of the New York Academy of Sciences* 933, 222–234.

DeNapoli, J. S., Dodman, N. H., Shuster, L., Rand, W. M., Gross, K. L. (2000). Effect of dietary protein content and tryptophan supplementation on dominance aggression, territorial aggression, and hyperactivity in dogs. *Journal of the American Veterinary Medical Association* 217, 1012–1012.

Dodman, N. H. et al. (1996). Effect of dietary protein content on behavior in dogs. *Journal of the American Veterinary Medical Association* 208, 376–379.

Duffy, D. L., Hsu, Y., Serpell, J. A. (2008). 'Breed differences in canine aggression.' Applied Animal Behaviour Science 114(3): 441–460.

Fatjó, J., Ruiz-de-la-Torre, J. L., Manteca, X. (2006). The epidemiology of behavioural problems in dogs and cats: a survey of veterinary practitioners. Animal Welfare, 15: 179–185.

Gershman, K. A., Sacks, J. J., and Wright, C. (1994). 'Which Dogs Bite? A Case-Control of Risk Factors.' *Pediatrics* 93: 913–17.

Gilchrist, J., Sacks, J. J., White, D., D., Kresnow, M-J. (2008). 'Dog Bites: Still a Problem?' *Injury Prevention: Journal of the International Society for Child and Adolescent Injury Prevention* 14(5): 296–301. www.ncbi.nlm.nih.gov/pubmed/18836045 (14 November 2014).

Graham, J. E., Robles, T. F., Kiecolt-Glaser, J. K., Malarkey, W. B., Bissell, M. G., Glaser, R. (2006). Hostility and pain are related to inflammation in older adults. *Brain, Behavior, and Immunity* 20, 389–400.

Guy, N. C., Luescher, U. A., Dohoo, S. E., Spangler, E., Miller, J. B., Dohoo, I. R., Bate, L. A. (2001). 'Risk factors for dog bites to owners in a general veterinary caseload.' *Applied Animal Behaviour Science* 74(1): 29–42.

Hiby, E., Rooney, N., Bradshaw, J. (2004). 'Dog training methods: their use, effectiveness and interaction with behaviour and welfare.' Animal welfare (South Mimms, England) (13): 63–69.

Howe, L. M., Slater, M. R., Boothe, H. W., Hobson, H. P., Holcom, J. L., Spann, A. C. (2001). 'Long-Term Outcome of Gonadectomy Performed at an Early Age or Traditional Age in Dogs.' *Journal of the American Veterinary Medical Association* 218(2): 217–21. http://avmajournals.avma.org/doi/abs/10.2460/javma.2001.218.217

Langley, G. (2012). *Inquiry into dog attacks on postal workers.* www.royalmailgroup.com/sites/default/files/Langley_Report.pdf

Martin, S. T. (2001). 'Is There a Correlation between Puppy Socialization Classes and Owner-Preceived Frequency of Behaviour Problems in Dogs?' University of Guelph.

McGreevy, P. D., Masters, A. M. (2008). 'Risk factors for separation-related distress and feed-related aggression in dogs: additional findings from a survey of Australian dog owners.' Applied Animal Behaviour Science 109(2): 320–328.

Messam, L. L. M., Kass, P. H., Chomel, B. B., Hart, L. A. (2008). 'The human-canine environment: A risk factor for non-play bites?' Veterinary Journal 177(2): 205–215.

Newman, J. (2012). Human-directed dog aggression; a systematic review. MPhil Thesis, University of Liverpool.

Overall, K. L. (2003). Medical differentials with potential behavioral manifestations. *Veterinary Clinics of North America: Small Animal Practice* 33, 213–229.

Overall, K. L., Love, M. (2001). Dog bites to humans – demography, epidemiology, injury, and risk. Journal of the American Veterinary Medical Association, 218: 1923–1934.

Perez-Guisado, J., Munoz-Serrano, A. (2009). 'Factors linked to dominance aggression in dogs.' Journal of Animal and Veterinary Advances 8(2): 336–342.

Porta, M. (2008), *A dictionary of epidemiology*, 5th edn. Oxford University Press, Oxford,

Reisner, I. R., Houpt, K. A., Shofer, F.S. (2005). 'National survey of owner-directed aggression in English Springer Spaniels.' Journal of the American Veterinary Medical Association 227(10): 1594–1603.

Reisner, I. (1991). The pathophysiologic basis of behavior problems. *Veterinary Clinics of North America Small Animal Practice* 21, 207–224.

Rosado, B., García-Belenguer, S., León, M., Palacio, J. (2007). 'Spanish Dangerous Animals Act: Effect on the Epidemiology of Dog Bites.' *Journal of Veterinary Behavior: Clinical Applications and Research* 2(5): 166–74. http://linkinghub.elsevier.com/retrieve/pii/S155878780700202X (14 November 2014).

Sackett, D. L. (1979). 'Bias in analytic research.' J Chronic Dis 32(1–2): 51–63.

Saetre, P. et al. (2006). The genetic contribution to canine personality. *Genes Brain Behav* 5, 240–248, doi:DOI 10.1111/j.1601-183X.2005.00155.x.

Shetty, M. R. A, Chaturvedi, S., Singh, Z. (2005). 'Profile of Animal Bite Cases in Pune.' *J. Commun. Dis.* 31(1): 66–72.

Shuler, C. M., DeBess, E. E., Lapidus, J. A., Hedberg, K. (2008). 'Canine and Human Factors Related to Dog Bite Injuries.' *Journal of the American Veterinary Medical Association* 232(4): 542–46. www.ncbi.nlm.nih.gov/pubmed/18279087

3

SIGN. 'Scottish Intercollegiate Guidelines Network.' www.sign.ac.uk/guidelines/fulltext/50/annex oldb.html (15 October 2015).

Strandberg, E., Jacobsson, J., Saetre, P. (2005). Direct genetic, maternal and litter effects on behaviour in German shepherd dogs in Sweden. *Livestock Production Science* 93, 33–42, doi:DOI: 10.1016/j. livprodsci.2004.11.004.

Svartberg, K. (2002). Shyness–boldness predicts performance in working dogs. *Applied Animal Behaviour Science* 79, 157–174.

Szpakowski, N. M., Bonnett, B. N., Martin, S. W. (1989). 'An Epidemiological Investigation into the Reported Incidents of Dog Biting in the City of Guelph.' *Canadian Veterinary Journal* 30: 937–42.

Wake, A. A. F., Stafford, K. J., Minot, E. O. (2006). 'The Experience of Dog Bites: A Survey of Veterinary Science and Veterinary Nursing Students.' *New Zealand veterinary journal* 54(3): 141–46.

Winter, J. (2015). 'Provisional Monthly Topic of Interest: Admissions Caused by Dogs and Other Mammals.' *Health and Social Care Information Centre*. www.hscic.gov.uk/catalogue/PUB17615/prov-mont-hes-admi-outp-ae–April 2014 to February 2015-toi-rep.pdf.

## 10.8 Further reading

Newman, J. (2012). Human-directed dog aggression; a systematic review. MPhil Thesis, University of Liverpool.

Villaroel, A. (2015). Practical clinical epidemiology for the veterinarian. Wiley Blackwell, Ames, Iowa.

Thrusfield, M. (2007) Veterinary Epidemiology, 3rd Edition. Blackwell Science Ltd, Oxford, UK.

Shuler, C. M., DeBess, E. E., Lapidus, J. A., Hedberg, K. (2008). 'Canine and Human Factors Related to Dog Bite Injuries.' *Journal of the American Veterinary Medical Association* 232(4): 542–46. www.ncbi.nlm.nih.gov/pubmed/18279087

# CHAPTER 11

# Fatal Dog Attacks

## *Wim Van de Voorde and Dingeman Rijken*

**This chapter contains graphic photographs that some readers may find distressing.**

## 11.1 Introduction

The vast majority of dog bites are non-fatal. Epidemiological studies indicate that most dog bites are of minor severity, yet it is believed that up to half the reported bites leave permanent scars and one-third of these may cause disability (Berzon et al., 1974). Fatal dog bites, fortunately, are rare with an incidence of 7.2 deaths per 100 million population per year in the United States (Sacks et al., 1996b). From 1979 to 1998, only 238 deaths were reported in the United States (Sacks et al., 2000).

A clear relationship exists between the victim's age, severity of injuries, and the body part injured. The highest rate, in terms of injury and mortality, is attributed to children less than twelve years old and elderly females (Shields et al., 2009). Victims of fatal dog attacks are reported to be under the age of twelve in 85% of the cases and less than ten years old in 70%, with one-third of all deaths occurring among infants less than one year old (De Munnynck et al., 2002). In one report, of all the dog bite deaths reported in a five-year period, 31% of the victims were infants in the first twelve months of their lives, who were left unattended in a crib (Mathews et al., 1994). Newborns are reported to be 370 times more likely to die from a dog bite than adults aged thirty to forty-nine years (Sacks et al., 1989), whereas elderly women aged sixty-five to ninety-two years may be twice as likely to succumb to a dog bite-related fatality compared with elderly men of the same age (Shields et al., 2009).

Young children (as opposed to babies) may be at increased risk of attack from domestic dogs for a variety of reasons, because they are small and often run around quite rapidly, possibly simulating some of the characteristics of small prey to a watching dog. They would not be able to escape from a predatory dog as they are not fast enough to outrun the animal and lack an understanding of the need to rapidly distance themselves from danger (see Chapter 30). Children may also not be strong enough to offer effective resistance if an animal begins to attack, particularly if the dog is larger or heavier than the victim. Children may also be curious about dogs and may inadvertently or deliberately hurt or provoke an animal; for example, by making direct eye contact or by interfering with pups. It is not generally believed that fatal attacks are motivated by hunger (Tsokos et al., 2007). In this chapter we review what is known about fatal dog attacks and the need for their careful investigation, since our knowledge is based largely on case reports, some of which are reported in the scientific literature.

## 11.2  Understanding fatal dog attacks

In general, most dogs involved in biting or attacks are known to the victim and a good proportion, perhaps about one-third, belong to the victim's family (Sacks et al., 1996a). Pet dogs account for 93% of bites to children under four years old and for 75% of bites to children four to sixteen years old. The family dog is reported to be involved in nearly 70% of the fatal attacks (Jarrett, 1991). Although chaining or fencing in a dog may seem a good way to prevent bites, many bites occur while the dog is restrained in some way. A previous report showed that of 227 human dog bite-related fatalities, 24% involved unrestrained dogs away from their owner's property, 58% involved unrestrained dogs on their owner's property, 17% involved restrained dogs on their owner's property, and fewer than 1% involved restrained dogs away from their owner's property (Sacks et al., 2000). Perhaps surprisingly, stray dogs are usually involved in less severe bite incidents (Wright, 1991). Whereas attacks by pet dogs may often lead to wounds in the head and neck region, stray dogs commonly deliver bites to the hands and legs. The fact that people behave differently towards their own dogs than towards stray dogs may, at least partly, explain this difference (De Munnynck et al., 2002).

Fatal incidents are not simply an extreme sample of bite incidents. It is important to distinguish the risk of a bite from the risk of a potentially fatal bite. Recent studies have stated that, contrary to public opinion, so-called 'dangerous breeds' are not necessarily the most frequent contributors to bite incidents (De Keuster et al., 2006) and more 'friendly' breeds, including the Siberian Husky, Chow, or Dachshund are known to have killed children (Wiseman el al., 1983; Bux et al., 1992; Clark et al., 1991; Tsuji et al., 2008). For a total of 264 fatal dog attacks in the United States and Canada from 1982 to 2006, the supposed breeds causing the deaths were, in descending order of reported frequency: Pit Bull Terrier (104), Rottweiler (58), Wolf hybrid (18), Husky (13), German shepherd (7), German shepherd mix (6), Bull Mastiff (Presa Canario) 6, Chow (6), with various other breeds making up the remainder. Although there may be questions over the reliability of breed reporting (Chapter 7) and the risk associated with breed cannot be separated from confounds related to the type of person who might tend to keep such a dog and how they might keep it, the American Pit Bull Terrier may pose a higher risk than some other breeds because of the strength of its bite (Chapter 12) and a tendency to hold on to its victim (Souviron, 2011).

Dogs acting as a pack, although less common, are far more dangerous than the same animals individually (Kneafsey et al., 1995; Avis, 1999). A study of human dog bite-related fatalities over a twenty-year period showed that of 238 deaths, 67.2% involved one dog,

20.6% two dogs, and 12.2% involved three or more dogs (Sacks et al., 2000). Dog pack attacks with human predation appear to be extremely rare, accounting for only 6.9% of all fatal dog attacks (Pomara et al., 2011). Although individually benign, the same dogs when part of a group can become more dangerous. Packs of dogs not only inflict a greater number of wounds as compared to attacks by single dogs, pack-related behavioural influences (the 'pack instinct') may act to prolong and/or escalate the attack (Santoro et al., 2011). Shields et al. (2009) described a pack attack of nine dogs against a three-year-old boy weighing 14kg. The victim was no match against Rottweiler and Chow dogs weighing between 16 and 36kg. It has been suggested that in a pack situation, once an aggressive act is initiated, whether as a playful nip or a serious bite, the others may join in, so the problem may escalate until the victim is killed or the dogs are driven off (Kneafsey et al., 1995). They can become excited and bleeding may exacerbate the problem further. Other factors that are suggested to facilitate the initiation of fatal attacks on humans by dogs include a possible genetic predisposition, male gender, intact reproductive status, poor health, late and inadequate training and socialisation, lack of supervision, defence of territory or puppies, hunger, predatory experience, pack-dog experience, age, size, and behaviour of victims; and absence of other people in the vicinity (Raghavan, 2008). Most these factors remain hypothetical, as there are insufficient data to test these hypotheses.

## 11.3  Forensic pathology

An animal bite can be defined as any break in the skin caused by an animal's teeth, regardless of the intention and three patterns have been observed:

1.  Non-fatal dog bite wounds that can be light, severe or life-threatening, e.g. due to prolonged bleeding.
2.  Dog bites that directly or indirectly (through infection and sepsis) lead to the victim's death.
3.  Post-mortem lacerations of the victim's body (Pollak et al., 1989).

The classical dog bite presents either as a four-point puncture wound from the canines or as tearing of the tissue in more severe attacks (Whittaker, 2008). To identify a lesion as a dog bite wound it should have ragged and irregular wound edges; show multiple, parallel, linear scratches or drying scuff abrasions; and include a puncture wound and sometimes an avulsion with irregular borders resembling a dental arch print (Grellner et al., 1998).

It is usually relatively easy for a dentist to distinguish between a human and an animal bite because of the size of the dental arch, and more particularly the arrangement and size of the teeth – a dog has large canines and diminutive incisors in both the upper and lower jaws (Whittaker, 2008).

The morphology of dog bite wounds is explained by some very specific dental and maxillofacial features [Figure 11.1] and more detail on the anatomy of dog bite wounds can be found in Chapter 16. However, it is important to appreciate the features of both the bite and its location, which contribute to variation in the wound sustained.

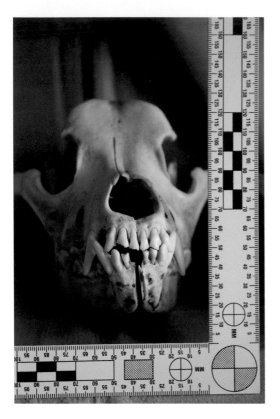

**Figure 11.1** Skull with canine dentition (Rottweiler, case De Munnynck et al., 2002).

## 11.3.1 Dog-related features affecting type of wound

The shape of the bitemark caused by a dog bite is a narrow, almost rectangular, arch at the front with conspicuous pointed markings from the canines on the corners of the rectangle. The morphologic presentation of dog bite wounds depends on the size and the breed of the dog as well as the surface bitten; and will differ whether or not the full dentition was used to produce them.

Only in ideal circumstances will a complete impression of all frontal teeth be found and often only a prominent canine impression can be seen (Pollak et al., 1989). The injuries caused involve a combination of biting, crushing and tearing that results in a characteristic pattern of punctures, lacerations and avulsions of skin and soft tissue (Tong et al., 1965; Prahlow et al., 2001).

The canine masseter-pterygoid complex is short and strong and its insertion on the mandible provides a powerful mechanical advantage. The force an adult dog can exert with its jaws is often 7.5–10kg/cm$^2$, sometimes leading to extensive bruising around the bitemark. This may increase to 20kg/cm$^2$ in some breeds of dog. Vertical forces exceeding 32kg/cm$^2$ have been measured during a dog attack, which is sufficient to penetrate sheet metal (Miller et al., 1993). The Pit Bull has been suggested to have the most powerful jaws described for any breed of dog described (95kg/cm$^2$) compared to the Rottweiler (53kg/cm$^2$) and the German shepherd (40kg/cm$^2$) (Souviron, 2011). However, relative bite strength indicates that, for their size, other breeds may pose a relatively greater risk (Chapter 12).

Forensic pathologists have noted multiple torn wounds with adjacent puncture wounds in many dog bites: the so-called a-hole-and-a-tear combination (Gershman et al., 1994). The puncture wound, a round hole, is made by a canine tooth and serves as an anchorage, while the other teeth cut into the flesh, causing stretch lacerations in the process of biting, shaking and tearing [Figure 11.2]. This should be considered pathognomonic for dog bites, especially when accompanied by tissue defects and claw marks, the latter being narrow, superficial linear abrasions arranged parallel to each other, four or five in number and found usually in the vicinity of the bite. This pattern allows differential diagnosis with bites of other animals that are not accompanied by pulling and shaking nor by the usage of the prominent canine, and with stab wounds caused by sharp instruments (Tong et al., 1965; Mittmeyer et al., 1976; Prahlow et al., 2001).

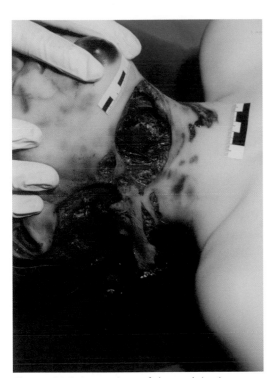

**Figure 11.2** Lacerations of the neck in six year old girl killed by three Rottweilers (case De Munnynck et al., 2002).

### 11.3.2 Location-related features affecting type of wound

Bite marks differ in appearance depending on whether they are on the skull, arms, legs, back, lips, or neck. Especially on the arm bruising is seen. A bite mark pattern on the neck may vary greatly in size and in shape depending on the bite mark recipient's head and neck movement (flexion, extension, rotation, etc.), the animal's dentition, and its head movements. Given that the back is a relatively flat surface, a dog is unable to open its jaw sufficiently wide to obtain contact with the canines on the skin. The bite mark pattern is markedly different from those on the arm, the neck, and the skull (Souviron, 2011).

### 11.3.3 Bite marks in fatal attacks

In severe to fatal attacks extensive soft tissue loss on the head, neck, and torso with loss of viscera and extremities may be observed as the dog moves its head vigorously (De Munnynck et al., 2002). Clothing can be shredded. Extensive scalp avulsions were also observed in most of the cases. Avulsions or partial avulsions of the ears were another common finding. Amputation is also possible. Fractures of the facial bones and/or calvarium are common. Depressed skull fractures and cranial perforations are possible in a child. The forces exerted by the animal may be strong enough to snap the vertebral spine, or even cause decapitation (Loewe et al., 2007).

Lesions involving blood vessels and/or organs of the neck may result in exsanguination

(Figure 11.2). Extensive injuries can mimic homicidal sharp-force trauma (Shkrum et al., 2007).

Most fatal lesions are located in the head and neck region involving soft tissue laceration, laryngeal crushing as well as opening or compression of the extracranial vessels, causing death by means of asphyxia, haemorrhage or air embolism (Reuhl et al., 2001; Kneafsey et al, 1995; Clark et al., 1991; Miller et al., 1993; Tsokos et al., 2007). Calkins et al. (2001) reported eight cases with life-threatening injuries including a (depressed) skull fracture, subdural hematoma, pneumothorax, intima tear of the axillary artery, internal carotid artery injury with middle cerebral artery infarction, spinal cord injury, cavernous sinus laceration, pneumothorax, and laceration of oesophagus and trachea. Also, extensive fatal abdominal injuries have been described (Clark et al., 1991).

Septic shock has also been reported as possible cause of death (Reuhl et al., 2001). Infections of dog bites (Chapter 20) are especially dangerous in those who are innately or therapeutically immunosuppressed or have undergone splenectomy.

Apart from the head and neck region, the extremities may also be involved in dog bites because these are used in defence movements. One death by pulmonary embolism has been reported after calf cellulitis complicating a dog bite (Falconieri et al., 1999).

## 11.4 Forensic investigation of fatalities involving dog bites

A forensic approach to a fatal dog attack should include a detailed assessment of the scene, the victim and the dog (De Munnynck et al., 2002) (See Chapters 14 and 15).

It is, of course, important to make the distinction between pre- and post-mortem bites, which is usually not difficult. The latter tend to be yellowish with no or minimal blood. Classically, post-mortem damage to a body by a dog usually involves an elderly recluse who has not been seen for some time. In such cases coming to the forensic pathologist's attention, death is often due to an underlying medical condition, and the domestic dog, commonly motivated by hunger, has eaten portions of the deceased. The body is often putrefied and the injuries may be parchmented, with little or no blood loss (Tsokos et al., 2007). In post-mortem feeding dogs tend to target the face and neck: stripping skin and subcutaneous tissues. This might complicate visual identification (Figure 11.3). They may also target genitalia, which might make a case look very strange at the onset, with the possibility of mimicking some form of sadistic sexual murder (Rossi et al., 1994; Rothschild et al., 1997). Dogs can also gnaw through bone. Bone tissue damage caused by carnivores is ragged, and leaves behind a series of tooth-sized pits and indentations along the margin (Santoro et al., 2011).

One must be aware that dogs may be falsely accused of attacking or biting children. Boglioli et al. (2000) reported the supposedly fatal attack by a German shepherd on a six day old baby. Forensic investigation brought to light that the dog did not kill the child. Instead, the father had killed the infant after he was urinated on during a nappy change. He then dismembered the infant and fed his remains to the family's dog.

Victims of dog attacks can be found completely undressed, which may erroneously suggest a sexual assault rather than a dog bite setting. On the other hand, rape of humans by dogs has also been reported and canine sperm can be detected both microscopically and with

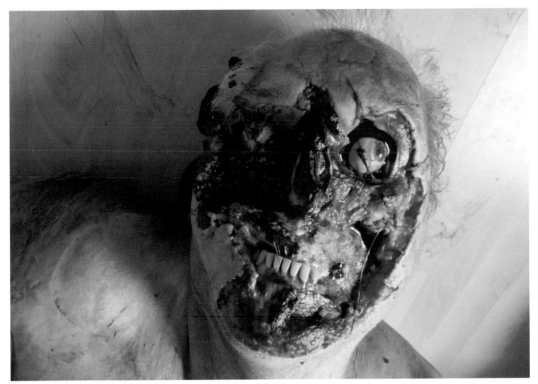

**Figure 11.3** Post-mortem predation by pet dog (shepherd).

DNA analysis (De Munnynck et al., 2002). An example of this was when a five-year-old boy had gone into the bush to have a bowel movement when a neighbour's large dog sexually assaulted him. Witnesses pulled the dog off the child. Following the attack, the child complained of abdominal pain and was noted to pass blood per rectum. Surgery disclosed a discrete anterior rectal wall perforation and a faecal pelvic peritonitis. After surgical treatment the child made a full recovery (Wiseman et al., 1983), but such a condition could easily become fatal if not treated promptly and appropriately.

## 11.5 Case reports of fatal dog bites

The following range of case reports (Table 11.1) illustrate the diversity of situations and injuries associated with fatal attacks. This series highlights that many of the dogs appear to be otherwise healthy and that, although several seem to involve encroachment on the dog's territory or activity, there is perhaps no such thing as the typical fatal dog attack.

While it may be possible to identify the cause of death, the reasons why the dogs have killed in this particular incidence often remains a mystery, commonly because this is not reported and/or investigated. Patronek and colleagues report on the co-occurrence of potential risk factors in USA dog bite fatality cases from 2000–09 (Patronek et al., 2013) and they conclude that these cases often pertained to: absence of an able-bodied person to intervene; incidental or no familiar relationship of victims with dogs; owner failure to neuter dogs;

**Table 11.1** Case reports of fatal dog attacks

| Victim Features | Circumstances of Incident | Nature of Injury | Cause of Death | Reference and other information |
|---|---|---|---|---|
| Ten year old boy | Threw a stone at the dog. | Multiple puncture wounds and laceration wounds all over the body including the scalp. Nose and upper lip were avulsed. Anterior aspect of upper jaw showed gnawing and bite marks. | Exsanguination | Sharif, 1977 |
| Three year old boy (15kg) | Boy crawled unwitnessed under a fence into an enclosure occupied by four husky sled dogs. | Twelve deep cervical lacerations, extending down to the cervical vertebrae with extensive deep cervical haemorrhage secondary to a tear of the right internal jugular vein. Lacerations in lumbosacral region, buttock and thigh. | Exsanguination | Wiseman et al., 1983 |
| Seventy-one year old woman (55.3kg) | Victim found dead in her house with her 40kg Chow dog. | Multiple bite marks on body with associated perforations, lacerations, contusions and abrasions. Perforations of the left femoral vein and the right external pudendal vein in the groin. Bite marks patterns found to left chest and 60% of the lower lobe of the left lung was contused. | | Bux et al., 1992<br><br>Bite mark analysis revealed patterned wounds identical to the dental pattern of the Chow dog. |
| Family of four individuals | Family ventured to an island to pick berries. The island was inhabited by a pack of 8 Labrador Huskies used as sled dogs that had been placed there for a summer to roam free. While picking berries the father and two children became separated from the wife. | | | Avis, 1999<br><br>All dogs were in good health and had a good layer of subcutaneous tissue. All had identifiable human remains in their stomach.<br><br>Testing for rabies was negative. |
| Wife – 44 year old | | Extensive soft tissue loss to the lower face, neck and thorax as well as extensive tissue loss to the right thigh and left upper arm. The right upper limb was absent. Chest cavity had been exposed and all viscera were absent. Numerous bite marks were present on the body. | | |
| Son – 10 year old | | Extensive tissue soft tissue loss to head, neck, thorax and upper limb which had been amputated at the scapula. Body cavities were intact. Numerous bite marks present over entire body. | | |
| Husband – 49 year old and son – 8 year old | They were alerted by her screams and found her pinned to the ground by a number of dogs which were biting her in the head and neck area. The husband and children scared the dogs away by throwing rocks. Upon approaching the woman it became apparent that she was dead. The eldest child ran back to the boat to get matches to build a fire in an attempt to keep the dogs away from the body | | | |

| Victim Features | Circumstances of Incident | Nature of Injury | Cause of Death | Reference and other information |
|---|---|---|---|---|
| | while they went for help. The dogs then attacked and killed the child. By the time the father and surviving child arrived at the boat the dogs had begun feeding on the body.<br><br>The survivors once again threw rocks at the dogs, which this time attacked them. Both had to run into the water to escape. When the rescue team arrived on the island, the dogs were feeding on the female body. | | | |
| Six year old girl (22.9kg) | Child was left alone in the garden with three large adult male non-neutered Rottweilers. | Punctures, lacerations and claw marks to head and neck region. Back of head showed a large avulsion of the scalp. Abrasion of the face with bruised lips and petechial conjunctival haemorrhages. Several large lacerations of the face and deep gaping wound under chin exposing the perforated thyroid cartilage, with deep laceration of the musculature, a small tear of the right jugular vein and avulsion of the right lateral processes of the cervical vertebrae C1 and C4. | Asphyxia and external bleeding | De Munnynck et al., 2002<br><br>Post-mortem examination of three dogs was negative for any disease or other peculiarities that could explain the violent behaviour. No human tissue was found in the mouth or gastric contents. |
| Married couple<br>Seventy-six year old man | Man was found in the garden behind the house, lying face down on the bloodstained ground. His trunk was naked with numerous shards of clothes scattered in the vicinity.<br><br>Family owned four dogs, a Maremma sheepdog and three Cane Corso, which were roaming through the garden. | Injuries to the head, neck, trunk and upper limbs. Scalp was almost totally absent. The frontal part of the temporal, parietal and occipital bones lay bare. Left lower eyelid and left zygomatic region showed a stretch laceration with exposure of the underlying bones. Soft tissue loss from the left ear. Numerous lacerations on the right side of the neck, with the main being a deep irregular shaped gaping wound that exposed part of mandible and a deep laceration of the musculature and vessels. Numerous gaping wounds to the left arm and similar injuries to the right upper arm. All these torn wounds presented ragged and irregular margins with adjacent puncture wounds. | Exsanguination | Di Donato et al., 2006<br><br>Swabs collected from the mouth and teeth of the Cane Corso revealed the presence of DNA of both spouses. |
| Seventy year old woman | Woman was found naked and covered in blood lying on her back in front of the house. | Similar wounds over the head, neck, trunk and upper and lower extremities. | Exsanguination | |

3

| Victim Features | Circumstances of Incident | Nature of Injury | Cause of Death | Reference and other information |
|---|---|---|---|---|
| Three month old male infant | Boy was found dead on the floor in the living room. He had been in his father's arms on the sofa when his mother went out shopping. The father had been severely intoxicated and sleeping. The family's Dachshund was roaming around freely. There were some bloody pools resembling bloody vomit or excreta on the floor of other rooms of the house. | Soft tissue loss at the right side of the face with the ear missing and visible brain matter. | Exsanguination | Tsuji et al., 2008<br><br>The gastric contents of the dog did not include human tissue, but the victim's DNA was isolated from the paws, mouth and gastric/duodenal contents. |
| Two month old male infant | The infant was attacked by the family Pit Bull, which was previously stray and recently acquired by the family. | Decapitation with bite marks surrounding the ragged wound margins on the neck. | Decapitation | Loewe et al., 2007<br><br>Examination of the gastric contents of the dog revealed multiple fragments of bone, skin and soft tissue, the nose, 1 eye globe and both ears of the infant. |
| One year old boy | Boy was placed on the kitchen floor by his grandmother. During a short absence of the grandmother the family Pit Bull attacked the child. | Multiple lacerations and sets of puncture wounds to the face, neck and arms. Extensive scalp and facial avulsions. Internal findings included a punctured right internal jugular vein and a fracture dislocation of the vertebral spine at the level of C7-T1. There were also punctures, lacerations and a crushing injury to the larynx. | | Loewe et al., 2007 |
| One year old boy | Playing in the front yard of his home, attacked by two freely roaming Pit Bull dogs. | Gaping wound on the right side of neck with numerous puncture wounds to the underlying main carotid artery and jugular vein, as well as the oesophagus and trachea. | | Loewe et al., 2007 |
| Six year old girl | While walking to school she was attacked by two family Pit Bull dogs and dragged into her backyard of the dwelling. | Numerous lacerations, puncture wounds and avulsions to the face and neck (67 in total). Brush burn abrasions consistent with drag marks. Multiple fragments of skull bone absent and/or separately received with the body including the left orbit and left maxilla. | | Loewe et al., 2007 |

| Victim Features | Circumstances of Incident | Nature of Injury | Cause of Death | Reference and other information |
|---|---|---|---|---|
| Forty-four year old woman | Woman was attacked by two Pit Bulls that resided at an occupied dwelling while walking down the street. The subject was observed lying on the ground with both dogs attacking the body. | Multiple clusters of abrasions, deep lacerations, and puncture wounds distributed over the face, the front and back of the neck the arms, the lower back, and the legs. There was complete avulsion of the left ear and partial avulsion of the right ear. Extensive scalp avulsions were also noted. There was complete transection of the left brachial artery, the left basilic vein, and the right common carotid artery. There was a bone defect in the T1 vertebra and dislocation of the first right rib. | | Loewe et al., 2007 |
| Ninety-one year old woman | Woman was attacked by her own family Pit Bull dog at home. | Multiple extensive scalp avulsions with exposure of the calvarium and subgaleal haemorrhage. Numerous lacerations were present on the eyes, cheeks, mouth, lower face, left upper neck, ears, and the left side of the head. Many paired puncture wounds were noted. Two of the lacerations on the face were deep and associated with absence of the lip, skin, facial muscle and soft tissue, right maxilla, and zygoma, resulting in exposure of the sinuses and oropharyngeal cavity. There were fractures of the bilateral zygoma, bilateral maxillary bones, the palatine bone, and the right mandible with loss of several upper and lower teeth and laceration of the tongue. A closed right hip fracture was also present. | | Loewe et al., 2007 |
| Six year old boy (22kg) | Boy was playing football on a school ground with his classmates when two unrestrained American Staffordshire Terriers, the male weighing 37.5kg and the female 26kg, began to chase the ball. The dogs then attacked the boy. The attack lasted for 10 minutes and observers were unable to stop the dogs. | Defleshing of the face and scalp with skeletonisation of the head. The left jugular vein had been severed. Other injuries consisted of scattered bites with scratches of the shoulders. | Death was due to exsanguination with evidence of air embolism | Tsokos et al., 2007 Post-mortem examination of the dogs revealed no underlying organic diseases; toxicology was negative; and rabies tests were also negative. Fragments of the victims' face and scalp were present within the male dog's stomach. |

3

| Victim Features | Circumstances of Incident | Nature of Injury | Cause of Death | Reference and other information |
|---|---|---|---|---|
| Ten year old girl | Girl had been playing in a garden, opened an enclosure containing a family friend's 2 German shepherd dogs (both male). She was observed by a friend to play with the dogs and then to fall over, initiating an attack by both animals. | Marked full-thickness defleshing of the face and scalp, with no significant injuries elsewhere. | Exsanguination | Tsokos et al., 2007 |
| Eleven year old girl | Girl had been playing in a garden with her family dogs (2 German shepherds, 1 male and 1 female, weighing 31 and 27kg) was found dead with the dogs attacking the body. | Marked defleshing and skeletonisation of the face, with scattered non-lethal bites of the upper arms and thighs. | Exsanguination | Tsokos et al., 2007 <br> The dogs were euthanised. Fragments of soft tissue from the victim were found in the male dog's stomach. <br> Both dogs tested negative for rabies. |
| Three week old male infant | Baby was left sleeping on a sofa, with the family dog (a large male mixed-breed terrier weighing 42kg) in the house. When checked, the infant's headless body was found on the floor of the lounge room, with bloodstaining of the sofa where he had been sleeping. | Decapitation and several puncture wounds of the neck. | Death was attributed to decapitation | Tsokos et al., 2007. <br> Necropsy of the dog revealed no underlying organic diseases, toxicology was negative, and rabies tests proved negative. The victim's entire fragmented head, with associated scalp and neck skin, was found within the dog's stomach. |
| Seventy-nine year old woman | Woman was found lying face down on the street. She was covered in blood. The neighbour's dog, a Japanese Tosa, was licking around the victim's neck. | Lacerations over the neck with a severed right internal jugular vein and vertebral artery. The C5 vertebral transverse process was fractured. Contusions and abrasions over the left side of the chest. Multiple valve-type wounds located over the left legs. | Exsanguination | Oshima et al., 2008 |
| Three year old boy | Boy was attacked by two female Rottweilers in a fenced yard. | Extensive avulsion of the scalp and facial soft tissues, including lacerations of the left carotid artery, left jugular vein, and extremities as well as maxillary, mandibular, nasal, and orbital fractures. | | Shields et al., 2009 |

| Victim Features | Circumstances of Incident | Nature of Injury | Cause of Death | Reference and other information |
|---|---|---|---|---|
| Three year old boy | Boy was found deceased in a residential yard with 10 Rottweiler and Chow dogs weighing between 16kg and 36kg. The owner of the dogs claimed that the deceased child was placed in the yard after another unidentified dog had killed the boy. | Lacerations of the scalp, right subclavian vein, left common carotid artery, oesophagus, liver, left common iliac artery, perianal area, and extremities; diffuse cerebral oedema with herniation; and pulmonary, adrenal, and renal haemorrhage. | | Shields et al., 2009

Dental alginate impressions were made of the dogs and examined. The result was that some dogs could be implicated. No dog could be conclusively linked to a particular bite mark. |
| Three year old boy | Boy was mauled by a 38kg Rottweiler in his grandmother's yard. The Rottweiler had been playing unrestrained with a ball in the yard. Investigators surmised that the boy had attempted to play with the ball when he was attacked, as bloody handprints covered the ball. | Subtotal avulsions of the scalp and ears, gaping full thickness lacerations of the posterior neck, abraded punctures of the back and right buttock, abraded contusions and puncture lacerations of the upper and lower extremities, multiple excoriations of the right lateral chest, acute subendocardial haemorrhage, and mild cerebral oedema. Among many distorted and avulsed injuries, one showed a substantial, relatively undistorted maxillary and mandibular component that could be directly compared with the resected dog's jaws. | | Shields et al., 2009.

The mandibular teeth of the Rottweiler fit quite precisely into the penetrating lacerations made by the canine teeth. He was an older dog with unusual wear patterns of his lower incisors, including loss of a left central incisor. The bite wound showed a pattern of abrasions of the incisor teeth that reproduced the distinctive patterns of the Rottweiler. Distinctive spacing between maxillary premolar teeth was also reflected in the maxillary mark. |
| Five year old boy | Boy was fatally attacked by his neighbour's intact, male Wolf hybrid (90kg). Investigators were informed that the dog's owners starved the animal to 'make him meaner.' | The boy was admitted to the ICU where he remained for 2 days prior to death. The autopsy revealed evidence of lacerations of the vertebral arteries bilaterally, compression of the carotid arteries, cerebral oedema, and a puncture wound through the foramen magnum. | | Shields et al., 2009 |

3

| Victim Features | Circumstances of Incident | Nature of Injury | Cause of Death | Reference and other information |
|---|---|---|---|---|
| Thirty-two year old man | Man died from bacterial sepsis secondary to a dog bite. The man had presented to the emergency room with fever, nausea, vomiting, and diarrhoea 2 days after being bitten by a Pit Bull dog. | The hospital blood culture was positive for Capnocytophaga species, and the ante-mortem laboratory studies were consistent with disseminated intravascular coagulation (DIC) associated with the sepsis. | | Shields et al., 2009 The victim underwent a splenectomy 5 years before his death after a motor vehicle collision. |
| Fourteen month old girl | Girl was attacked by the family's Pit Bull when she approached the dog while feeding. The dog jumped upwards and grabbed the child in the occipital region, gripping firmly until witnesses were able to remove the dog forcibly. | Large gaping defect involving the scalp and skull with exposure, laceration, and pulpifaction of underlying brain tissue. | Open craniocerebral trauma | Shields et al., 2009 The dog's dentition was examined and the intercuspid distance measured 5cm, which compared with the perforating cuspid marks on the skull of the child. |
| Sixty year old man | Man was mauled by two Pit Bulls as he walked in an alley. Witnesses attempted unsuccessfully to thwart the dogs' attack by blowing car horns and throwing objects. | Puncture wounds of the right internal jugular vein; fractures of the hyoid bone, and thyroid cartilage; cutaneous facial avulsion and traumatic absence of the right ear; and puncture wounds, abrasions, and avulsions of the extremities, buttocks, and chest. | | Shields et al., 2009 |
| Six year old boy (27 to 29 kg) | Boy sustained traumata after an unwitnessed attack and mauling by a domestic Akita (57 to 68 kg). The victim and other children had used sticks to tease the dog, who would subsequently display aggressive behaviour. | Multifocal cutaneous lacerations and puncture wounds of the head and neck, trunk, pelvis, and extremities. | Exsanguination | Shields et al., 2009 |
| Forty-five year old man | Man was found dead on the grounds of an abandoned military base. His body was discovered lying face down with signs that the body had been dragged. A dog pack was known to live in the vicinity of the scene. | Extensive soft tissue loss of the face. The facial muscles were exposed on the left side and the scalp was almost completely missing. A deep laceration of the face revealed a left mandible; the nose was severely lacerated. The wound's edges revealed many small, parallel, partially curved superficial notch marks. Only a few other bite marks were identified on the remainder of the body. The bite marks were excised and analysis of the samples revealed evidence of ripping and shredding of skin and muscle tissue. Analysis of the skull revealed numerous indentations and striations, which were particularly evident on the peripheral area of the missing scalp. | | Santoro et al., 2011 A comparison was made between the cutaneous samples, where the injuries were located, and the dental casts in order to verify the compatibility of the marks and to possibly identify which of the dogs bore the greatest responsibility for the injuries sustained. |

| Victim Features | Circumstances of Incident | Nature of Injury | Cause of Death | Reference and other information |
|---|---|---|---|---|
| Eighty-three year old woman | Woman was found unconscious outside the farm where she lived with her sons and her 27 dogs. She was still alive when found and rushed to the nearest hospital. | She was unconscious on arrival due to haemorrhagic shock and died shortly afterwards. Post-mortem examination showed large lacerations of the scalp with exposure of the underlying bone and several puncture wounds on the neck. Lacerations, multiple small puncture wounds, and abrasions were observed on the whole body (upper and lower extremities, thoracic and abdominal regions, back). Clusters of 4 to 5 superficial linear parallel abrasions between puncture wounds (single or in pairs) were seen, especially on upper and lower extremities. Internal examination showed a crushed left brachial biceps and lacerated left brachial artery. | Exsanguination | Pomara et al., 2011 |
| Twenty-seven year old woman | Woman was found dead in her home with signs that the body had been dragged. Her clothes were intact except for a scarf around the neck showing multiple tears. The victim had a history of epilepsy and the dog was known to assist her when she was having a seizure. | Extensive avulsion of the scalp exposing the bone. The wound's edges revealed many small parallel, partially curved superficial notch marks. The left ear was missing. Numerous indentations and striations were present on the skull. There were multiple puncture wounds and lacerations over the neck. Internal findings included a crushed right sternocleidomastoid muscle and lacerated right internal jugular vein and vertebral artery. The C5 vertebra was fractured and there was a disjunction between the second and the third cervical vertebrae. The thyroid cartilage and the laryngeal cartilage were fractured. | Exsanguination | Salem et al, 2013

Dental examination of the involved dog was carried out. Inter-canine and inter-incisal distances were recorded and were in concordance with the bite marks. A DNA analysis showed the presence of the victim's blood on the dog canines. |

3

compromised ability of victims to interact appropriately with dogs; dogs kept isolated from regular positive human interactions versus family dogs; owners' prior mismanagement of dogs; and owners' history of abuse or neglect of dogs. However, it must be remembered that this is simply a case series description, with no denominator comparison in order to actually attribute evidence of risk. It does, however, generate hypotheses for testing in future studies.

## 11.6 Conclusion

Clearly some types of dog are more capable of inflicting the extensive damage commonly associated with a fatal attack, but other factors must play a role. Victims are often the young and elderly and there is an over-representation of certain breeds. However, whether or not this relates to some biological breed-related characteristic or owner characteristic is not clear. These dogs are not typically physically ill, nor is there consistent evidence of some form of psychological disease afflicting these animals. There is a need for thorough and systematic investigation of the victim, scene of the incident and the dog if we are to learn more about these rare but important events, so we can reduce future risk.

## 11.7 References

American Board of Forensic Odontology, Inc. (2013). Guidelines for bite mark analysis. In: *Diplomates Reference Manual; Section III: Policies, Procedures, Guidelines & Standards.* Page 110–126.

Avis, S. P. (1999). Dog pack attack: Hunting humans. *The American Journal of Forensic Medicine and Pathology* 20(3): 243–246.

Berzon, D. R., DeHoff, J. B. (1974). Medical costs and other aspects of dog bites in Baltimore. *Public Health Reports* 89(4): 377–381.

Boglioli, L. R., Taff, M. L., Turkel, S. J., Taylor, J. V., Peterson, C. D. (2000). Unusual infant death: dog attack or post-mortem mutilation after child abuse? *The American Journal of Forensic Medicine and Pathology* 21(4): 389–394.

Bux, R. C., McDowell, J. D. (1992). Death due to attack from chow dog. *The American Journal of Forensic Medicine and Pathology* 132: 305–308.

Calkins, C. M., Bensard, D. D., Patrick, D. A., Karrer, F. M. (2001). Life threatening dog attacks: a devastating combination of penetrating and blunt injuries. *Journal of Pediatric Surgery* 36: 1115–1117.

Clark, M. A., Sandusky, G. E., Hawley, D. A., Pless, J. E., Fardal, P. M., Tate, L. R. (1991). Fatal and near fatal animal bite injuries. *Journal of Forensic Sciences* 36: 1256–1261.

De Keuster, T. D., Lamoureux, J., Kahn, A. (2006). Epidemiology of dog bites: a Belgian experience of canine behaviour and public health concerns. *The Veterinary Journal* 172: 482–487.

De Munnynck, K., Van de Voorde, W. (2002). Forensic approach to fatal dog attacks: a case report and literature review. *International Journal of Legal Medicine* 16: 295–300.

Di Donato, S., Ricci, P., Panarese, F., Turillazi, E. (2006). Cane corso attack two fatal cases. *Forensic Science, Medicine, and Pathology* 2(2): 137–141.

Falconieri, G., Zanella, M., Malannino, S. (1999). Pulmonary thromboembolism following calf cellulitis: report of an unusual complication of dog bite. *The American Journal of Forensic Medicine and Pathology* 20: 240–242.

Gershman, K. A., Sacks, J. J., Wright, J. C. (1994). Which dogs bite? A case-control study of risk factors. *Pediatrics* 93: 913–917.

Grellner, W., Meyer, E., Fechner, G. (1998). Vortäuschung eines versuchten Tötungsdelikts durch Hundefraß bei Bewußtlosigkeit. *Archiv für Kriminologie* 201: 165–171.

Jarrett, P. (1991). Which dogs bite? *Archives of Emergency Medicine* 8: 33–35.

Kneafsey, B., Condon, K. C. (1995). Severe dog-bite injuries, introducing the concept of pack attack a literature review and seven case reports. *Injury* 26: 37–41.

Lauridson, J. R., Meyers, L. (1993). Evaluation of fatal dog bites: the view of the medical examiner and animal behaviourist. *Journal of Forensic Sciences* 38: 726–731.

Lessig, R., Wenzel, V., Weber, M. (2006). Bite mark analysis in forensic routine case work. *Experimental and Clinical Sciences Journal* 5: 93–102.

Loewe, C. L., Diaz, F. J., Bechinski, J. (2007). Pitbull mauling deaths in Detroit. *The American Journal of Forensic Medicine and Pathology* 28: 356–360.

Mathews, J. R., Lattal, K. A. (1994). A behavioural analysis of dog bites to children. *Journal of Developmental and Behavioral Pediatrics* 15: 44–52.

Miller, S. J., Copass, M., Johansen, K. et al. (1993). Stroke einer Fragebogenaktion. *Rechtsmedizin* 11: 4–11.

Mittmeyer, H. J., Staak, M., Kraemer, R. (1976). Über Verletzungsmuster und Identifizierungsprobleme bei Hundbissen. *Archiv für Kriminologie* 157: 172–178.

Oshima, T., Mimasaka, S., Yonemitsu, K., Kita K., Tsunenari, S. (2008). Vertebral arterial injury due to fatal dog bites: a case report. *Journal of Forensic and Legal Medicine* 15: 529–532.

Patronek, G. J., Sacks, J. J., Delise, K. M., Cleary, D. V., Marder, A. R. (2013). Co-occurrence of potentially preventable factors in 256 dog bite–related fatalities in the United States (2000–2009). *Journal of the American Veterinary Medical Association*, 243(12), 1726–1736.

Pollak, S., Mortinger, H. (1989). Tödliche Hundebißverletzungen. *Beiträge zur gerichtlichen Medizin* 47: 487–495.

Pomara, C., Errico, S. D., Jarussi, V., Turillazzi, E., Fineschi, V. (2011). Bite mark analysis in a fatal dog pack attack. *The American Journal of Forensic Medicine and Pathology* 32: 50–54.

Prahlow, J. A., Ross, K. F., Lene, W. J. W., Kirby, D. (2001). Accidental sharp force injury fatalities. *The American Journal of Forensic Medicine and Pathology* 22: 358–366.

Raghavan, M. (2008). Fatal dog attacks in Canada, 1990–2007. *The Canadian Veterinary Journal* 49: 577–581.

Reuhl, J., Bratzke, H., Feddersen-Petersen, D. U., Lutz, F. U., Willnat, M. (1998). Tod durch 'Kampfhund'-Bisse, ein Beitrag zur aktuellen Diskussion. *Archiv für Kriminologie* 202: 140–151.

Reuhl, J., Urban, R., Bratzke, H., Willnat, M. (2001). Tödliche Hundebisse im Sectionsgut rechtsmedizinischer Institute: Ergebnisse einer Fragebogenaktion. *Rechtsmedizin* 11: 4–11.

Rossi, M. L., Shahrom, A. W., Chapman, R. C., Vanezis, P. (1994). Postmortem injuries by indoor pets. *The American Journal of Forensic Medicine and Pathology* 15(2): 105–109.

Rothschild, M. A., Schneider, V. (1997). On the temporal onset of post-mortem animal scavenging: 'motivation' of the animal. *Forensic Science International* 89: 57–64.

Sacks, J. J., Sattin, R. W., Bonzo, S. E. (1989). Dog-bite related fatalities from 1979 through 1988. *Journal of the American Medical Association* 262: 1489–1492.

Sacks, J. J., Lockwood, R., Hornreicht, J., Sattin, R. W. (1996a). Fatal dog bites, 1989–1994. *Pediatrics* 97: 891–895.

Sacks, J. J., Kresnow, M., Houston, B. (1996b). Dog bites: how big a problem? *Injury Prevention* 2: 52–54.

Sacks, J. J., Sinclair, L., Gilchrist, J., Golab, G. C., Lockwood, R. (2000). Breeds of dogs involved in fatal human attacks in the United States between 1979 and 1998. *Journal of the American Veterinary Medical Association* 217: 836–840.

Salem N. H., Belhadj, M., Aissaoui, A., Mesrati, M. A., Chadly, A. (2013). Multidisciplinary approach to fatal dog attacks: a forensic case study. *Journal of Forensic and Legal Medicine* 20: 763–766.

Santoro, V., Smaldone, G., Lozito, P., Smaldone, M., Introna, F. (2011). A forensic approach to fatal dog attacks. A case study and review of the literature. *Forensic Science International* 206: 37–42.

Sharif, S. M. (1977). Dog bite death. *Forensic Science* 9: 151–153.

Shields, L. B., Bernstein, M. L., Hunsaker, J. C., Stewart, D. M. (2009). Dog bite-related fatalities: a 15-year review of Kentucky Medical Examiner cases. *The American Journal of Forensic Medicine and Pathology* 30: 223–230.

Shkrum, M. J. and Ramsay, D. A. (2007). Penetrating trauma. In: *Forensic Pathology of Trauma*. Humana Press, Totowa, New Jersey (US). Page 357–403.

Souviron, R. R. (2011). Animal bites. In: Dorion, R.B.J. (editor). *Bitemark evidence* (second edition). CRC Press, Boca Raton, Florida (US). Page 209–240.

Thompson, P. G. (1997). The public health impact of dog attacks in a major Australian city. *Medical Journal of Australia* 167: 129–132.

Tong, G. T. F., Pang, T. C. (1965). Unusual injuries: savaged to death by dogs. *Medicine, Science and the Law* 5: 158–160.

Tsokos, M., Byard, R. W., Püschel, K. (2007). Extensive and mutilating craniofacial trauma involving defleshing and decapitation. Unusual features of fatal dog attacks in the young. *The American Journal of Forensic Medicine and Pathology* 28: 131–136.

Tsuji, A., Ishiko, A., Kimura, H., Nurimoto, M., Kudo, K., Ikeda, N. (2008). Unusual death of a baby: a dog attack and confirmation using human and canine STRs. *International Journal of Legal Medicine* 122: 59–62.

Whittaker, D. (2008). The dentist's role in child abuse and neglect. In: Busuttil, A., Keeling, J. W. (editors). *Paediatric Forensic Medicine & Pathology*. Hodder Arnold, London, United Kingdom. Page 420–434.

Wiseman, N. E., Chochinov, H., Fraser, V. (1983). Major dog attack injuries in children. *Journal of Pediatric Surgery* 8: 533–536.

Wright, J. C. (1991). Canine aggression toward people. Bite scenarios and prevention. *Veterinary Clinics of North America: Small Animal Practice* 21: 299–314.

# CHAPTER 12

# Jaw Structure and Bite Potential

## *Samantha Penrice and Marcello Ruta*

## 12.1 Introduction

Domestication has produced some of the most extreme cases of variation within species, as shown by domestic dog breeds, where body size variation exceeds that of any other terrestrial mammal (Boyko et al., 2010), and cranial shape diversity is greater than that of all other carnivores (Drake and Klingenberg, 2010). This great range of shapes extends to the lower jaw of the dog, so it would be reasonable to think that different shapes of jaws might affect the way it can function. The relationship between form and function in dog breeds is relevant to our understanding of dog bites, when we consider the diversity of potential jaw structures. The dog's jaw works like a lever, the rate at which the lever can lift the load (how much force the dog can create by closing its mouth) is influenced by the physical properties of the lever and the load. Imagine you are fishing and you catch a fish and want to lift it out of the water. How quickly you can do this is affected by the size of the fish (the load), the length and width of the rod (the beam), and how strong you are (the physical effort). Bigger fish will need a bigger effort, so will a longer rod. A dog bite is much the same; all of the effort comes from the back of the jaw, and the jaw must be lifted in order for a bite to happen.

The shape and proportions of both the jaw and the jaw-closing muscles are expected to correlate with bite strength but also, and equally importantly, with biomechanical performance, i.e. the modality, speed, and effectiveness of bite delivery. The strength of these muscles is not the sole factor responsible for the maximum bite force or the damage that dogs can inflict. Similarly important are the relative positions of the muscle insertions and of the position of the jaw joint in relation to the tooth row. Bite force is only one aspect of jaw function. Other physical characteristics of a dog's jaw have the potential to increase the damage caused by bite, including its ability to slice or hold prey, to withstand pressure without deformation, or to close rapidly. If a small dog has the same shape jaw as a large dog, then if it bites something that is comparatively smaller, in theory this could cause the same relative damage as the large dog. In contrast, a large dog may not cause as much damage if its jaw does not have the physical features to do so.

Comparatively little attention has been devoted to the general biomechanical performance of jaws, regardless of their absolute size. Long-term studies have sought to establish the underlying causes of dog bites such as breed, personality, and triggers (Shuler 2008; Schalamon et al., 2006; Overall and Love, 2011). Retrospective studies provide insight into common factors, but they do nothing to suggest the potential bite damage from different breeds.

In vivo studies of bite forces are challenging (Lindner et al., 1995; Ellis et al., 2008, 2009). Most importantly, the practical aspect of measuring bite forces directly may be riddled with difficulties, both at the level of experimental design and in light of ethical aspects associated with the use of animals in this context. Bite forces can be assessed through a series of measurements taken from the skull and the jaw (Ellis et al. 2009; Anderson et al., 2013; Wroe et al., 2005). Existing work in this area tends to emphasise absolute bite force, with inevitable attention paid to large and/or dog breeds/types of a perceived temperament. Ellis et al. (2008, 2009) found that bite force increases with skull size, and that within categories of small, medium and large, shape has an effect on bite force in the latter two, and there is a greater pressure exerted from the molars than the canines. The influence of size on these models leads to a clear bias towards large animals having a greater force and the effect of shape in dogs is limited to broad categories (Ellis et al., 2009).

A number of questions remain. How comparable are the potential biting abilities of different dog breeds when the effect of size is removed such that only shape is taken into account? Does a small breed have the ability to cause the same relative damage as a large breed? To answer these questions we have undertaken a preliminary analysis that we report here for the first time.

## 12.2  Assessing shape and function

We have used a two-fold approach to assess the lower jaw of the dog and its physical ability to bite and cause damage. The first is geometric morphometrics, a shape analysis method that looks at the overall morphology of the jaw. The second is a functional analysis, a series of measurements taken from the lower jaw that take into account the biomechanics of biting. The way both of these methods work means the effect of size and genetic similarity is removed. As we remove size as an influencing factor, it means that the shape and proportions are the focus here. If a small dog bites something small, then can it cause a lot of damage? Do the breeds that bite most frequently have a jaw that can cause the most damage with their bite?

To answer this we photographed the side view of lower jaws belonging to seventeen breeds of dog. All specimens represent adults from the vertebrate osteological collections of the University of Lincoln's School of Life Sciences. The jaws were chosen with the aim of encompassing a small, but representative range of breed shapes, sizes, and types (categorised according to their uses; see Table 12.2). The breeds include: Basset Hound, Beagle, Boston Terrier, Boxer, Chihuahua, Chow Chow, Cocker Spaniel, Dachshund, German shepherd, Great Dane, Great Pyrenees, Labrador Retriever, Labrador, Pekingese, Schnauser, Shetland Collie and St Bernard.

## 12.2.1 Shape analysis

Geometric morphometrics quantifies the shape variation and subsequent similarities and differences between individuals. This means we can see the relationships between breeds based solely on their lower jaw. Fifteen points ('landmarks') were selected on the original photographs of the jaws (Figure 12.1) and turned into a series of XY co-ordinates that were used for Principal Component Analysis. This is used to show the breed positions in 'morphospace', which is their position in relation to each other based on their jaw shape (Figure 12.2). The values on these axes are arbitrary; we are only interested in where the breeds fall on the axes. We also created deformation grids (Figure 12.3) that show us which parts of the lower jaw differ the most from the average shape of all seventeen breeds.

The Principal Components (PCs) that form the axes in Figure 12.1 are variables that account for more than 75% of the shape variation in our seventeen breeds. When looking at Figure 12.2, if two breeds are close on the graph, they have similarly shaped jaws.

Across the PCs (Figure 12.3) the Labrador Retriever and German shepherd are consistently close to each other in morphospace. The Cocker Spaniel, Beagle, Basset Hound and Shetland Collie are consistently found close together. The Boxer and Chihuahua are the furthest apart breeds in PC1 v PC2 and PC1 v PC3 (Figure 12.2). The Boston Terrier is consistently positioned at the positive end of all PC axes. The St Bernard has a positive position on PC1 but not 2 or 3 (Figure 12.2).

Now, if we look at the deformation grids we can see that the Boxer, St Bernard and Boston Terrier have the tallest jaws (landmark 9), the Chihuahua has the shortest. The lowest point of the jaw (landmark 1) is further forward and higher in the Chihuahua than in the Boxer. The Boston Terrier and Pekinese both have jaws that curve upwards at the front, the opposite of the 'flat' jaws of the Labrador and German shepherd. We can also see

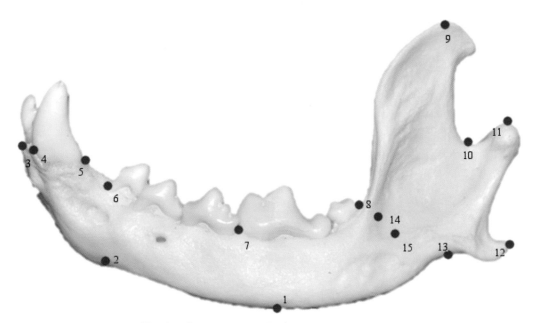

**Figure 12.1** Placement of landmarks on a Boston Terrier.

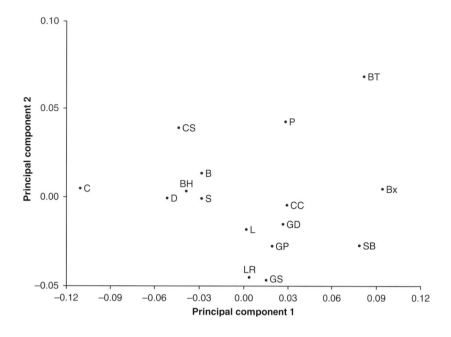

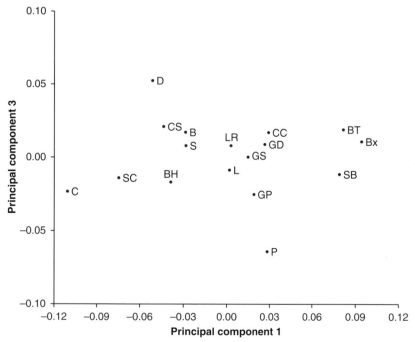

**Figure 12.2** Occupation in morphospace and shape changes A) Breed positions in morphospace along PC1 and PC2 B) Breed positions in morphospace along PC1 and PC3.

Abbreviations are as follows; Basset Hound (BH), Beagle (B), Boston Terrier (BT), Boxer (Bx), Chihuahua (C), Chow (CC), Cocker Spaniel (CS), Dachshund (D), German shepherd (GS), Great Dane (GD), Great Pyrenees (GP), Labrador Retriever (LR), Labrador (L), Pekinese (P), Schnauser (S), Shetland Collie (SC), St Bernard (SB).

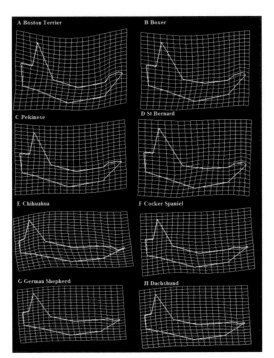

**Figure 12.3** Deformation grids representing morphospace deviations from the mean shape for A Boston Terrier, B Boxer, C Pekinese, D St Bernard, E Chihuahua, F Cocker Spaniel, G German shepherd, H Dachsund.

that the topmost position of the jaw is furthest forward in the Dachshund, and furthest backward in the Pekinese.

### 12.2.2 Functional analysis

Many things can influence the effect of a dog's bite. A dog's jaw can be seen as a third order lever (a lever where the force is between the fulcrum and the load) and the physical proportions of the jaw will determine the efficiency of that lever, in this case, the biomechanical properties of the dog's bite.

To assess biting potential of our seventeen breeds, seven metrics of biomechanical performance were adapted from Anderson et al. (2013) (Figure 12.4). These are ratios calculated from two linear measurements (X and Y), taken from the original photographs of the jaws and are detailed below. We used these ratios to plot the breeds in 'functional space', again using PCA scores on X and Y axes, showing which breeds are functionally most similar. In Figure 12.5, as with the morphospace, if two dogs are close together on the graph, their jaws have similar biomechanical functions.

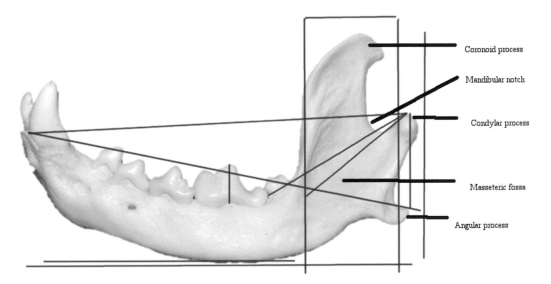

**Figure 12.4** Measurements used for bite mechanic ratios. See Table 12.1 for further explanation.

Table 12.1 Measurements and their biomechanical significance.

| Measure | Function | X | Y |
|---|---|---|---|
| **Anterior mechanical advantage** | A high ratio means a high bite force at the front of the jaw. The lowest potential mechanical advantage along the jaw ramus. | The top of the condylar process, to the bottom of the masseteric fossa. | The top of the condylar process to the front of the canine socket. |
| **Posterior mechanical advantage** | A high ratio means a high bite force at the back of the jaw. The highest potential mechanical advantage (Anderson et al., 2013). | The top of the condylar process, to the bottom of the masseteric fossa. | The top of the condylar process to the front of the most posterior molar socket. |
| **Jaw depth/length ratio** | A high ratio means a high resistance, a stronger jaw. The jaw's resistance to bending loads acting along an up and down direction during biting. | The greatest distance from the top of the coronoid process to the bottom of the jaw ramus (jaw depth). | The back of the angular process to the front of the jaw (excluding incisors) along a horizontal line (jaw length). |
| **Molar depth/jaw depth ratio** | Comparatively larger and taller teeth are better for holding and slicing prey, or inflicting wounds. The size of the largest tooth (relative to the rest of the jaw) changes the efficacy of holding or biting prey. | The greatest depth of the first molar. | The top of the coronoid process to the bottom of the jaw ramus (jaw depth). |
| **Relative length of the masseteric fossa** | Large muscles can produce large forces. A proxy for the cross sectional area of the muscle, which in turn approximates the force exerted by the masseter muscle during jaw closing. | The point where the condylar process meets the mandibular notch to the anterior margin of the fossa. | The back of the angular process to the front of the jaw (excluding incisors) along a horizontal line (jaw length). |
| **Relative tooth row length** | The outcome of biting is localised at the level of the teeth making contact with an object, the length of the tooth-bearing section of the jaw can approximate the effectiveness of the slicing/holding action and is an indirect measure of functional variation in the teeth. | The distance between the front of the most posterior molar socket to the front canine socket. | The back of the angular process to the front of the jaw (excluding incisors) along a horizontal line (jaw length). |
| **Condylar offset** | The jaw joint relative to the tooth row effects jaw occlusion. If the joint is aligned with the dental row, then the teeth occlude like scissors from the back to front of the jaw. If the joint is offset relative to the tooth row, then the teeth occlude simultaneously (or nearly so) in a wrench-like fashion. | The perpendicular distance between that auxiliary line and the dorsalmost extremity of the condylar process. | The back of the angular process to the front of the jaw (excluding incisors) along a horizontal line (jaw length). |

**Table 12.2** Ratio of seven functional indices of bite mechanics of seventeen dog breeds, highest and lowest ratios are highlighted in bold.

| Breed | Type | Ant. Mech. Adv. | Post. Mech. Adv. | Condylar Offset | Relative Depth | Relative Molar Size | Relative Masseteric Fossa | Relative Tooth Row |
|---|---|---|---|---|---|---|---|---|
| Basset Hound | Scent Hound | 0.301 | 0.873 | 0.091 | 0.515 | 0.187 | 0.213 | 0.658 |
| Beagle | Scent Hound | 0.290 | 0.863 | 0.093 | 0.495 | 0.201 | 0.219 | 0.645 |
| Boston Terrier | Mastiff | 0.354 | 0.843 | 0.224 | **0.595** | 0.206 | 0.224 | 0.699 |
| Boxer | Mastiff | **0.437** | 0.941 | **0.240** | 0.542 | **0.120** | **0.269** | **0.553** |
| Chihuahua | Toy | **0.264** | 0.875 | **0.044** | **0.348** | **0.359** | 0.212 | 0.704 |
| Chow | Spitz | 0.358 | 0.914 | 0.136 | 0.510 | 0.148 | 0.287 | 0.601 |
| Cocker Spaniel | Spaniel | 0.275 | **0.837** | 0.119 | 0.504 | 0.211 | 0.196 | **0.721** |
| Dachshund | Scent Hound | 0.281 | 0.894 | 0.060 | 0.412 | 0.220 | 0.228 | 0.685 |
| German shepherd | Herding | 0.361 | 0.914 | 0.106 | 0.516 | 0.138 | 0.216 | 0.597 |
| Great Dane | Mastiff | 0.359 | 0.877 | 0.116 | 0.505 | 0.128 | 0.209 | 0.581 |
| Great Pyrenees | Herding | 0.364 | 0.868 | 0.114 | 0.588 | 0.147 | 0.224 | 0.591 |
| Labrador Retriever | Retriever | 0.347 | 0.911 | 0.085 | 0.515 | 0.164 | 0.235 | 0.605 |
| Labrador | Retriever | 0.349 | 0.872 | 0.109 | 0.503 | 0.137 | 0.225 | 0.651 |
| Pekinese | Toy | 0.373 | 0.951 | 0.168 | 0.552 | 0.149 | 0.223 | 0.592 |
| Schnauzer | Herding | 0.334 | 0.974 | 0.091 | 0.448 | 0.155 | 0.221 | 0.654 |
| Shetland Collie | Herding | 0.281 | 0.868 | 0.046 | 0.375 | 0.260 | 0.199 | 0.642 |
| St Bernard | Mastiff | 0.426 | **0.978** | 0.144 | 0.560 | 0.131 | **0.289** | 0.565 |

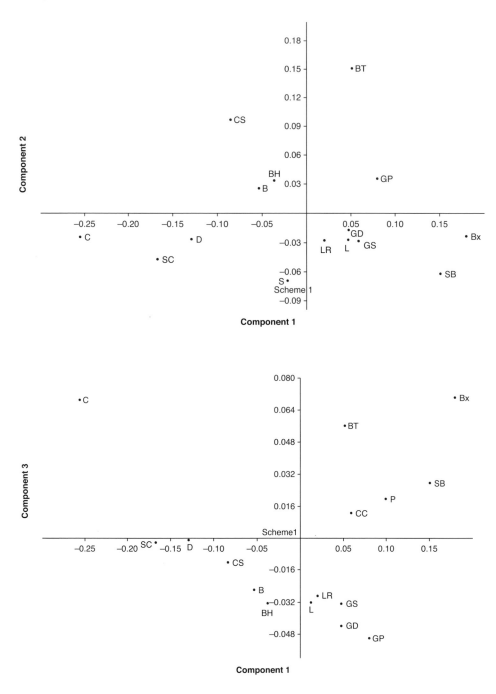

**Figure 12.5** Occupation in functional space and PC loadings A) Breed positions in functional space along PC1 and B) Breed positions in functional space along PC1 and PC3.

Abbreviations are as follows; Basset Hound (BH), Beagle (B), Boston Terrier (BT), Boxer (Bx), Chihuahua (C), Chow Chow (CC), Cocker Spaniel (CS), Dachshund (D), German shepherd (GS), Great Dane (GD), Great Pyrenees (GP), Labrador Retriever (LR), Labrador (L), Pekinese (P), Schnauser (S), Shetland Collie (SC), St Bernard (SB).

The similarities and differences between jaw function of breeds can be seen in Figure 12.5. The first three principal components account for more than 90% of the variance in function. The ratios tell us about the differences between each of the seven function measurements, but the principal components tell us about the overall biomechanical differences of the breeds.

The Chihuahua and the Boxer are placed distantly from each other in 'functional space' (i.e. on the graph). If we take a closer look at the biomechanical ratios we can see that these two breeds have the highest and lowest anterior mechanical advantages; a high ratio means a tall and short jaw that can produce a high bite force at the front. The Chihuahua also has the lowest condylar offset, meaning that of all the breeds, the back of its jaw will close first, like a pair of scissors. A high condylar offset ratio means that the front and back of the jaw close at a more similar time, as seen in the Boxer. Interestingly, the Chihuahua also has the largest relative molar size, so when it bites the first contact is with a large, slicing tooth.

The Boston Terrier stands alone, driven largely by its high relative depth, which provides a strong anchor for its small, curved jaw. Although it does not have a high initial bite force, the loading capacity is fairly high. In other words, it can resist breakage. The Labrador Retriever, German shepherd and Great Dane are consistently placed together and all have fairly unremarkable biomechanical measurements. None of them have the most dominant features to cause the most damaging bite. Their jaws are of a medium height and long and shallow. These jaws do not have a high resistance to the objects they bite because they lack strong anchors (height) to create large forces and the shallow nature of the jaws means that they have a lower loading capacity.

The Dachshund and Shetland Collies have similar biomechanical properties, and also have no distinct biomechanical features. The deformation grid for the Dachshund shows a long, flat and shallow jaw, and they have larger molars and a longer tooth row, both features that help to hold prey, compared to the German shepherd group.

Surprisingly, the St Bernard is closely associated with the Pekinese. The St Bernard has the greatest posterior mechanical advantage and relative masseteric fossa; it has a large muscle pocket and can create a large bite force at the back of its jaw. The Pekinese scores highly on these measures as well. This shows us that, once size is removed, two breeds that on the surface seem very different – one a toy breed, another a Mastiff – have actually got comparable bite potential.

## 12.2.3 Relationship between shape and function

Can we determine a dog's bite potential just by looking at the shape of their jaw? In short, yes. There are two ways to assess the relationship between shape and function; distance and position. We found that there is a significant relationship in both cases (distance-Mantel test p = 0.0002; position Procrustes p = 0.0002). This means that if two breeds are very distant/different in shape, then they are very different/distant in biomechanical function. It also means that their position in relation to other breeds is consistent. Ultimately, this means that we can use shape as a predictor for physical bite potential.

## 12.3  Bite potential

The shape of the lower jaw in the domestic dog can be used as a predictor of relative bite force. If two dogs have similarly shaped jaws then they will have similar relative bite abilities. We have used several ways of measuring potential bite ability because the overall initial force does not necessarily mean that it will be the most damaging bite.

The Chihuahua and Boxer consistently show up as being separated in both shape and biomechanical function spaces. The shape can be seen in the deformation grids (Figure 12.3), the Boxer having a deeper and more compact jaw than the Chihuahua.

The relative bite force ratios show that the boxer has the largest value for anterior mechanical advantage, suggesting it is able to produce the greatest force of all of the breeds studied at the anterior point of its jaw.

The Chihuahua exhibits the lowest value for the same ratio, so even before accounting for size, its bite at the front of the jaw is among the weakest of the breeds studied, but not necessarily the least dangerous.

The relationship is not quite so straightforward, since other factors may also come into play, Boxers do not necessarily produce the most damaging bite as the masseteric fossa, molar and tooth row are the smallest values across the breeds and bite forces have been shown to be lower at the canines than the molars in an in vivo study (Ellis et al., 2009). This means that although the initial bite is hard, the dentition and bite hold is not the most damaging. A large molar will allow for prey holding and slicing and an extended tooth row means that the contact area between dentition and object is large. The small masseteric fossa shows that the muscle attachment site is minimal in the Boxer. In contract, the Chihuahua has the largest relative molar, potentially making up for its weak loading ability (depth to length ratio) and initial bite (anterior mechanical advantage). The large condylar offset in the Chihuahua shows that its jaws occlude like a pair of scissors, so this large molar is the first point of contact in a bite from this breed. Hence, Chihuahuas could cause damaging, scissor-like bites if their molars are engaged with the subject.

## 12.4  Damage potential

The object that is bitten will also obviously play a role in the potential damage of a bite as the force exerted must exceed the load, i.e. you must have a bite that is tougher than the object being bitten (Anderson et al., 2013). If you bite something that is hard, then you will cause less impact than if you bite something soft. What makes something 'hard' can include the initial material (soft skin verses tough leather), or the overall size of something e.g. biting a twig or biting a branch, you could break the twig, but you won't break the branch even though they are both wood. Skin quality may vary with age and so the damage inflicted by the same bite may also vary with age, regardless of other factors. Children are common victims of dog bites (Shuler et al., 2008; Schalamon et al., 2006; Overall and Love, 2011) and so the potential damage by a small dog should not be dismissed. A small dog biting a small finger could cause the same or more damage as a much bigger dog biting an arm, depending on the jaw structure of the biter.

The Boston Terrier is consistently placed as an 'outlier' in both shape and function spaces.

On closer inspection of the deformation grids and the PC ratio loadings, it appears that a deep (tall) and short jaw is the reason for their outlying positions. The depth to length ratio is a representation of flexural stiffness. The theory of the second moment of area states that the strength of a beam (i.e. a jaw) will increase as the depth increases and that the strength will also increase if a beam of a consistent depth is shortened; in other words, a short and thick jaw will be stronger than a long and thin jaw. So, a dog with a short face might not be able to bite quickly, or with a large initial force, but it can exert a large pressure on an object because its jaw is stronger. This means that, in relative terms, the Boston Terrier's jaw will be able to bite proportionally harder objects than a German shepherd or a Dachshund. Interestingly this breed is descended from both 'bull' and 'terrier' lines, which might be predicted to need the hardest bite, and so this heritage seems to have been maintained in the breed's jaw conformation.

Two of the three scent hounds in the sample, Beagle and Basset Hound, are regularly found in close proximity in both shape and function. These breeds are genetically close (vonHoldt et al., 2012) and so this may not be surprising, but the Dachshund, also a scent hound, is not consistently placed closer to Beagle and Basset Hound, and debate has been had about whether it should be considered a hound. From these results, it can be suggested that 'breed type' is not a good predictor of jaw shape and bite performance. This is further supported by the distant placements among 'Mastiff' types, namely the Boxer, Boston Terrier, Great Dane and St Bernard in both shape and function.

German shepherd dogs are consistently reported as being responsible for a high proportion of dog bite incidents (Shuler et al., 2008; Schalamon et al., 2006; Overall and Love, 2011) and they plot out close to Labrador Retrievers in shape and function, suggesting the bites from both might be similar. The position of these two breeds in both shape and function spaces are close to the mean configurations. However, behaviour and triggers for biting are not factored into this subject and so it seems reasonable to suggest that, given their biomechanical similarities, these breeds do genuinely bite with different frequencies, but whether this difference is genetic or ontogenetic remains unknown. One might speculate that if a mixed breed dog had the higher tendency to bite of a German shepherd, and had the jaws of a Chihuahua or a Boxer (both of which have the potential to cause significant damage with their bites), then the likelihood of an even more severe injury would increase.

## 12.5 Conclusion

This work highlights the importance of considering more than the size of a dog when considering the anatomical features of a breed that relate to the risk of a damaging bite, and the damage that can be caused by that bite. A large dog is not inevitably going to be more damaging because it is large, and a small or short-faced dog is certainly capable of causing lasting harm. The initial bite force might not be the worst part of a bite. If a dog has a long tooth row, it can hold its prey, if it has a large molar it can slice, a short and deep jaw can withstand a lot of pressure so it can bite harder objects. A puncture wound caused by a Boxer jaw could be less devastating in terms of scarring than a slicing wound of a Chihuahua. Some small dogs could cause life-changing injuries when biting something small, such as an infant.

The association between jaw shape and the biomechanical properties of a bite means that we can infer the potential bite damage of a dog based on the shape of its lower jaw. The information here can also be applied to dogs of mixed breed, by comparing their jaws with those of known breeds. The main benefit of this work is that it can be carried out on living dogs with minimal intervention and without veterinary expertise, providing owners with more information on their dogs. We do not have to rely on bite incident reports or the limited published studies to know the potential damage an individual can cause.

## 12.6 Acknowledgements

We thank Julian Bartrup, Ciara Casey and Marco Perez Tanchez for kindly allowing us to examine specimens in their care. We also thank Christopher Penrice for his technical expertise. We appreciate the generous help and assistance provided by Barbara Burgess through all stages of completion of this work.

## 12.7 References

Anderson, P. S. L., Friedman, M., Ruta, M. (2013). Late to the table: Diversification of tetrapod mandibular biomechanics lagged behind the evolution of terrestriality. *Integrative and Comparative Biology*, 53(2), pp.197–208.

Boyko, A. R. et al. (2010). A simple genetic architecture underlies morphological variation in dogs. *PLoS Biology*, 8(8), pp.49–50.

Drake, A. G., Klingenberg, C. P. (2010). Large-scale diversification of skull shape in domestic dogs: disparity and modularity. The American Naturalist, 175(3), 289–301.

Ellis, J. L. et al. (2008). Calibration of estimated biting forces in domestic canids: Comparison of post-mortem and in vivo measurements. *Journal of Anatomy*, 212(6), pp.769–780.

Ellis, J. L. et al. (2009). Cranial dimensions and forces of biting in the domestic dog. *Journal of Anatomy*, 214(3), pp.362–373.

Lindner, D. L., Marretta, S. M., Pijanowski, G. J., Johnson, A. L., Smith, C. W. (1995). Measurement of bite force in dogs: a pilot study. *Journal of veterinary dentistry*, 12(2), 49–52.

Overall, K. L., Love, M. (2011). Special Report Dog bites to humans – demography, epidemiology, injury, and risk. *Javma*, 218(112), pp.1923–1934.

Schalamon, J. et al. (2006). Analysis of dog bites in children who are younger than 17 years. *Pediatrics*, 117(3), pp.e374–e379.

Shuler, C., DeBess, E. Lapidus, J., Hedberg, K. (2008). Dog bites in Multnomah County, *Javma* 232 (5), pp.1–5.

Wroe, S., McHenry, C., Thomason, J. (2005). Bite club: comparative bite force in big biting mammals and the prediction of predatory behaviour in fossil taxa. *Proceedings. Biological sciences/The Royal Society*, 272(1563), pp.619–625.

# Section 4
# Investigative and Legal Issues

In Section 4, we consider the investigative and legal issues surrounding dog bites. In the absence of clear guidelines in these areas, world-leading experts in their fields present best practice standards, sometimes for the first time. To introduce this subject, Fiona Cooke, in Chapter 12, guides us through the myriad of dog-related legislation in a range of countries and the key principles in which they connect and differ. She concludes that there is clearly no gold standard simple legislative mechanism in use, and a new trend towards repealing breed-specific legislation for being deemed ineffective.

When a dog bite incident occurs, a thorough investigation will provide evidence not only for any legal repercussions, but also to help society to understand why dog bites occur in the first place. The quality of this investigation is varied, if it occurs at all. In Chapter 14, James Crosby presents a gold standard approach for investigating dog bite incidents and managing the scene for the purpose of gathering evidence. He clearly points out that when a bite occurs it is not a 'done deal' and the dog is in fact a crucial part of the evidence. This is further emphasised by Anna Maria Passantino in Chapter 15, who focuses on the specific forensic procedures used for investigating dog bites and suspects, in order to establish who has inflicted the bite. In Chapter 16, James Crosby takes a deeper look at the unique and identifying anatomy of dog bite wounds. This information can be critical to the rapid exclusion of the supposed perpetrator of a bite, who may not even be a dog, and it is for this reason that we include the chapter in this section. However, this information is also an essential primer for understanding some of the health- and medical-related issues that are discussed in the next section. Continuing with the legal theme, in Chapter 17 UK dog law expert Tina Wagon provides guidance on choosing a dog bite expert for the courts. Although the chapter is focused on the demands and needs of the UK legal system, the key messages are transferable to other countries. The best practice protocol for assessing 'dangerous dogs' for the courts is then presented in Chapter 18 by leading UK expert witness Kendal Shepherd. She highlights the importance of a thorough behavioural examination if we are to understand why the bite may have occurred, and thus the risk of recurrence. This offers a humane and compassionate approach to risk reduction that considers the needs of both owners and victims in a mature way.

# CHAPTER 13

# Canine Aggression and the Law – an International Perspective

*Fiona Cooke*

## 13.1 Introduction

There is a plethora of legislation that attempts to address dog aggression internationally. To understand dog law in an international context, it is crucial to recognise that not only do legal systems around the world vary but so do views on dogs. In addition, the legal interpretation of information about what constitutes a dangerous or aggressive dog is affected by a number of factors, including influences on the development of law at the time of enactment (passing of the law). There are considerable differences in how the law approaches the management and control of dogs that have either demonstrated they are dangerous or are presumed dangerous. Countries across the world demonstrate high levels of variability, not only in the content and structure of dog-related legislation, but also in the focus of that legislation.

This chapter examines some of the responsibilities and restrictions placed on dogs and their owners by legislative regimes internationally.

There are two types of legislation concerning supposedly dangerous dogs. Those that:

1. Address incidents of aggression in any individual dog
2. Address concerns regarding breeds or types of dogs.

Due to the extensive variation within and across countries around the world, this chapter will highlight key issues, providing an insight into the present situation. Two major themes arising throughout this chapter are:

- Dog licensing/registration regimes
- 'Breed-specific legislation' (BSL).

Both topics are controversial, inviting much debate.

## 13.2 Licensing

In an attempt to maintain records of dogs kept, type of dogs and ownership, dog licensing/registration regimes have been implemented for many years in a number of countries. These regimes have been more effective in some countries than others. Twenty-three countries in Europe have a dog licensing/registration scheme (Tasker, 2007). There is presently discussion of reinstating dog licensing/registration in a number of other countries (RSPCA, 2010).

## 13.3 Breed-specific legislation

Breed-Specific Legislation (BSL) specifies individual breeds or 'types' of dog that are covered by certain legislative regimes. Internationally, similarity is evident between the types and breeds of dogs included under BSL:

- These dogs are often identified by their physical characteristics, and are considered by some to pose greater risks to public safety than other breeds (see Chapter 7).
- Specific regulations and requirements are created for these breeds (or 'types') of dogs, placing restrictions on management, ownership, breeding and sale, often with the aim of eradicating that breed in the country, district or state. In some countries, ownership of some breeds or types of dogs is illegal, while in others special dispensation must be sought from local or central government.

A number of countries have attempted to address incidents of dog aggression through the enactment of BSL, including the UK, France, Ireland, Germany, Italy, Spain, Austria, Switzerland (DeMeester, 2004), the USA, Canada, Australia and Japan.

## 13.4 Civil/criminal offences

Internationally, a distinction is often made between public law (governing the relationship between individual citizens and the state), and private law (governing relationships between individuals and/or between private organisations). However, for purposes of discussion here, the significant practical distinction is between civil law and criminal law:

- **Civil law** regulates relationships between individuals, or organisations, or between the two, usually with the aim of remuneration or compensation.
- **Criminal law** is about society, and the punishment of offences that go against the laws of that country. For this reason, the majority of criminal cases are prosecuted by the state.

The standard of proof required for different types of judicial processes can vary, but it is fundamental to have an agreed standard in order to 'mark a point between […] two extremes: a mere conjecture at one end, and absolute certainty at the other' (Del Mar, 2011).

In criminal law systems such as those in the UK and USA, a case is required to be proven against the defendant 'beyond a reasonable doubt', while the evidential burden in civil law is lower than this, requiring the balance of probability standard (Wilkinson, 2012). In civil law judicial systems such as in Germany and France, the standard of proof is 'beyond rea-sonable doubt' in all cases. However, this judicial standard will not be applicable at all times internationally due to complex individual legal structures. Dog-related legislation can fall into either the criminal or civil category, dependent on the aims of the legislation and the legislative structure of the individual country.

## 13.5  Reversal of the burden of proof

There are some discrepancies in the way that evidence must be provided under certain judi-cial systems, in contrast to the usual criminal law requirements. In the usual course of legal proceedings, the onus is on the prosecution to prove that an offence has been committed. This is often explained in criminal law using the terminology 'innocent until proven guilty'. Some of the legislation discussed in this chapter, however, reverses the burden of proof in criminal law, which presents an anomaly in the approach. The reversal of the burden of proof is a peculiarity pertaining to dangerous dog legislation in the UK and Denmark, among other countries. In UK law, the DDA s.1 reverses this burden of proof requirement in an unusual departure from the standard expectation that the prosecution has a case to prove. As a result, the owners of an alleged s.1 type dog must prove that the dog is not of 'type'. This usually involves the employment of expert witnesses, who are experienced in identi-fying dogs of 'type'. The reversal of the burden of proof for identifying allegedly dangerous types of dog is reflected in Denmark in its restricted breed legislation.

## 13.6  Variations in legislation between countries

### 13.6.1 UK

By far the most controversial legislation encompassing dogs in the UK is the **Dangerous Dogs Act 1991 (DDA) (as amended 1997)** and the equivalent legislation in Scotland and Northern Ireland. The DDA was enacted as a 'knee-jerk reaction' (Lord Redesdale, 2009) to a number of tragic incidents involving dogs and children in the late 1980s and early 1990s.
   There are two main parts to this Act:

**Section 3 of the DDA** allows for legal action to be taken against the person respon-sible for any dog that is 'dangerously out of control' in a public place. The definition of 'dangerously out of control' includes causing 'reasonable apprehension' in a person (s.3(b)). Recent legislative developments in England have resulted in the recently enacted Anti-social Behaviour, Crime and Policing Act 2014 Part 7: 'Dangerous Dogs'. This legislation extends the reach of the DDA s.3 to private places and attacks on Assistance Dogs (s.2(a)(i)(ii)).

**Section 1 of the DDA**, an extremely controversial element, applies to 'dogs bred for fighting'.

- This section prohibits four types of dog that are alleged to be inherently dangerous or aggressive (see Table 13.1). The reason that these dogs are defined as 'type' rather than breed is because type is determined on the basis of physical characteristics (R v Knightsbridge Crown Court ex p Dunne; Bates v DPP [1993]).

- It is an offence to own or keep any such dog unless it is on the Index of Exempted Dogs. Registration. This index imposes stringent requirements on owners for the management of their dogs, including being insured, muzzled and on a lead in all public places (this definition is applied strictly – for example it includes locked cars parked in public places (Bates v DPP [1993]).
- Any dog of these types, whether or not on the Index of Exempted Dogs, cannot be legally bred from, sold, exchanged or gifted.
- In 2012, 477 dogs were placed on the Exempted Index in England, Scotland and Wales (Hansard, Commons Debate, 2013). There are very few Tosas, Filas and Dogos in the UK; any reference made to s.1 dogs is almost always directed towards Pit Bull Terrier types.

**Table 13.1** Table of dog bans and restrictions.

| Country or State | Banned/Restricted breeds |
| --- | --- |
| **UK** | Pit bull<br>Japanese Tosa<br>Dogo Argentino<br>Fila Brasileiro |
| **Germany** | Alano espanol<br>American Bulldog<br>American Staffordshire Terrier<br>Bandog<br>Bull mastiff<br>Bull terrier<br>Cano Corso Italiano<br>Doberman<br>Dogo Argentino<br>Dogue de Bordeaux<br>Fila Brasileiro<br>Kangal<br>Kaukasischer Owtscharka<br>Mastiff<br>Mastin Espanol<br>Mastino Napoletano<br>Perro de Presa Canario<br>Perro de Presa Mallorquin<br>American Pit Bull Terrier<br>Rottweiler<br>Staffordshire Bull Terrier<br>Tosa Inu<br>Bull Terriers<br>Rottweilers<br>Cross-breeds of the above |
| **Austria** | Bandog<br>Ridgeback<br>Bull Mastiff<br>Mastiff |

Mastin Espanol
Bordeauxdogge
Bull Terrier
Mastino Napoletano
Fila Brasileiro
Pit Bull Terrier
Rottweiler
Tosa Inu
Dogo Argentino
Staffordshire Bull Terrier
Crossbreeds of the above

**Denmark**

Pit Bull Terrier
Tosa Inu
Dogo Argentino
Kangal
Boerboel
Caucasian Shepherd Dog (Ovtcharka)
Central Asian Shepherd Dog (Ovtcharka)
Tornjak
Sarplaninac
American Staffordshire Terrier
Crossbreeds of the above

**Switzerland (Canton-dependent)**

American Pit Bull Terrier
American Staffordshire Terrier
American Bull Terrier
Pit Bull Terrier
Crossbreeds with 10% or more bloodline of any of the above
    breeds

**Zurich**

Rassetypen List 2 (banned with exceptions):
American Pit Bull
American Staffordshire Bull Terrier
Bandogs
American Bull Terrier
Bull Terrier
Crosses of the above

Rassetypen List 1 (training classes mandatory):
Any dog over 45cm and 15kg
Molloserhunde
Doberman
Schaferhunde
Sweiz. Sennenhunde
Nordische Hunde (eg. husky)
Apportierhunde (eg. Labrador)
Triebhunde
Schnauzer (excepting small)
Large Terriers (e.g. Airedale)
Eurasier (e.g. Akita Inu)
Urtypenhunde (e.g. Podenco)
Laufhunde (large only e.g Bloodhound)
Schweisshunde (large only, eg. Dalmation, Rhodesian
    Ridgeback)
Vorstehhunde (e.g Irish Setter)
Windhunde (e.g. Afghan Hound)

| France | Category 1 (without Pedigree papers):<br>Staffordshire Terrier<br>Pit Bull Terrier<br>Boerbull<br>Tosa Inu<br><br>Category 2 (with Pedigree papers of cross-breeds of pedigree dogs):<br>Staffordshire Bull Terrier<br>Tosa Inu<br>Rottweiler (pedigree, crossbreed or appearance thereof) |
|---|---|
| **Australia**<br>**Victoria** | American Pit Bull Terriers<br>Dogo Argentino<br>Fila Brasileiro<br>Japanese Tosa<br>Presa Canario<br>Or crossbreeds of the above<br>American Staffordshire Terrier (if no pedigree certificate or if not certified by vet)<br>Greyhound (unless exempted by assessment) |
| **Canada, Ontario** | Pit Bull |
| **Japan** | Any dog over 55cm tall<br>American Pit Bull Terrier<br>Japanese Tosa |
| **Netherlands** | Now repealed:<br>Pit Bull Terrier<br>Rottweiler |
| **Italy** | Previously 92 breeds, now repealed |

Grant (2008) found that the UK DDA is widely considered to be a failure and the debates about whether or not it is effective in managing dog attacks continue.

Scotland recently enacted the **Control of Dogs (Scotland) Act 2010**, with the aim of addressing potential incidents of dog aggression or dangerous behaviour proactively.

- The Act allows authorised officers to act to educate and support owners who have a dog demonstrating concerning behaviour to prevent future more serious incidents.
- This legislation, despite focusing on the responsibility and actions of dog owners, did not repeal the DDA s.1, which means that these types of dog are still prohibited in Scotland.

It used to be the case that there was a registration system for dogs across the UK, yet it now only remains in Northern Ireland. There has been a lot of recent discussion about reintroducing dog registration in England and Wales, but despite a lot of support for this from stakeholders and researchers (RSPCA, 2010), this has not as yet transpired. The expectation is that registration would allow tighter controls of dogs as well as allowing for higher rates of traceability regarding aggressive incidents. However, this would only be effective if it was enforced efficiently, and at present there are a number of serious shortcomings in the enforcement of companion animal welfare legislation in the UK, which would have to be addressed prior to any such scheme having the infrastructure to be effective (Cooke, 2013).

### 13.6.2 Germany

In Germany all dogs must be registered with their local council under the national dog licensing scheme. The fees for this registration are set by the local council and can vary dependent upon the type of dog, training class attendance and local breed restrictions. Germany has a long history of dog registration (Upton et al., 2010), which is often argued to be one of the reasons for low stray dog rates in the country.

BSL varies across different states (Bundestaaten) in Germany, although import and trade of Pit Bull Terriers is prohibited by German federal law (unless the owner applies for local permission to own a restricted breed, which can be extremely costly and is not an option available to those holding criminal records). In Germany, permission must be sought to acquire any dog classified as 'dangerous'; classifications depend upon the individual state.

Categorisation of Kampfhunde (fighting dog) is quite regularly seen across German states, with the focus of BSL being on Kampfhund breeds and cross-breeds. The restriction of breeds in Hamburg followed the same pattern as in the UK; as a result of tragic incidents involving dogs and children.

In Lower Saxony, BSL was enacted in 2000 but was later ruled to be void as not based on scientific evidence, because a number of studies regarding temperament assessment tests suggested there was no scientific basis for increased aggression in specific breeds (Schalke et al., 2008).

In Hamburg a number of breeds are restricted, with breeds and cross-breeds thereof always considered 'dangerous' (see Table 13.1). Other breeds are identified as 'dangerous' dogs, however they can be exempted from this categorisation on passing temperament tests (see Table 13.1). A number of breeds are required to undergo mandatory temperament tests. In Hamburg, dogs that will be categorised as 'dangerous' will not be subject to the requirements to wear a muzzle before they are nine months old.

In Germany a dangerous dog not of specific type is defined in many states as a dog that has 'ever attacked humans or other animals' and training dogs to attack humans is prohibited. Owners of any dangerous dog, whether breed-specific or otherwise, must be over eighteen years old, insured, keep the dog contained safely and pass an exam to demonstrate their knowledge of dog handling. Owners who commit other crimes such as drink-driving or drug offences may automatically lose their dangerous dog licence in a number of states. For example, in Bavaria, any dog that has undergone training in order to increase aggressive or dangerous behaviour may be classified as a Kampfhund, and owners of these dogs may be fined heavily and required to adhere to muzzle and lead restrictions (Category 1). Owners with dogs with Category 2 classification are required to attend mandatory training and may be able to remove restrictions upon their dogs by providing a behavioural assessment demonstrating that the dog does not have aggressive tendencies.

### 13.6.3 Austria

Austria's dog registration model requires all dog owners to have a licence for their dog. As with the majority of states in Germany, Austria identifies Kampfhunde as restricted breeds due to alleged inherent aggressiveness (see Table 13.1). States do not all have the same list of 'dangerous dogs', but there are a number of similarities across states.

In Austria there has been a concerted effort to integrate dog registration and the control of potentially dangerous dogs. All Kampfhund owners, including all household members aged over sixteen, must take mandatory theory and practical tests to demonstrate competency in dog ownership (if the test is failed three times the dog will be seized by the authorities (Art 68, TschV). If owners of non-restricted breeds take a voluntary exam with their dogs they are eligible for a reduction in licence fees.

## 13.6.4 Denmark

A relatively unique element of Danish dog law is the recently added description of what constitutes a 'savage' dog (Dog Act 2010, as amended 2014). Any dog found to have savaged a person or another dog must be euthanised, however the new provisions also allow the owner of the attacking dog to request an expert assessment of the case.

Breed-specific legislation applies in Denmark, with legislation in 1991 banning (with possible exemptions) two breeds. In 2010, legislation added eleven further restricted breeds to this list (see Table 13.1). These breeds and any cross-breeds thereof must be kept on short leads and wear muzzles when off the owner's property.

## 13.6.5 Switzerland

Switzerland has a national dog registration scheme for Hundereglement (dog regulation). Dogs must be registered with their council under Cantonal laws, which can also specify particular requirements of dog owners. A relatively unique aspect of dog ownership in Switzerland is that all dog owners, regardless of what breed or type of dog they intend to own, must take a theory test prior to acquiring a dog. This must then be followed by the successful completion of a practical test of competent dog ownership within one year of acquisition of the dog. However, these requirements are currently under review and may be dropped.

There are a number of banned breeds throughout Switzerland (see Table 13.1) and any cross-breeds thereof with more than 10% bloodline of these banned breeds. These were considered in a recent examination of the legislation to pose a greater danger than other breeds (on the basis of their body strength, bite strength and hold type) and it was considered impracticable to assess each individual temperament (Schweizerisches Bundesgericht, 136 I 1). The twenty-six Cantons are able to designate their own banned breeds or breed restrictions, with wide variation across the country in how these are structured.

In Zurich, there are two lists of breed types that have additional legislation applicable to them. These are Rassetypenlisten (breed type lists) 1 and 2 (see Table 13.1). List 2 types are banned (with the exception of a thirty-day maximum stay per year). Owners of List 1 types must attend Government-approved training classes with their dog for a minimum of four fifty-minute sessions when between the ages of eight and sixteen weeks. If these training sessions are missed, at least ten to twenty approved training classes must be attended at a later date if the owner is to keep the dog.

In contrast to Zurich and a number of other Cantons in Switzerland, Bern does not have a restricted breeds list or a specification of 'dangerous dogs'. If an individual dog is considered to be 'bissig' (biting), having injured a person or dog, then it must wear a muzzle

(Hundegesetz/BE, Art.7(5)) and is subject to restrictions including neutering and specific handlers. There are also specific areas designated in which all dogs must be on a lead, and this can be extended for individual dogs (Hundegesetz/BE, Art.7(1)).

### 13.6.6 France

In France, there are two legally specified categories of restricted dogs; 'Attack' dogs (category 1) and 'Guard' dogs (category 2) (see Table 13.1). Dogs with pedigree papers are exempt from the restrictions under Category 1 legislation; however, they will still fall under Category 2. In order to legally be in possession of a Category 1 or 2 dog, owners must be registered with their town hall and must carry their licence (Permis de dètention d'un chien de 1er ou 2ème categorie) with them at all times when with the dog. In order to be granted such a licence, owners must permit their dog to undergo a behavioural assessment performed by a vet. A passed behavioural assessment must be accompanied by insurance, certification from an approved training course (including training, behaviour, control and accident prevention) and dog ID. No one under the age of eighteen or with a criminal record is eligible for a licence for a Category 1 or 2 dog. In addition, all Category 1 dogs must be neutered.

If a dog of any breed or type bites a person in France it must be reported to the local council. This is in accordance with rabies prevention regulations, but also creates cause for the mandatory clinical and behavioural assessment of the dog, providing opportunities to assess any risk it may pose.

### 13.6.7 Australia

In Australia, there is a wide variation between the dog legislation enacted in various jurisdictions. Throughout Australia, all dogs must be registered with the local council, microchipped and contained securely when on a property (Domestic Animals Act 1994).

In Victoria, there has been compulsory registration of dogs since 1970. The Domestic Animals Act 1994 (as amended 2014) is state legislation, implemented by municipal councils. S.3(1) of the Act specifies Restricted Breed Dogs (see Table 13.1). License fees are breed-dependent and can be reduced by neutering. The Dangerous Dogs Act 1994 specifies 'types' of dogs that must be registered with the local authority, wear visible collars and there must be signs on the property at which they live. Since 2005 (Domestic Animals Regulations 2005), courts have been able to request DNA samples to support 'typing'. American Staffordshire Terriers will not be considered to be restricted breed dogs if the owner has an accepted pedigree certificate or veterinary declaration stating that the dog is of this breed. Any dogs designated as restricted breed must have been in Victoria prior to September 2010 and registered before 2011 (as any breed) in order to be able to be kept under the prescribed conditions, including neutering and microchip implantation.

Victoria also places restrictions on owners of greyhounds, with regulations requiring them to be muzzled when outside their owner's premises (Domestic Animals Act 1994). A greyhound will only be exempted from these requirements if it has passed through Greyhound Racing Victoria's Greyhound Adoption Program (GAP), in which case a specially designed green collar must be worn by the dog at all times to identify it as having such an exemption. All greyhounds must be kept on lead at all times outside their owner's property. All dog ownership laws also apply to greyhounds.

A broadly accepted classification structure for dangerous dogs (of any breed) is similar across a number of jurisdictions in Australia. Independent of any breed restrictions, there are also categories of 'dangerous' for individual dogs dependent upon behaviour displayed. Classes vary across states, but often include 'dangerous' or 'menacing'. For example, in New South Wales, dogs that have 'without provocation' attacked or killed a person or animal, or have threatened or displayed aggression to them, are categorised as dangerous. Any dog kept for the purposes of hunting is also considered dangerous. South Australia classifies dogs as 'dangerous', 'menacing' or 'nuisance' when they behave in a specific way, including the dog attacking, harassing or chasing a person, animal or bird. In Tasmania the dog must either have caused serious injury to a person or animal, or there must be reasonable cause to believe it would do so, to classify it as 'dangerous'.

## 13.6.8 USA and Canada

The USA and Canada both demonstrate the massive variation evident across countries and their states in development of dog law. Some states have long lists of restricted or banned breeds, while others do not have any breed-specific legislation. All states have legislation covering dogs of any breed behaving dangerously, for example in Maine, USA, a dog is considered 'dangerous' if it assaults or threatens imminent bodily injury to a person or domesticated animal (dangerous dog Maine Code 2005 (§3952)). In Maine, it is lawful to kill a dog if necessary to protect a person or domesticated animal in an unprovoked, sudden assault (s.3951). If the dog is found to be dangerous following the report of an incident, the court can order the dog to be muzzled, restrained and confined to the owner's premises, or a secure enclosure. If a dog has 'killed, maimed or inflicted serious bodily harm upon a person' the court can order the dog to be euthanised (1997, c. 690, §35).

In Ontario, Canada, BSL was introduced as recently as 2005 (Dogs Statute Law Amendment Act 2005). This legislation prohibited individuals from owning, breeding, transferring, importing or training a Pit Bull to fight. Dogs of this type may be kept under restrictions if owned prior to 2005 (these dogs are considered 'grandfathered' or 'restricted' Pit Bulls), including being kept on a lead and muzzled when off the owner's property and neutered. The expansion of the legislation relating to any breed of dog was created by the Dog Owner's Liability Act 1990 (as amended 2005), whereby if a dog has bitten or attacked, behaved in a manner that poses a menace to the safety of persons or domestic animals or the owner did not exercise reasonable precautions as to prevent this, the dog may be declared dangerous and either made subject to control measures or euthanised depending on the nature of the offence.

In Calgary, Canada, there is no BSL legislation, as the intention is to prevent dog bites using licensing and enforcement. Under the Responsible Pet Ownership Bylaw (23m2006), all cats and dogs residing in the City of Calgary must have a City of Calgary licence by the age of three months.

It is recognised that the majority of classifications and identifications of dangerous dogs, with the exception of BSL, are essentially after the fact (Australian Veterinary Association, 2012). Multnomah County in Oregon USA implemented a 'potentially dangerous dog' classification in 1989 in an attempt to address this. This programme categorises dogs that have come to the attention of the authorities from Level 1–5 and places restrictions upon them.

At Level 1, which encompasses a dog displaying threatening or aggressive behaviour, the dog must be restrained securely. Level 5, where a dog has caused serious physical injury or death of a person or has been used as a weapon, stipulates that the dog must be euthanised and that the owner may have their right to own a dog suspended.

### 13.6.9 Japan

In Japan, all dogs must be registered with the local city office under the official nationwide dog registration system. There are specific laws covering 'fighting dogs', as with a number of the countries discussed above. However, in Japan any large dog over 55cm is covered by this legislation regardless of breed or type, as well as named 'fighting breeds' (see Table 13.1). Fighting breeds are not prohibited, but they do attract restrictions. These types of dogs must be kept in a cage, for which the key must remain with the owner, unless being trained, transported or exercised (in a way that prevents danger to people, animals or property). Fighting dogs must always be supervised when off the owner's property, and a lead and muzzle should be attached to prevent bite incidents when away from the owner's property. If there is a fighting dog on the premises, there should be visible notification to the public of this. There is no legislation against breeding such dogs in Japan, however any dogs classified as fighting dogs but not intended for use as breeding stock should be neutered.

### 13.6.10 South Africa

There is no centralised BSL in South Africa. Region-specific dog law is focused primarily on the safety of the person. In Cape Town, for example, it is an offence to '... urge any dog to attack, worry or frighten any person or animal unless in self-defence' (Animal By-Law 2010 s.6(b)). All dogs in Cape Town must be registered with the local council. In the Emalahleni Municipality, dogs may not be 'a source of danger' (By-Laws Relating to the Licensing of and Control Over Dogs, s.9), which is further clarified as being 'wild or vicious' or having 'acquired the habit of charging passing vehicles, bicycles or persons' (s.10(a)(b)).

Similarly, in Johannesburg, the focus is on the behaviour of the dog. No dogs that are 'wild, dangerous or ferocious' or that are in the habit of chasing people or vehicles are permitted in public places (By-Laws Relating to Dogs & Cats s.6(a)(b)). Courts may make certain directions in respect of injuries caused by animals (Animal Matters Amendment Act, 1993).

## 13.7 Wolf–dog hybrids

A number of countries have specific regulations with regard to wolf–dog hybrids (a domestic dog crossed with a wolf). The generation of wolf–dog hybrid can affect whether or not it is considered to be a Dangerous Wild Animal or a domestic dog, and the resulting restrictions on such dogs. These definitions are country-specific, with a few examples provided below.

In the UK, The Dangerous Wild Animals Act 1976 (as modified by The Dangerous Wild Animals Act 1976 (Modification) (No.2) Order 2007) regulates the keeping of certain kinds of dangerous animals. Licences are required for the keeping of any animal appearing in the schedule to the Act (subject to certain exemptions, for example those kept by zoos or for scientific procedures), or any hybrid thereof. Wolves are specified in the schedule as requiring a licence. In addition, under the Act any animal with at least one parent as such a hybrid requires a licence. However, the second generation following a wolf–domestic dog hybrid does not require a licence if neither parent is such a hybrid, therefore where an animal is third generation (or any generation thereafter) no licence is required under the legislation.

In Maine, USA, ownership of a wolf hybrid is banned unless the owner holds a permit to hold a wild animal in captivity (s.3921-B). There are specific regulations concerning wolf hybrids, with owners or keepers of a wolf hybrid found at large committing a civil violation under the Uncontrolled Dogs legislation (s.3911-B).

## 13.8  Repealed BSL

In the Netherlands BSL prohibiting Pit Bull Terriers and Rottweilers was introduced in 1993. However, in 2008 after careful assessment of the legislation and research into the impact of breed on dog bite risk and whether BSL had mitigated the number of dog bites recorded (Cornelissen and Hopster, 2010), BSL was repealed and there are now no restricted dog breeds or types in the Netherlands. Italy used to have one of the largest restricted dogs lists, with ninety-two breeds originally named on it. This was reduced to seventeen breeds and then in 2009, all legislation restricting breed types was repealed. There is now also a growing trend in the USA for the rejection of BSL (National Canine Research Council, 2014).

## 13.9  Conclusion

In summary, most legislation considered above focuses on retrospective rather than proactive action on dog aggression. This is usually after the fact, which is tragically too late for the victims. In contrast, some countries are using measures to address the issue of responsible dog ownership and attempt to proactively deal with potential dog aggression in order to prevent bites before they occur. Even though this is also the intention of BSL, it has been repealed in a number of countries due to doubts about its effectiveness. Whether the number of attacks would be even higher without it, or more significant due to the capacity of restricted-type dogs to cause more serious injury when they do bite, is a source of debate. This chapter highlights potential dangers associated with some of the legislation aimed at controlling dog bites, and the need to treat each dog as an individual. Clearly there are cultural factors that need to be considered in controlling risk as well as a demand for educating dog owners properly, if we are to address the defects in much of the present legislation and genuinely minimise the risk to citizens from dogs.

## 13.10  References

Animal Matters Amendment Act 1993. Available at: www.gov.za/sites/www.gov.za/files/Act42of1993.
    pdf (accessed 5 March 2016).
Anti-social Behaviour, Crime and Policing Act 2014. Available at: www.legislation.gov.uk/
    ukpga/2014/12/contents/enacted/data.htm (accessed 5 March 2016).
Bates v DPP (1993). 157 JP 1004.
Control of Dogs (Scotland) Act 2010. Available at: www.legislation.gov.uk/asp/2010/9/contents
Cooke, F. (2013). The application, implementation, enforcement and development of companion

animal welfare in local authorities in Great Britain. In: *All Parliamentary Group for Animal Welfare Sub-Group for Dogs: Review and Recommendations for Developing an Effective England-wide Strategy for Dogs* (2014).

Cornelissen, J. M. R., Hopster, H. (2010). Dog bites in the Netherlands: A study of victim, injuries, circumstances and aggressors to support evaluation of breed specific legislation. *Veterinary Journal* 186(3): 292–298.

Dangerous Dogs Act 1991. Available at: www.legislation.gov.uk/ukpga/1991/65/contents (accessed 5 March 2016).

Dangerous Dogs Amendment Act 1997. Available at: www.legislation.gov.uk/ukpga/1997/53/contents (accessed 5 March 2016).

Danish Act on Dogs 2010 (as amended 2014. Available at: www.foedevarestyrelsen.dk/english/ImportExport/Travelling_with_pet_animals/Pages/The-Danish-dog-legislation.aspx (accessed 5 March 2016).

DeMeester, R. (2004). Critical review of current European legislation regarding the issue of dangerous dogs. In Heath, S., Osella, C. (eds) *Proceedings of the 10th European Congress on Companion Animal Behavioural Medicine*, Cremona, Italy. Pp.38–42.

Del Mar, K. (2011). The International Court of Justice and Standards of Proof, in: Bannelier, Chistakis, Heathcote (eds), *The ICJ and the Development of International law. The Lasting Impact of the Corfu Channel case*, Routledge.

Dog Control Bill (HL) 2nd Reading, 24 April 2009, vol 709, col 1689. Lord Redesdale. Available at: www.publications.parliament.uk/pa/ld200809/ldhansrd/lhan64.pdf (accessed 5 March 2016).

Dog Owners' Liability Act R.S.O. 1990 (as amended 2005). Available at: www.ontario.ca/laws/statute/90d16 (accessed 5 March 2016).

Dogs Statute Law Amendment Act 2005. Available at: https://www.ontario.ca/laws/statute/S05002 (accessed 5 March 2016).

Emalahleni Municipality: Local Government Notice: By-Laws Relating to the Licensing of and Control over Dogs. Available at: www.emalahlenilm.gov.za/documents/By-Laws/DOG%20CONTROL%20BY-LAW.pdf (accessed 6 March 2016).

Grant, D. (2008). *Briefing document on dangerous dogs and their owners as experienced by the RSPCA Harmsworth Hospital Holloway*, London. Unpublished.

HC Written Answers, Hansard, 5 Nov 2013: col 107W. Environment, Food and Rural Affairs: *Dangerous Dogs*. George Eustice. Available at: www.publications.parliament.uk/pa/cm201314/cmhansrd/cm131105/text/131105w0001.htm (accessed 5 March 2016).

Hundegesetz/BE, Bern. Available at: http://skn.li/downloads/hundegesetz-2013.pdf (accessed 9 January 2015).

Maine Code: Agriculture and Animals: Dangerous Dogs 2005. Available at: http://legislature.maine.gov/legis/statutes/7/title7sec3907.html (accessed 5 March 2016).

National Canine Research Council. (2014). *Breed-Specific Legislation is on the Decline.* http://nationalcanineresearchcouncil.com/uploaded_files/tinymce/Breed%20specific%20legislation%20on%20the%20decline.pdf (accessed 5 January 2015).

RSPCA (2010). *Improving Dog Ownership: The economic case for dog licensing.* RSPCA. Available at: file:///C:/Users/Bill/Downloads/Dog%20registration%20report%20(7).pdf (accessed 5 March 2016).

R. v. Crown Court at Knightsbridge ex parte Dunne; Brock v. Director of Public Prosecutions [1993] 4 All ER 491.

Schalke, E., Ott, S.A., von Gaertner, A. M., Hackbarth, H., Mittman A. (2008). Is breed-specific legislation justified? Study of the results of the temperament test of Lower Saxony. *Journal of Veterinary Behaviour* 3: 97–103.

Schweizerisches Bundesgericht, BGE 136 I 1. Available at: http://relevancy.bger.ch/php/clir/http/index.php?lang=de&zoom=&type=show_document&highlight_docid=atf%3A%2F%2F136-I-1%3Ade (accessed 5 March 2016).

Tasker, L. (2007). *Stray Animal Control Practices (Europe)*. WSPA and RSPCA. Available at: http://www.fao.org/fileadmin/user_upload/animalwelfare/WSPA_RSPCA%20International%20stray%20control%20practices%20in%20Europe%202006_2007.pdf (accessed 6 March 2016).

The Australian Veterinary Association (2012). *Dangerous dogs – a sensible solution: Policy and model legislative framework*. St Leonards. Available at: https://www.ava.com.au/sites/default/files/AVA_website/pdfs/Dangerous%20dogs%20-%20a%20sensible%20solution%20FINAL.pdf (accessed 6 March 2016).

Upton, M., Bennett, R., Wismore, T., Taylor, N., Hanks. J., Allison, K., Pflug, S. (2010). *Dog licensing and registration in the UK*. Reading University. A Report to the RSPCA.

Wilkinson, S. (2012). Standards of Proof in International Humanitarian and Human Rights Fact-Finding and Inquiry Missions. Geneva Academy of International Humanitarian Law, Geneva, Switzerland.

# CHAPTER 14

# The Investigation of Dog Bite Incidents and Procedures for Gathering Evidence

*James Crosby*

## 14.1 Introduction

In-depth investigation of dog bite incidents has, in the past, been relatively rare. Especially in the US, Law enforcement officials have too often adopted the attitude, 'The dog did it – we are done'. This has been understandable: when confronted with an apparently mauled victim and a bloody dog the most common (and probably logical) reaction is to assume the dog is guilty, take the dog and have it destroyed, so no further investment of resources is needed.

Why does the lack of investigation matter? A half-hearted approach fails to address core concerns and needs of trainers, owners, the public, and the legal system, which at the very least might help us develop an evidence-based approach to prevention. Clearly if the dog is dead, it will not reoffend, but the destruction of the dog does not help us understand why the event happened and so prevent similar events with different dogs. Behaviour experts want to know why a particular dog bit, and why it was as serious as it was, in order to design protocols and methods of reducing or preventing such behaviour. Owners are concerned as to how to avoid having their dog bite at all, and whether a dog that has bitten can be remediated or whether they should destroy their family companion. The public in general, dog owning or not, wants to know it is secure and safe. The legal system has its own increasing demands. Criminal and civil liability may well attach to even a simple dog bite, and as the bite progresses in severity so do the potential consequences.

We must consider the disposition of an involved animal(s). Are they just to be killed? Is there a need for or value in training, rehabilitation, or management measures to be applied for public safety? How can we increase public safety and security while being humane and fair in a way that is lawful and practical? How do the needs for private and public safety co-ordinate or conflict with resource allocation?

Dogs have existed closely with us for at least 15,000 years, perhaps more (Clutton-Brock, 1995). With this kind of extensive history it is clear that dogs are not, as a matter of course, a constant threat to humans. Although they do bite, dogs typically live out their lives without physically harming anyone seriously, at least to the extent that any victim feels the dog should be disposed of.

   Dogs bite for a reason (see Chapter 1). That reason may not be immediately apparent to us as humans, and must be sought using a dog's frame of reference. To find that reason is part of the duty of the investigator. We must insist on thorough, detailed, and professional investigations into dog bite-related injuries and deaths, based on carefully collected evidence (see Chapter 14). We must establish standards for best practice to give those investigating these incidents the tools needed to properly investigate dog bite-related injuries. This chapter describes the general procedures that should be followed to give all professionals involved in an incident the greatest opportunity to achieve their goals successfully. It seems that all too often the interests of one group may override that of others to the detriment of progress on this issue.

## 14.2  First response

Response to an emergency involving an apparent dog attack must start with safety and security. The needs of the victim are primary: aid must be rendered, and safely. The dog(s) may be loose, and if so must be contained to allow emergency responders to assist the victim. Note that containment does not mean death – a dead dog can provide little evidence.

- **Observation is key.** Supervising personnel should immediately begin observing the scene and the dog(s) involved. A chaotic scene is difficult to tame, with emotions high. Notes made on scene and as soon as possible are most valuable.
- **Containment of the dog(s) involved is an immediate need.** If the scene is a closed garden or building then existing barriers can be used. Doors can be closed, fences latched, or makeshift barriers erected to limit the motion of the dogs to small areas so that they are no longer an immediate risk. Specific animal officers (including from other organisations) may respond quickly, and if so they can use their tools and skills to contain the animals safely. In a serious case, when taken by animal officers, the dog(s) should be secured and transported in clean cages, free from contamination and with multiple dogs separated from each other. Evidence shed by the dogs, such as blood, vomitus, faeces or tissue must be collected, labelled, and preserved.
- **Positive identification of the dog(s) involved is critical.** At the scene the dog should be photographed and labelled clearly. Many dogs look similar, so in the interest of chain of evidence, implanting or reading of a microchip can provide positive, unalterable and unique identification. This can be implanted at the scene by qualified personnel if the dog is amenable, or can be implanted at a veterinarian's practice while en route to secure containment. If the dog is chipped at the veterinarian immediately on removal from the scene, the veterinarian can use the opportunity to assist in the collection of necessary physical evidence from the dog such as blood samples, DNA swabs, stomach contents, etc. The microchip number should be used in addition to case numbers to positively identify samples and their source if there are multiple dogs.

- **Even dogs killed on scene for safety reasons should be implanted with micro-chips** or scanned to confirm existing identification. This allows better accountability and identification of samples, and helps later verification if a defendant's legal team requests independent examination of the body.

## 14.3 Initial investigation

Once the animal is secure and the victim either treated or secured (in case of death) the collection of evidence begins. Evidence in an investigation can be broken down into four basic categories:

1. Circumstantial
2. Testimonial
3. Physical
4. Behavioural

After the collection of circumstantial and testimonial evidence, the investigator is free to search for and collect physical evidence. Circumstantial and testimonial evidence must be supported by the physical evidence. Appearances can deceive, testimony can change, and opinion can replace observations. Physical evidence is less prone to waiver or be subject to personal interpretation or agenda.

### 14.3.1 Circumstantial evidence

Circumstantial evidence is simply the nature of the scene and conditions observed and noted by the investigator.

- Where was the dog first seen?
- What were its actions on arrival of responders?
- Where were the victim and any other people on site?
- Were there any other dogs or animals present and where were they?
- What were they doing?

The essential circumstantial evidence in a dog-related incident must also include welfare issues. These are discussed in more detail later.

### 14.3.2 Testimonial evidence

The investigator speaks to people. Initial statements are taken. Witnesses may say that they saw the incident. The witnesses may have, to them, a clear picture of the incident, but there are cautions that will be addressed below. Further, detailed questioning later, after emotion has waned, will produce more data.

Testimonial evidence must be used with caution. The unreliability of eye witnesses in high stress incidents is well documented in criminal justice literature (Lezak, 1974; Schmechel et al., 2006). In a high stress encounter there are cautions the investigator must be aware of in using testimony.

- **One of the first concerns with witness testimony is if the witness actually saw the incident**. Helpful citizens often believe they saw a series of events when in reality they may have seen only parts. The human mind connects these parts into what seems, to the witness, to be a coherent whole. The investigator must press to determine exactly what the witness did see and check to make sure they could have seen what they report from their position. A dog attack is over quickly. Sound and assumption can easily fill visual gaps.
- **The agenda of witnesses must also be considered**. What do they have to gain, or lose, from their report? Do they have a vested interest in the outcome? Are they reliable? What level of experience with dogs do they possess? The past experiences of the witness have a direct impact on their perception of an incident. Are they experienced animal owners who recognise normal and abnormal behaviour in dogs or do they have little or no dog-focused background, since this can affect the way they process human and dog interactions (Kujala et al., 2012).

### 14.3.3 Physical evidence

Physical evidence collection begins with extensive photography. As much of the scene and the surrounding area possible should be included. Details in photographs that may be missed by investigators caught up in the event are preserved for later. In today's technological environment this may include the macro level with satellite imagery. Overall photography, close-ups, and photos from the dog's level assist reconstructing the scene. Dogs see the world differently than we do. They may have a wider field of view, have altered colour vision, are often short-sighted (Miller et al., 1995; McGreevy et al., 2003) and are not at human eye level. I have personally found that a walk-through with a small, action-type video camera with a wide angle lens placed at dog level can aid understanding a dog's perceptions. Standard crime scene measurements and a full diagram are essential for documentation and orientation of photos later.

Collection and preservation of physical evidence is a developed science that continues to mature. Procedures for the collection and preservation of physical evidence have been established and standardised to a great extent, as shown by many training programmes at university level (e.g. BScs in Forensic Science). Chain of custody issues should be followed fully as with any criminal investigation. If a victim is dead the case is a homicide, like any other homicide. The only difference here is that the instrument of the crime is a live, decision-making creature. Collection and documentation should be to normal standards, but there are evidence issues peculiar to dog bite investigations that an investigator must consider. The types of physical evidence in dog bite investigations can be broken into two general tiers (1. animal and victim, 2. environment and scene).

Specific examples of Tiers 1 and 2 range from the obvious (blood spatter and bites) to more detailed items such as DNA from both the suspect and the victim's injuries; drag and ground disturbance; scent factors that may have influenced the dog; perceptive factors such as lighting or weather. These bits of data help the investigator construct a fuller picture of the physical event.

14.3.3.1  TIER 1: Actual physical evidence collected and documented from victims and
          animal suspects

Box 14.1 summarises examples of this type of evidence. This is the traditional physical evidence common to many investigations, but with a spin targeting dog-specific issues.

---

### Box 14.1 Physical Evidence Tier 1 – Animal and Victim – Canine Cases

- Hair and tissue
- Baseline DNA – dog and victim
- DNA from dog's mouth/fur
- Blood spatter and transfer patterns
- Blood samples collected on scene, including blood transfer to scene and objects
- Dog stomach contents
- Dog faeces recovered after related incident
- Dog blood toxicology
- Dog urine toxicology
- Dog physical condition
- Medical (scarring or injury)
- Dentition documentation or mould from the dog
- Injuries to victim (photo documentation)
- Victim clothing items
- Human toxicology from autopsy
- Training/containment tools (leashes, collars, etc)
- Scene surface disturbances such as footprints, drag marks, etc
- Toys or objects in scene.

---

Tier 1 is considered hard evidence. Much of it is common to many crime scenes. Hair, tissue, and blood evidence are documented and gathered. Reference DNA must be collected from both the suspect dog(s) and from the victim. Much as with the human victim, toxicology should be conducted on the dog.

Obviously the related incident will have resulted in an injury, an apparent bite. We will define, for working purposes, a bite as contact between teeth and skin that causes an injury. The injury in a bite is disruption of the skin, with accompanying damage to the vascular system, muscles, bones, and other organs.

The bite is evidence and must be documented (see Chapters 14 and 16 for full details on this process). Teeth can leave distinctive marks. The marks can be documented with detailed photographs. Initial photos should be taken on scene, before any clean up or alteration by movement, or, if practical in the case of a live victim, treatment. Further documentary photos can be taken either in hospital during or after treatment or during autopsy. These photos, including proper scale, can then be compared to potential sources, and particular sources can be included or excluded (see Chapters 12 and 14). Evidence can be gathered from within the bite itself. When a dog bites there is potentially transfer of DNA in both directions, i.e. a dog both takes and leaves a DNA trace. Canine DNA is individually identifiable (Clarke and Vandenberg, 2010) and it can be proved clearly that a certain dog had contact with a victim.

Clothing items of the victim should be seized and preserved for both DNA collection and to match defects in the clothing to bite wounds on the victim. In some cases clothing is removed by the dog's actions during an incident. Presence or absence of corresponding clothing can help determine the order of bites and possibly the flow of events during an incident.

### 14.3.3.2  Tier 2: Physical evidence specific to canine incident cases consisting of environmental and situational data

An investigator must attempt to gather all the available information about the incident and the actions of all involved directly before the event (see Box 14.2). Situational evidence includes setting, context, and actions preceding the incident. These factors must be viewed as they apply to the unique experience and world view of the dog. Analysing all the actions that, added together, became the incident, along with physical and environmental factors, assist the investigator in determining the reason for an apparent bite.

---

**Box 14.2  Physical Evidence Tier 2 – Environment and Scene – Canine Cases**

- Nature of the scene (residence, indoors, etc.)
- Sensory issues (hearing, eyesight) of dog
- Attractions or distractions in the area
- Lighting and weather
- Level of activity at the time of the bite
- Movement of participants in the incident
- Presence, condition, and behaviour of other dogs at the scene or nearby
- Non-canine animals present in the scene
- Presence of food source
- Humans other than the victim(s) and their actions
- Possible scent sources outside primary scene
- Wind direction
- Familiarity of dog with the environment
- Familiarity of the dog with humans on scene
- Normal environment and experience of the dog.

---

## 14.3.4  Behavioural evidence

The basic behaviour may seem to be obvious: a dog bit a person and caused injury. But the *why* behind the bite affects both prosecution and public safety considerations. Was this a 'dangerous' dog or was this an accident? Did this dog act 'on its own' or was the dog's behaviour shaped by the action, or inaction, of a person? Can, or should, such a person be held responsible?

In the context of a dog incident investigation, the investigator is not looking to predict what a dog may do in the future (which may be useful in other circumstances such as a seized breed, see chapter 18). The investigator is looking for behaviours that may be diagnostic in determining what the dog did in the past. Total reconstruction of an incident is usually impossible, but an evaluator can look for sensitivities and triggers that may have contributed to a particular action by the dog. To do this an investigator needs to gather detailed information of how the dog lived and acted before the incident. This information is part of the testimony gathered. How did the dog behave on a daily basis? What level of socialisation with people and other animals did the dog have? What was the purpose of the dog? Was it a family member or a 'resident dog'? Had the dog received training, if so from whom, and what training methods were used? This information gives us a general structure, a perception of what behaviour was expected from the dog.

Firstly, background witness statements are valuable in determining the past behaviour of a dog. Neighbours may not have filed formal complaints but may have observed the dog interacting with other dogs or people. They may have knowledge of past conflict. Veterinary staff may have experience with the dog and be able to provide observations and documents of both the physical condition and behaviour of a dog as seen in their setting. There may be local trainers, groomers, veterinarians or other professionals that have had contact with the subject dog. All of these pieces add up to a more detailed picture of the animal, just as background witnesses add to the profile of a human offender. In a dog-inflicted injury case these factors can help establish whether the owner could have reasonably anticipated dangerous behaviour from the dog and can show whether remediation was attempted.

Nonetheless, direct behavioural evidence is essential. A process involved in gathering direct behavioural evidence from the dog for the courts is covered in Chapter 18, but will be described briefly here for this specific context. As said before, the investigator is not looking to *predict future behaviour*. The investigator is looking to assess behaviours and triggers present, documented with quantifiable, direct observation, to establish the dog's behaviour post-incident and thereby attempt to reconstruct causes or contributing factors to the actions of the dog at the time of the incident. This is imperfect: experiences may have occurred since the incident that have changed the dog's reactions to circumstances, including the effects of the incident itself. Yet clues can be gathered that help the investigator look deeper into the dog's reasons for action. Is this a dog that startles easily? Did the victim of the incident surprise the dog and approach suddenly? Is the dog unusually sensitive to approach by a specific class of person (such as children)? Was the victim an unfamiliar child?

The investigator should be looking for some specific behaviours as they apply to the incident. Some of these specific behavioural factors are:

* Reaction to startle (sudden noise)
* Recovery from startle
* Reactivity to other dogs
* Reactivity to non-canines
* Resource guarding (food, toy, person, location)
* Reaction to 'friendly stranger'
* Reaction to 'threatening stranger'

- Reaction to classes of people
- Reaction to physical contact
- Social contact with humans – willing or reticent?
- Ability to respond to redirection when aroused
- Territorial behaviour.

Any behaviour evaluation used should possess certain qualities. The evaluation must be reproducible, be consistent, and should go from general to specific behaviours. One begins with overall observed behaviour –what is the dog doing? How does the dog respond to the evaluator's approach? These general observations lead to more specific situations, and ideally lead closer to the actions and environment reported immediately before the incident. If possible and safe, after a general evaluation an attempt to recreate as much of the situation that preceded the bite may reveal other specific behaviours. If the target of the incident was an infant, the use of a crying baby doll may elicit a notable response, but may not be a reliable predictor alone. *Caution should be used in assuming that a recreation will produce an identical response*: the recreation is not likely to reproduce exactly the entirety of the situation, especially since involving real victims and the real owner are not advisable. With that in mind, a reasonable approximation of the incident may be useful.

During an examination an ultimate single cause may not emerge. What the investigator may discover, though, is that a number of individual factors added up to produce a particular reaction. This is called 'trigger stacking' (Hedges, 2015). The individual triggers or stimuli may be, in isolation, insufficient to produce an overt reaction. However, as they are added together, the effect is cumulative. A dog that, for example, is not socialised to children, has high levels of prey/toy 'drive' and has a protective predisposition, may face each of those factors individually without reaction. Have a small child run loudly and quickly at the dog on its own property past the dog's food bowl and the additive effect of the separate risk factors may precipitate a strong response. Assessing all the factors and determining the parts of the additive result is one purpose of the evaluation.

The other purpose of determining triggers has to do with accountability and prosecution. Were the risk factors evident to the owner/caretaker? Were the triggers created or reinforced by the owner? Were attempts ever made to minimise the risk associated with the triggers or risk factors, or did the owner manage the dog properly to reduce the risk? Did the owner, or should the owner, have perceived that the triggers and resulting behaviours were likely to result in the injury or death of another person?

A behaviour evaluation must be recorded. Multi-viewpoint video has proven best to establish both the actions of the dog and the interplay between the dog and the evaluator. Fine details such as eye contact and facial expressions matter since these details are basic to canine communication. Further, an evaluator may not observe quick signals directly, or may be distracted by safety and other concerns. Observing video post-evaluation has often revealed signalling that the author has missed while in the midst of an evaluation.

A behaviour evaluation should occur as soon as practically possible. The longer the time that lapses between the incident and the evaluation, the greater the chance that other influences have changed the dog's behaviour. A dog mistreated originally may respond profoundly to humane and kind treatment in a shelter, and after some months of positive treatment this may change the dog's responses (see Chapter 28). Although remediation of problem behaviour is generally a good thing, this change may obscure triggers that were causally linked to the apparent bite incident.

### 14.3.5 Health and circumstantial evidence

The health of a dog involved in an incident is of evidentiary value and should be assessed by a veterinary surgeon. The first set of factors to examine are overall physical well-being and defects. Problems such as eyesight, hearing, limits to mobility and injury need to be documented. Any deficits should be identified as being acute or chronic. Chronic, untreated pain can establish certain patterns of aggressive behaviour (Barcelos et al., 2015), whereas acute onset of a painful condition such as an ear infection or injury can increase the risk of an aggressive response in a normally placid individual. Illness can cause discomfort, disorientation, sensitivity to noise or light. Chronic problems such as hyperthyroidism, possibly related to diet, can underlie inappropriate expression of aggression (Köhler et al., 2012). A full blood chemistry panel with toxicology can reveal whether a dog has been administered analgesics (possibly for or as a result of fighting) or given hormone supplements (steroids) to achieve body condition, strength, or an aggressive predisposition. A dog's reproductive status also affects behaviour. An intact male may act aggressively to protect his reproductive access to an in-oestrus female, or be affected by the scent of a nearby receptive female.

As an adjunct to the veterinary examination of the dog to collect evidence, the dog's condition and the environment it was kept in must be evaluated considering its welfare impact, since they may affect its aggressive predisposition. Does the dog appear to be fed adequately (a malnourished dog may be more willing to take risks over accessing food)? Was it sheltered properly? Did it have access to adequate, fresh water? The investigator will need to discover if the dog had been allowed appropriate exercise, social interactions, and expression of normal behaviour. Had the dog received required vaccinations and does the dog appear free from discomfort or disease? How have the dog's needs been met, and is the standard of care shown in accord with recognised minimum standards. In many incidents deficits are discovered upon investigation. Poor nutrition, substandard veterinary care, and lack of socialisation with conspecifics or humans can all contribute to creating a situation where the dog cannot show healthy, placid behaviour (Miklosi, 2007). These deficiencies must be recognised, documented, and considered when evaluating the human responsibility attached to an event. How did these deficits play into the circumstances of the incident?

The five freedoms as established by the Brambell Commission (Ohl, 2012; Brambell, 1965) must be considered:

- **Freedom from hunger or thirst** by ready access to fresh water and a diet to maintain full health and vigour
- **Freedom from discomfort** by providing an appropriate environment including shelter and a comfortable resting area
- **Freedom from pain, injury or disease** by prevention or rapid diagnosis and treatment
- **Freedom to express (most) normal behaviour** by providing sufficient space, proper facilities and company of the animal's own kind

- **Freedom from fear and distress** by ensuring conditions and treatment which avoid mental suffering.

## 14.4 The question of warning and provocation

Often we hear that a dog 'snapped' without warning. Our examination of the testimony may allow us to see if warnings were given, and/or if the person failed to appreciate them (see Chapter 2). This takes detailed questioning of the people who may have witnessed the incident or, if none survive, testimony of past incidents may prove illuminating.

Dogs have an extensive vocabulary of communication tools (Chapter 2). Some of these are audible, but many are non-verbal. The signals that a dog uses to convey fear or frustration can seem similar to humans. Growling, snarling, barking – these are all audible signals whose true richness of content may not be fully appreciated (Pongrácz et al., 2006). Superficially someone may not distinguish a bark saying 'You are bothering me' from 'You are threatening me/You are frightening me', and may even perceive it erroneously as a direct challenge to be responded to with greater human force, when non-escalation and withdrawal would be the sensible option.

Our questioning must focus not only on the overall chain of events, but the events immediately before the incident. What was happening a minute before? Thirty seconds? Ten seconds? When given general 'what happened' questions witnesses tend to give general answers. 'Nothing', or, 'the dog just snapped' are common answers. By dissecting the incident moment by moment we often pull out information that otherwise would have been lost in the overall fog of the crisis.

We also have to address concerns of provocation. Normally one considers provocation from a human perspective. Did someone poke, hit, torture, or otherwise mistreat a dog to precipitate an incident? Might the person be perceived to 'deserve' the attack? Although subjective, examining the perceptions and beliefs surrounding an incident can shed light on how (and if) the bite may have possibly been prevented; however, it must be noted that human perceptions of blame and provocation in regards to dog bites may have little to do with how events actually occur and are more related to perceived knowledge/experience levels and relationships between the individual animals and people involved (Westgarth et al., 2015).

## 14.5 Synthesis

Once all of the evidence is collected and the subject dog(s) has/have been evaluated it is time to put the whole picture together. Physical evidence, testimony and behavioural evaluation all help assemble the picture that answers the investigator's questions:

- What happened
- Why it happened
- Whom (if anyone) is responsible.

What did the physical evidence show? The sheer number of bites is always of prurient interest to media, but we are more concerned where, when, and from what direction they occurred. Was the incident frontal or did the dog pursue a fleeing victim? Where does the issue of provocation enter? Do we have the right dog? Are there other 'suspects' at large? Is there a risk to public safety beyond the incident at hand?

Is the testimony received consistent, and does the physical evidence back it up? Does this particular incident make sense in the context of prior behaviour by this particular dog, and if so should, or did, the owner know there was a problem? What if any remedies did he or she pursue, and were these strategies reasonable considering the prior behaviour seen?

Dogs, although undoubtedly capable of independent action, do not usually depart far from prior behaviours. As owners and caretakers of domestic dogs, humans are ultimately responsible for their care and supervision. Failure to appropriately supervise dogs' actions and monitor problematic behaviour must be placed firmly on the caretaker, and the results of said failures must be borne by the responsible humans. The investigator has a duty to both the humans and the animals to search for contributing factors and assign that responsibility. Only a complete investigation will provide the data needed to fulfil that duty.

## 14.6 References

Barcelos, A. M., Mills, D. S., Zulch, H. (2015). Clinical indicators of occult musculoskeletal pain in aggressive dogs. *Veterinary Record*, 176(18), 465–465.

Brambell, F. W. R. (1965). Report on the Technical Committee to enquire into the welfare of livestock kept under intensive conditions.

Clarke, M. and Vandenberg, N. (2010) Dog attack: the application of canine DNA profiling in forensic casework. *Forensic Science and Medical Pathology* 6, 151–157.

Clutton-Brock, J. (1995). Origins of the dog: domestication and early history. In Serpell, J. (ed). The Domestic Dog; its evolution, behaviour and interactions with people. Cambridge University Press, pp.7–20.

Hedges, S. (2015). Advanced approaches to handling dogs in practice *The Veterinary Nurse* 6(6), 308–315

Köhler, B., Stengel, C., Neiger, R. (2012). Dietary hyperthyroidism in dogs. *Journal of Small Animal Practice*, 53(3), 182–184.

Kujala, M. V., Kujala, J., Carlson, S., Hari, R. (2012). Dog experts' brains distinguish socially relevant body postures similarly in dogs and humans. *PloS one*, 7(6), e39145.

Lezak, M. D. (1974). Some psychological limitations on witness reliability. *Wayne Law Review* 20.1 (1973-1974): 117–134.

McGreevy, P., Grassi, T. D., Harman, A. M. (2003). A strong correlation exists between the distribution of retinal ganglion cells and nose length in the dog. *Brain, Behavior and Evolution*, 63(1), 13–22.

Miklosi, A. (2007). Dog Behaviour, Evolution and Cognition Oxford University Press.

Miller, H. C., DeWall, C. N., Pattison, K., Molet, M. Zentall, T. R. (2012). Too dog tired to avoid danger: Self-control depletion in canines increases behavioral approach toward an aggressive threat. *Psychonomic bulletin & review*, 19(3). 535–540.

Miller, P. E., Murphy, C. J. (1995). Vision in dogs. *Journal-American Veterinary Medical Association*, 207, 1623–1634.

Ohl, F., van der Staay, F. J. (2012). Animal welfare: At the interface between science and society. *The Veterinary Journal*, 192 (1) 13–19.

Pongrácz, P., Molnár, C., Miklósi, Á. (2006). Acoustic parameters of dog barks carry emotional information for humans. *Applied Animal Behaviour Science*, 100(3), 228–240.

Schmechel, R. S., O'Toole, T. P., Easterly, C., Loftus, E. F. (2006). Beyond the Ken? Testing jurors' understanding of eyewitness reliability and evidence. *Jurimetrics Journal*. 46, 177–214.

Westgarth, C., Watkins, F. (2015). A qualitative investigation of the perceptions of female dog bite victims and implications for the prevention of dog bites. *Journal of Veterinary Behavior-Clinical Applications and Research,* 10, 479–488.

## Supplementary: Suggested Investigative/Response Checksheet

### Investigative outline – bite investigation protocol
Immediate actions for first responders

1.  Secure the scene from contamination. Exclude unnecessary personnel. Identify condition of victim and of suspect animal(s). If animal(s) are alive, contain safely.
2.  Identify and secure potential witnesses. Separate them from each other and from the immediate scene.
3.  Exclude media from filming victim or actual scene until after all processing and removal is complete.

## Initial response – animals

1.  Observe animal(s) demeanour while handling immediate tasks. Take notes. How are they acting towards responders? Others? Each other? Are they aggressive, fearful, or quiet? Watch for unusual behaviours – excessive salivation, chewing on selves or unusual objects. Vomiting? Try to prevent animal(s) from eating or drinking before capture and testing.
2.  Physically capture/secure the animal(s) and separate. MAKE SURE YOU ARE FULLY GLOVED BEFORE YOU TOUCH THE ANIMAL TO AVOID CONTAMINATING WITH HUMAN DNA. Do not secure multiple animals in same kennel. Ensure they are placed in clean kennel.
3.  If animal(s) vomited or defecated at the scene, collect for analysis.
4.  The next priority is sample collection. Animal(s) may have to be sedated to handle safely – if so document type and dosage of sedative. Once animal(s) is safely restrained and docile, collect DNA swabs of upper and lower jaw area of each animal. Examine animal for visible signs of blood or fluids on fur. If any is seen, either use swabs to collect or cut and collect fur in the stained areas. If possible re-examine for further stains or fluids using ultraviolet lamp. Have a veterinarian evacuate the stomach of each animal and save the contents separately for testing for human tissue or DNA. Document any pieces of tissue visible in the stomach contents safely – suggest labelling as 'potential tissue – unknown origin' unless you are absolutely sure it is human tissue. The tests will positively identify it later. Have blood samples from each dog collected and preserved for testing. Two 5ml tubes for each animal should be sufficient.
5.  If the animal is deceased at the scene, the same samples must be collected. A veterinarian or medical examiner can dissect the stomach for contents, etc. Use a clean body bag to transport the animal after external samples are taken to avoid contamination. Try to avoid using simple rubbish bags, blankets, etc. If you have to cover the animal during scene processing, use a clean sheet from EMS and retain the sheet with the body after transport. Blood samples must also be collected from each animal and should be gathered by a veterinarian or technician using care to prevent contamination of the sample.
6.  Once samples are collected from the animal they must be identified securely. Check for microchipping. If animal is not microchipped, have veterinarian immediately microchip

each involved animal and use chip numbers to label all samples for continuity. Simple photos are not enough.

7.  If animal is alive, transport and secure properly at the appropriate facility. An animal involved or implicated in a fatality must not be allowed to remain in the custody of the owners during the investigation. These animal(s) must be contained securely and separately. Keep them apart from other animals and each other. Only a limited number of experienced personnel should be allowed direct contact with these animals.

8.  If at all possible, even if the owners request or permit euthanasia, keep the animals alive for evaluation by a behaviour expert. Observation and evaluation of the animals may give valuable information regarding recreating the incident. Don't be in a hurry to destroy the animals.

9.  If the animal is deceased at the scene and rabies testing is needed, request that the relevant laboratory use only the minimum brain tissue needed for testing and return the rest of the brain. Also ask it to retain and return the animal's head, keeping chain of custody, so that bite impressions and comparisons can be made. The animal's brain should be examined by a skilled veterinarian for evidence of lesion or physical abnormality that may have affected behaviour.

    a)  NOTE: If law enforcement personnel are forced to destroy the animal at the scene for safety reasons, please instruct them to shoot for the centre of body mass, not a head shot. Heads are a small, moving target, well armoured, and damage to the brain and jaw of the dog may limit information needed for full investigation.

## Initial response – human victim(s)

1.  Treat the scene like any homicide: control access, protect evidence, prevent contamination. REMEMBER – HUMAN HOMICIDE SUSPECTS MAY USE A DOG ATTACK/DOG CAUSED DAMAGE TO CONCEAL OTHER CRIMES.

2.  Take as many samples as possible on the scene before the body is disturbed. Seek blood, tissue, hair, and other fluids in the immediate surrounding area.

3.  Limit access to the body and the general scene until after photos have been taken. The disturbed ground around the scene may give clues to the event, such as fleeing footsteps, initial impact with the ground and subsequent dragging, etc. Document the physical scene in detail. Look for evidence that may indicate an additional animal involved, such as blood stains going up to a fence, etc.

4.  Collect samples of fluids, tissue, hair and fibres from the surrounding area. A person may actually be killed in one place and then dragged, sometimes by an animal that did not participate in the actual death.

5.  Have the medical examiner take swab samples from within the wounds. Canine DNA can be individually compared and identified, so the dog that inflicted a specific bite can be identified.

6.  Have detailed photos, including reference measurements, taken of all bite wounds. Such photos can be compared later with bite moulds and documentation to determine which dog bit where.

7. Ask the medical examiner to identify, as far as possible, the bite(s) that are the proximate cause of death, along with which bites are ante-mortem, and which tissue damage was post-mortem. A dog may have inflicted damage after death that did not participate in the actual killing. Cases have occurred wherein people were murdered, the body was placed with dogs and they were induced to bite the dead person to confuse or obscure the actual mode of death.

8. Document any scratches, dirt marks, or other non-fatal wounds to determine whether there are indicative of flight, defence, etc.

# CHAPTER 15

# The Forensics of Dog Bites

## Annamaria Passantino

## 15.1 Introduction

As has been discussed in other chapters, there are many different causes and 'risk factors' that may contribute to a bite event, but much may also be learned from the investigation of the dog bite itself. Indeed, in cases of fatal dog attacks, the bite may be the primary source of evidence in the case. This chapter examines the forensic process as it relates specifically to the examination of a bite from a dog per se; other chapters deal with the investigation of bites from other perspectives, such as a medical one to allow repair and reconstruction (Chapter 21), the wider forensic investigatory procedure that should follow a dog bite incident (Chapter 14), or the anatomy of the dog bite wound (Chapter 16).

## 15.2 Approaches for identifying the dog that has inflicted a bite

In most cases of non-fatal animal bites, the victim usually describes the circumstances and identifies the animal. While the cause of death may be readily apparent in cases of fatal dog attacks, an understanding of how and why the attack occurred still requires a complete investigation, and if there is more than one dog in the house, the role of different dogs in the fatality may not be immediately apparent. As with any death investigation, information (including videography, photographs and collection of trace evidence, if applicable) should be gathered at the scene.

Accurate photographic documentation of a crime scene is a crucial component of any venture into evidence collection, especially when it applies to recording potential bite marks inflicted on humans (Wright and Golden, 2010).

Table 15.1 describes a forensic approach to a fatal dog attack (De Munnynck and Van de Voorde, 2002) (see also Chapter 14).

**Table 15.1** Forensic investigation of fatal dog attack (Source: De Munnynck and Van de Voorde, 2002).

| Investigation | Stages | Evidence |
|---|---|---|
| Scene investigation | Information | Circumstances, witness, age of victims, dog breed, etc. |
| | Observation | Traces, environmental conditions, position of the body, etc. |
| | Collection | Trace evidence, blood samples, etc. |
| | Documentation | Photographs, sketches, diagrams, etc. |
| Examination of the victim | Information | Age, relationship to dog, health status, psychological profile, etc. |
| | External examination (preferably at the scene) | Bite marks (tear and hole), defence wounds, post-mortem changes, injuries, health status, etc. |
| | Internal examination | Collection of:<br>   – Trace evidence;<br>   – Samples for toxicological and DNA analysis<br>Cause/mechanism of death |
| | Toxicology | Identifications of dog hairs found on victim, etc. |
| | DNA analysis | Identifications of dog hairs found on victim, etc. |
| Examination of the dog | Information | Age, owner, previous behaviour, health history, relationship to victim, etc. |
| | External examination | Collection of trace evidence (blood, cloth, soil, hairs, etc.) |
| | Internal examination | Collection of oral and gastric contents, blood, brain tissue, urine, etc. |
| | Toxicology | Toxic substances, stimulating substances, etc. |
| | Microbiology | Exclusion of rabies, infections, etc. |

## 15.3  Bite patterns

If suspect dogs are available for examination, comparative bite mark analysis can be performed. In fact, a careful analysis of the dental characteristics and features of a bite mark may help to identify whether the biting injury was self-inflicted, caused by an aggressor, an animal, or at the very least may exclude a suspect (Pretty and Sweet, 2001).

Bites produced by dogs often cause much damage, with tissue laceration and avulsion of underlying muscle, damage to vasculature and, possibly, internal organs (Cowel and Penwick, 1989; Shamir et al., 2002), while human bites include a wide range of injuries from bruising, abrasions, lacerations and occasionally tissue avulsion. Each injury should therefore be evaluated to determine whether it was produced by human or animal teeth. The domestic dog (*Canis familiaris*) and humans have a notably distinct morphology of the teeth and arches. This distinction requires a comparative knowledge of dental anatomy of the two species (James, 2006). One parameter commonly considered helpful in identifying the origin of bite wounds is the distance between the canine teeth marks left on the victim. The distance between the upper canines in an adult human can range from 25 to 40mm.

According to some studies (Murmann et al., 2006) the intercanine distance may vary with the animal's breed and weight. This distance in the North American domestic dog ranges from 13.0 to 48.0mm in the maxilla, while for the mandible there is a range of 6.0 to 49.0mm. Thus, the distance may help exclude certain subjects when there are several suspects.

An accurate image is particularly important since the comparative analysis of potential suspects to the bite is entirely dependent on how skilfully the photographic images of the injury are recorded. For example, the bite site should be photographed using digital photography. Taking a picture of the lesion from a distance, showing the tissues around it, as well as close-up views for smaller lesions, with scales, is very useful for illustrating the description. A thorough documentation of the necropsy with pictures is very helpful, and a correct interpretation of the lesions, and use of correct terminology, is essential to be used in a court. All photographs must include the date, case number, and a scale/rule. The photographic procedures should be performed by the forensic odontologist or under the odontologist's direction to encourage accurate and comprehensive documentation of the bite site.

Scene investigation or 'locus' may be the best (or only) opportunity to establish the breed of the dog that bit. Examining a body within its scene is similar to taking a medical history; indeed the importance of the scene in forensic pathology is analogous to the importance of the medical history in diagnostic veterinary pathology. The process requires practice and skill, and the information should be critical, helpful, make a contribution, and it should not be wholly misleading.

- Detailed photographs (as outlined above) and body diagrams of the dogs as well as photographs of collars, scars and evidence of prior veterinary care are useful when the identity and owner are unknown. Information on whether or not the attack was witnessed will assist with conclusive identity of the aggressor. Further, the relationship of the dog to the victim, presence or absence of restraints, any history of aggressive behaviour, may be helpful in elucidating the reasons for the attack (for further investigation of this regard, see Chapter 14.).
- The examination of the victim should include identification of bite marks and defensive injuries. The American Board of Forensic Odontology has established specific guidelines to standardise the analysis of bite marks in the area of human identification, bite mark investigation and analysis. These standards and guidelines may evolve over time, and will be updated as necessary (for further details, see American Board of Forensic Odontology (ABFO) Inc. Guidelines for bite mark analysis. Diplomates Reference Manual Section III: Policies, Procedures, Guidelines & Standards Manual. 2009: 110–126).

Tables 15.2 and 15.3 describe the main examinations that are normally suggested during the investigation. However, the marks left behind do not always show the full arch and the distortions produced by the elasticity and retractility of tissues, movement and amount of contact can lead to misinterpretation. Punctures, lacerations and avulsions of skin and soft tissue are caused by a combination of biting, crushing and tearing. Forensic pathologists typically observe multiple tear wounds with adjacent puncture wounds, the so-called the 'hole-and-a-tear' effect. The puncture wound, a round hole, is made by the canine tooth of

**Table 15.2** Animal bite protocol.

Examine the animal for blood and visible transfer of evidence from the victim.
Gather the victim's DNA from the animal's claws.
Immediately take the animal to a veterinarian to induce vomiting.
Strain the contents and preserve tissue and cloth fragments or other foreign bodies found in the vomitus for comparison with victim and clothing.
Quarantine the animal for collection of faeces and compare the evidence of hair, tissue, bone, and clothing.
Take dental impression of the suspect animal; create and pour models in plastic.
Do a rabies test on both victim and animal since the animal's owner may later claim that the animal, unknown to him/her, may have been rabid.

**Table 15.3** Animal bite victim evidence.

Swab for animal saliva and DNA left on the victim.
Retain the victim's clothing for DNA analysis.
Analyse the clothing for teeth marks.
Follow ABFO guidelines for preservation of bite-mark evidence.

4

either the upper or lower jaw on one side that serves as an anchorage, while the other teeth cut into the flesh, causing stretch lacerations in the process of biting, shaking and tearing. This should be considered pathognomonic for dog bites, especially when accompanied by tissue defects and claw marks, the latter being narrow, superficial linear abrasions arranged parallel to each other, four or five in number and usually found near the bite. To identify a lesion as a dog bite wound it should have ragged and irregular wound edges, show multiple, parallel, linear scratches or drying scuff abrasions, include a puncture wound and sometimes an avulsion with irregular borders resembling a dental arch print. Analysing the clothing for teeth marks is also an important feature of the examination.

The oral cavity constitutes a key part of clinical examination of any animal that is involved in an attack. It is important in forensic work because bite wounds are often a cause of injury, infection or death in humans and other species. Furthermore, the effect of a bite is influenced by both the morphology of the oral cavity and the micro-organisms that it harbours (see Chapter 20). The oral cavity can provide other information as diet or health status. Moreover examination of the dog's oral and gastric contents may reveal blood, tissue and/or clothing from the victim. All animal-inflicted injuries must be differentiated into those that occurred ante-mortem and those that were caused post-mortem. The latter are the result of predation, for example, by dogs (Shepherd, 2003). Post-mortem predation is commonly characterised by lack of inflammation or other reaction and it tends to be concentrated on exposed, unclothed areas in humans (Cooper and Cooper, 2007).

The examination of the dog should be carried out for trace evidence that could link it to the victim (e.g. blood, urine, hair, clothing fibres) and that can help to reconstruct the event (e.g. soil, grass). If the dog suspected of having bitten has been destroyed it should be subjected to a post-mortem examination by an approved veterinary pathologist. This should note any pathological conditions (i.e. brain neoplasms, encephalitis, etc.) that might have affected behaviour (Munro and Munro, 2008). Factors to consider with regards to the decision to destroy the dog(s) include:

- Risk to public at and around scene
- Risk to officers handling the dog(s)
- Consent for destruction by owner
- Need to secure and preserve evidence, i.e., mouth and paw swabs, stomach contents, etc.
- Loss of evidence following destruction, i.e. physical conformation, behavioural assessment.

## 15.4  DNA examination

Deoxyribonucleic acid (DNA) analysis both of blood found on the dogs' coat or in their mouths, and of hairs found at the scene of the crime or on the victim's body, has gained importance in forensic investigations. In fact, the analysis of canine DNA from swabs and bandages directly from the wound and its surrounding area will provide stronger evidence of the identity of the perpetrator than other forms of evidence such as hair samples or blood and saliva stains found on the clothes of the victim (Eichmann et al., 2004). It is interesting to underline that,

> 'The remnants of canine saliva collected directly from the bite or the wound bandage need to be suitable for canine STR profiling. As observed in human DNA analysis, saliva has been recovered and successfully analysed from various substrates including human skin and human bite marks. Canine saliva should be best recovered from the area directly surrounding the human wound, where the dog's gums and flews contacted the skin of the bitten person.'

(Eichmann et al., 2004). The analysis could be prejudiced, for example, by the mixture with human blood in wound bandages, which potentially has adverse effects on the possibility of reconstruction of the canine-specific STR profile. There seems to be a correlation between the amount of blood – most likely of human origin – on the collected material and the ability to retrieve a canine-specific STR profile because of the amount of saliva surrounding the wound, as a consequence of the intensive contact (Eichmann et al., 2005). The study of hairs using mitochondrial DNA sequencing or analysis of the presence of canine-specific short tandem repeat systems using fluorescently labelled multiplex PCR has proved useful in reliably linking dogs to the scene of a crime or attack (von Wurmb-Schwark et al., 2009). The canine-specific DNA profiling of dog bite marks proved to be a promising way of investigation of forensic accidents involving dogs.

## 15.5  Other exams

Toxicological analyses may be performed if desired. For example, a urine sample should be examined for the presence of stimulating substances. Tissue may be submitted for microbiological analysis to rule out rabies and other infectious processes. With regard to rabies, it is necessary to remember that if the virus is isolated from saliva, positive immunofluorescent

**Table 15.4** Bite mark case report.

| Sections | Description |
| --- | --- |
| **Introduction** | This section provides the background information, the 'who, what, when, where and why' data related to the case. |
| **Inventory of Evidence Received** | This section lists all evidence received by the Forensic Pathologist/Odontologist/Veterinarian and details the source of the evidence. |
| **Inventory of Evidence Collected** | This section lists the nature, source, and authority for evidence collected by the Forensic Pathologist/Odontologist/Veterinarian. |
| **Opinion Regarding the Nature of the Patterned Injury or Injuries** | This section states the author's opinion as to whether the patterned injuries in question are bite marks. |
| **Methods of Analysis** | This section describes the analytic methods used for the patterned injuries determined to be bite marks. |
| **Results of Analyses** | This section describes the results of the comparisons and analyses. |
| **Opinion** | This section states the author's opinion of the relationship between one or more bite marks and a suspected biter or biters. |
| **Disclaimer** | Disclaimer statements may be included to convey that the opinion or opinions are based upon the evidence reviewed through the date of the report. The author may reserve the right to file amended reports should additional evidence become available. |

skin biopsies or virus neutralising antibody (from cerebrospinal fluid, or serum of a non–vaccinated patient) will indicate a diagnosis (Rupprecht, 1996).

Different bacteria can be isolated from dog bite wounds and in some situations these may also help through crossmatching to identify the dog that has delivered a specific injury. In the case of non-fatal attacks, the investigation of bacterial flora may have specific treatment value, and establish that a subsequent infection was indeed related to the bite rather than some other coincident event. The most common bacteria are *Staphylococcus aureus*, *Staphylococcus epidermidis*, various Streptococcus species, Corynebacterium, and Gram-negative such as E. coli. Other uncommon pathogens that should be considered include *Eikenella corrodens* (a cause of infection in human bites), *Bartonella henselae* (the cause of cat scratch disease), *Francisella tularensis* (the cause of tularemia), Leptospira spp. (which causes leptospirosis), *Pasteurella multocida* (it can cause very rapid cellulitis, local septic arthritis, osteomyelitis, tenosynovitis, bacteremia, etc.) *Streptobacillus moniliformis* and *Spirillum minus* (which causes rat bite fever) (Fleisher, 1999). Other severe infections can develop later after bites as a result of either hematogenous spread (e.g. sepsis, endocarditis, and meningitis) or undetected penetration of deeper structures (e.g. brain abscesses and septic arthritis). When fever occurs in immunosuppressed patients after a dog bite, the possibility of an infection with *Capnocytophaga canimorsus*, an invasive organism, should be considered. Capnocytophaga species were recovered from 4.7% of the wounds cultured by Talan et al. (1999). *C. canimorsus* can cause septic arthritis, endocarditis, renal failure, sepsis, and/or meningitis. See Chapter 20 for further details on the microbiology of dog bites.

A bite mark case report will be a useful outcome. The report may be structured into the sections reported in Table 15.4.

## 15.6 Conclusions

Biting injures are complex and the evidence collection, analysis and interpretation should be handled with caution. Generally, the courts require the forensic experts to identify which specific dog or human/other animal caused the damage or fatal bite in an effort to establish the owner/controller of the animal. For this reason, the forensic evaluation of a fatal dog attack requires an integrated approach in association with veterinary pathologists involving review of the circumstances of death, examination of the death scene, and autoptic examination of the victim. In certain cases, consultation with a veterinarian, wildlife officers, forensic pathologists, odontologists and anthropologists might prevent, reduce or correct misinterpretation of animal bites. A team approach provides the best opportunity for thorough documentation of circumstances, scene analysis, and proper photographic documentation.

## 15.7 References

Anon (2003). Non-fatal dog bite-related injuries treated in hospital emergency departments-United States, 2001. *Morbidity and Mortality Weekly Report* 52, 605–610.

Centers for Disease Control (2003). Nonfatal dog bite-related injuries treated in hospital emergency departments – United States, 2001. *Morbidity and Mortality Weekly Report* 52, 605–608.

Clark, M. A., Sandusky, G. E., Hawley, D. A., Pless, J. E., Fardal, P. M., Tate, L. R. (1991). Fatal and near fatal animal bite injuries. *Journal of Forensic Sciences* 36(4), 1256–1261.

Cleaveland, S., Fevre, E. M., Kaare, M., Coleman, P. G. (2002). Estimating human rabies mortality in the United Republic of Tanzania from dog bite injuries. *Bulletin of the World Health Organisation* 80, 304–310.

Cooper, J. E., Cooper, M. E. (2007). Introduction to Veterinary and Comparative Forensic Medicine. Blackwell Publishing, p.15.

Cowel, A. K., Penwick, R. C. (1989). Dog bite wounds: a study of 93 cases. *Compendium on Continuing Education for the Practicing Veterinarian*, 11: 313–320.

De Munnynck, K., Van de Voorde, W. (2002). Forensic approach of fatal dog attacks: a case report and literature review. *International Journal of Legal Medicine* 116, 295–300.

Duffy, D. L., Hsu, Y., Serpell, J. A. (2008). Breed differences in canine aggression. *Applied Animal Behaviour Science* 114(3-4), 441–460.

Eichmann, C., Berger, B., Steinlechner, M., Parson, W. (2005). Estimating the probability of identity in a random dog population using 15 highly polymorphic canine STR markers. *Forensic Science International* 151(1), 37–44.

Eichmann, C., Berger, B., Reinhold, M., Lutz, M., Parson, W. (2004). Canine-specific STR typing of saliva traces on dog bite wounds. *International Journal of Legal Medicine* 118, 337–342.

Fleisher, G. R. (1999). The Management of Bite Wounds. *The New England Journal of Medicine* January 340(2), 138–140.

Gershman, K. A., Sacks, J. J., Wright, J. C. (1994). Which dogs bite? A case-control study of risk factors. *Pediatrics* 93:913–917.

Gilchrist, J., Sacks, J. J., White, D., Kresnow, M. (2008). Dog bites: still a problem? *Injury Prevention* 14, 296–301.

Horisberger, U., Stärk, K. D. C., Rüfenacht, J., Pillonel, C., Steiger, A. (2004). The epidemiology of dog bite injuries in Switzerland–characteristics of victims, biting dogs and circumstances. *Anthrozoos* 17, 320–339.

James, H. (2006). Good bite mark evidence: a case report. *Journal of Forensic Odonto-Stomatology* 24, 12–13.

Kahn, A., Bauche, P., Lamoureux, J. (2003). Child victims of dog bites treated in emergency departments: a prospective survey. *European Journal of Pediatrics* 162, 254–258.

Keuster, T. D., Lamoureux, J., Kahn, A. (2006). Epidemiology of dog bites: A Belgian experience of canine behaviour and public health concerns. *The Veterinary Journal* 172, 482–487.

Kreisfeld, R., Harrison, J. (2005). Dog-related injuries. NISU Briefing. Australian Institute for Health and Welfare. Available at www.nisu.flinders.edu.au/pubs/reports/2005/injcat75.php. Accessed: 3 March 2015.

Mathews, J. R., Lattal, K. A. (1994). A behavioral analysis of dog bites to children. *Journal of Developmental & Behavioral Pediatrics* 15, 44–52.

Miller, S. J., Copass, M., Johansen, K., Winn, H. R. (1993). Stroke following Rottweiler attack. *Annals of Emergency Medicine* 22, 262–264.

Morgan, M., Palmer, J. (2007). Dog bites. *British Medical Journal* 334, 413–417.

Munro, R. and Munro, H. M. C. (2008). Animal Abuse and Unlawful Killing: Forensic veterinary pathology. Saunders Elsevier, *Edinburgh and London,* pp.86.

Murmann, D. C., Brumit, P. C., Schrader, B. A., Senn, D. R. (2006). A comparison of animal jaws and bite mark patterns. *Journal of Forensic Sciences* 51(4), 846 860.

Overall, K. L., Love, M. (2001). Dog bites to humans – demography, epidemiology, injury, and risk. *Journal of American Veterinary Medical Association* 218, 1923–1934.

Ozanne-Smith, J., Ashby, K., Stathakis, V. Z. (2001) Dog bite and injury prevention – analysis, critical review, and research agenda. *Injury Prevention* 7, 321–326.

Padar, Z., Angyal, M., Egyed, B., Furedi, S., Woller, J., Zoldag, L., Fekete, S. (2001). Canine microsatellite polymorphisms as the resolution of an illegal animal death case in a Hungarian Zoological Garden. *International Journal of Legal Medicine* 115, 79–81.

Pretty, I. A., Sweet, D. (2001). The scientific basis for human bite mark analyses - a critical review. *Science & Justice* 41, 85–92.

Rosado, B., Garcia-Belenguer, S., Leon, M., Palacio, J. A. (2009). Comprehensive study of dog bites in Spain, 1995-2004. *The Veterinary Journal* 179, 383–391.

Rupprecht, C. E. (1996). Chapter 61 Rhabdoviruses: Rabies Virus. In: Medical Microbiology. 4th edition. Baron, S., Editor. Galveston (TX): University of Texas Medical Branch at Galveston.

Sacks, J. J., Lockwood, R., Hornreich, J., Sattin, R. W. (1996). Fatal dog attacks, 1989–1994. *Pediatrics* 97, 891–895.

Sacks, J. J., Sattin, R. W., Bonzo, S. E. (1989). Dog Bite Related Fatalities from 1979 through 1988. *Journal of the American Veterinary Medical Association* 262(11), 1489–1492.

Sacks, J. J., Sinclair, L., Gilchrist, J., Golab, G. C., Lockwood, R. (2000). Breeds of dogs involved in fatal human attacks in the United States between 1979 and 1998. *Journal of American Veterinary Medical Association* 217, 836–840.

4

Savolainen, P., Lunceberg, J. (1999). Forensic evidence based on mtDNA from dog and wolf hairs. *Journal of Forensic Science* 44, 77–81.

Schneider, P. M., Seo, Y., Rittner, C. (1999). Case report: forensic mtDNA hair analysis excludes a dog from having caused a traffic accident. *International Journal of Legal Medicine* 112, 315–316.

Shamir, M. H., Leisner, S., Klement, E. Gonen, E., Johnston, D. E. (2002). Dog bite wounds in dogs and cats: a retrospective study of 196 cases. *Journal of Veterinary Medicine Series A* 49(2), 107–112.

Shepherd, R. (2003). Simpson's Forensic Medicine, 12th edn. Arnold, London, UK.

Sudarshan, M. K., Mahendra, B. J., Madhusudana, S. N., Narayana, D. H. A., Rahman, A., Rao, N. S., X-Meslin, F., Lobo, D., Ravikumar, K., Gangaboraia, H. (2006). An epidemiological study of animal bites in India: Results of a WHO sponsored national-multi-centric rabies survey. *The Journal of Communicable Disease* 38, 32–39.

Talan, D. A., Citron, D. M., Abrahamian, F. M., Moran, G. J., Goldstein, E. J. C. (1999). Bacteriologic analysis of infected dog and cat bites. *The New England Journal of Medicine* 340, 85–92.

von Wurmb-Schwark, N., Preusse-Prange, A., Heinrich, A., Simeoni, E., Bosch, T., Schwark, T., (2009). A new multiplex-PCR comprising autosomal and y-specific STRs and mitochondrial DNA to analyze highly degraded material. *Forensic Science International*: Genetics. 3, 96–103

Weiss, H. B., Friedman, D. I., Coben, J. H. (1998). Incidence of dog bite injuries treated in emergency departments. *The Journal of the American Medical Association* 279, 51–53.

Wiseman, N. E., Chochinov, H., Fraser, V. (1983). Major dog attack injuries in children. *Journal of Pediatric Surgery* 18, 533–536.

Wright, F. D., Golden, G. S. (2010). Forensic Dental Photography, Ch 11 in *Forensic Dentistry 2nd Ed.*, edited by Senn, D. R., Stimson, P. G. CRC Press – Taylor & Francis Group, pp.203–204.

# CHAPTER 16

# Anatomy of Dog Bite Injuries

## *James Crosby*

**This chapter contains graphic photographs that some readers may find distressing.**

## 16.1 Introduction

The description of dog bites can be a highly emotional issue, with perceptions of severity replacing objective standards. Establishing and applying consistent standards for the physical evaluation of a dog bite based on quantifiable, reproducible criteria is essential.

A bite mark can be generally defined as a pattern made by teeth in a substrate (Bernstein, 2005). A dog bite injury is a patterned injury. Patterned injuries represent a transfer of a pattern from one medium to another (Bernstein, 2005). In the case of dog bites, the pattern involved is that of the dog's teeth and jaw, as transferred to the tissue and/or bone of the victim. As in any patterned injury, the physical dimensions and characteristics of the injury can assist in determining not only the source of the injury, but can impart details such as direction and intensity of the injury-producing instrument (see Chapter 14).

In a dog bite, the instruments causing the injury are the dog's teeth – and to a lesser extent the jaw and skull as the framework that supports the teeth. Adult domestic dogs typically have forty-two teeth: twenty upper and twenty-two lower. These teeth engage in varying ways, depending on the angle and depth of the engagement. The orientation of the teeth in typical domestic canine dentition is illustrated in Figure 16.1. The teeth of a domestic canine engage differently, due to morphology, than human bites. Dorion (2005) describes the engagement of canine dentition by saying,

*'Tooth alignment along the dental arch from canine to the last molar does not follow a straight path … the dentition penetrates unevenly as a result of the different sizes of teeth, different horizontal heights of teeth, and the uneven anteroposterior alignment of teeth.'*

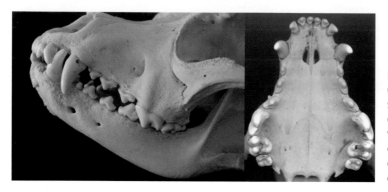

**Figure 16.1** Lateral view (left) of domestic canine skull showing longitudinal orientation of teeth: ventral view (right) of domestic canine maxilla showing grouping of teeth and orientation.

Thus, the examiner must keep in mind that a dog's dentition may penetrate irregularly depending on where in the dental arch primary contact occurs.

For analysis purposes the dental arch is broken into several groups of teeth, as can be seen in the two views shown in Figure 16.1:

- From the centre there are six incisors each, top and bottom. Incisors are generally elongated side to side, wedge-shaped front to back, and are designed for cutting and shearing.
- Next in line are four canines, two each top and bottom. The canines are rounded or oval in profile and extend approximately twice or more the length, gum line to tip, of typical incisors. The canine teeth perform several functions. As the longest teeth these are usually a dog's initial physical contact point with whatever object or item they encounter. The sharp, circular profile of these teeth allows a dog to pierce the target. The extension of these teeth beyond the level of engagement of the incisors allows the dog to moderate and control the level of damage done to a target. This limitation of damage is well illustrated by the Level 3 or moderated warning/communication bite (see Table 16.1) In this type of engagement there is a brief, inhibited contact with a target that results in either no puncture of the skin surface or at most limited, shallow puncture wounds that are unlikely to cause significant physical damage, though they may transmit infection.
- Past the canines are the premolars and molars. These teeth are generally for ripping and chewing food. In severe bites the forward-most of these teeth may engage the target. This usually involves the engagement of a limb such as an arm or smaller diameter leg that a dog may get deeply into its grasp. A large bite to softer, looser tissue such as in the abdomen, where fat and loose skin may be available, may also show deeper grasping and tearing, although most contact will still be centred on the forward teeth. Full engagement tearing by two opposing dogs struggling over possession of a child's body is shown in Figure 16.2. This assisted in confirming that both dogs in question participated in the attack.

## 16.2 Assessment of severity

In assessing a bite wound there are two sets of criteria that must be considered: the medical assessment of a bite as that assessment determines treatment (see Chapter 19 and 21) and the

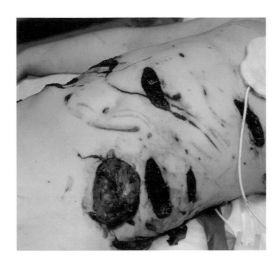

**Figure 16.2** Torn abdomen view of severe bite to human child. Extensive lateral tearing with full engagements of jaws by two large dogs contesting each other over possession of the child's body. Wounds inflicted ante-mortem and peri-mortem.

severity of the bite as seen from an investigative standpoint (see Chapter 14 and 15). These must be kept separate: they serve different purposes.

A surgeon may decide that a particular wound needs a particular treatment strategy. The treatment strategy can be dependent on factors beyond the dog. Placement of the wound (face v buttocks, for instance), age of the victim, likelihood of permanent scarring, infection, and others may well affect the clinical decision regarding sutures or reconstructive surgery (see Chapter 21).

For assessment that addresses behaviour and potential prosecution issues, and to compare separate bites dispassionately, a quantifiable tool and analysis must be adhered to apart from medical treatment decisions.

The severity of an attack depends on three factors: the intensity of the bite, the frequency of the bite, and the intent of the bite. In other words, how hard did the dog bite? How many times did the dog bite? What was the purpose of the bite? Did the dog bite once, with relative restraint, to gain space to flee from a frightening situation? Did the dog bite repeatedly but still hold back? Or did the dog bite once but very hard, with firm grip and tearing, shaking motions?

Assessment of bites based on quantifiable criteria is the purpose of Dr Ian Dunbar's Bite Assessment Tool, shown below in table form. This assessment tool ranks dog bites on six levels. The six levels, with the exception of Level 6, which is defined by result, are defined by the measurable engagement of teeth – how many, how deep, and how many bites.

## 16.3 Behaviour and bites

The purposes of bites are varied. They include establishing distance; settling social disagreements; control of the dog's environment; manipulation of objects; defence from a perceived threat; and predation (See Chapter 1).

The behavioural purpose of the bite can be related to the outcome scale of the bite as described below:

**Table 16.1** Dunbar bite scale. Dunbar, I. Dunbar dog bite assessment scale – official, available at: www.dogtalk.com/BiteAssessmentScalesDunbarDTMRoss.pdf

| | |
|---|---|
| Level 1 | Obnoxious or aggressive behaviour but no skin contact by teeth. | **Levels 1** and **2** comprise well over 99% of dog incidents. The dog is certainly not dangerous and more likely to be fearful, rambunctious, or out of control. Wonderful prognosis. Quickly resolve the problem with basic training (control) — especially oodles of Classical Conditioning, numerous repetitive Retreat n' Treat, Come/Sit/Food Reward and Back-up/Approach/Food Reward sequences, progressive desensitisation handling exercises, plus numerous bite-inhibition exercises and games. Hand feed only until resolved; do NOT waste potential food rewards by feeding from a bowl. |
| Level 2 | Skin contact by teeth but no skin puncture. However, may be skin nicks (less than one tenth of an inch deep) and slight bleeding caused by forward or lateral movement of teeth against skin, but no vertical punctures. | |
| Level 3 | One to four punctures from a single bite with no puncture deeper than half the length of the dog's canine teeth. May be lacerations in a single direction, caused by victim pulling hand away, owner pulling dog away, or gravity (little dog jumps, bites and drops to floor). | **Level 3:** Prognosis is fair to good, provided that you have owner compliance. However, treatment is both time-consuming and not without danger. Rigorous bite-inhibition exercises are essential. |
| Level 3b | Multiple bites at Level 3. | |
| Level 4 | One to four punctures from a single bite with at least one puncture deeper than half the length of the dog's canine teeth. May also have deep bruising around the wound (dog held on for N seconds and bore down) or lacerations in both directions (dog held on and shook its head from side to side). | **Level 4:** The dog has insufficient bite inhibition and is very dangerous. Prognosis is poor because of the difficulty and danger of trying to teach bite inhibition to an adult hard-biting dog and because absolute owner-compliance is rare. Only work with the dog in exceptional circumstances, e.g., the owner is a dog professional and has sworn 100% compliance. Make sure the owner signs a form in triplicate stating that they understand and take full responsibility that: 1. The dog is a Level 4 biter and is likely to cause an equivalent amount of damage WHEN it bites again (which it most probably will) and should, therefore, be confined to the home at all times and only allowed contact with adult owners. 2. Whenever children or guests visit the house, the dog should be confined to a single locked room or roofed, chain-link run with the only keys kept on a chain around the neck of each adult owner (to prevent children or guests entering the dog's confinement area.) 3. The dog is muzzled before leaving the house and only leaves the house for visits to a veterinary clinic. 4. The incidents have all been reported to the relevant authorities – animal control or police. Give the owners one copy, keep one copy for your files and give one copy to the dog's veterinarian. |
| Level 5 | Multiple-bite incident with at least two Level 4 bites or multiple-attack incident with at least one Level 4 bite in each. | **Level 5** and **6**: The dog is extremely dangerous and mutilates. The dog is simply not safe around people. I recommend euthanasia because the quality of life is so poor for dogs that have to live out their lives in solitary confinement. |
| Level 6 | Victim dead. | |

1. Dunbar suggests that Level 1 is a form of intimidation behaviour. This behaviour is often the initial negative contact between a human and a dog, and is probably the most common. A person, friendly or not, approaches a dog and the dog responds by growling, barking, and possibly lunging, and in general scares the target. Said human typically backs off immediately. This is a perfect example of clear and concise interspecies communication. For whatever reason, the dog is alarmed by the human's approach. The dog gives external signals, audible and visible, that he/she does not want any further advance by the human. The human acknowledges those signals and retreats.

2. Level 2 is the slightest level possible of physical contact between dog and human. Probably most 'aggressive dog' incidents never proceed past this point. Engagement of the dog's teeth is avoided. Scratches and/or bruising may be the result of the dog pushing back off the target, or from simple blunt snout contact.

3. Level 3 may best be termed 'engage and release'. In the 'engage and release' bite there is a single, very fast bite that is limited in force and usually strikes the closest target: a hand, an ankle, or a face in the case of a small child. The dog bites to drive back, or make a space to flee past a perceived threat. The substantive difference between a Level 2 bite and its escalation to Level 3 is the presence of clear, tooth-related injury. One or more canine teeth actually pierce the skin of the target. A Level 3b is more than one engagement of teeth at Level 3; the dog makes significant contact, but does not hold. There is no tearing or slashing, no clamping down; the victim is not dragged, pulled or shaken. There may be some surface (upper levels of the epidermis) tearing from a rapid withdrawal of the target (which is an understandable response, even if it makes matters worse), but it is strictly limited in depth. Withdrawal also shows clear directionality – the tear marks are directly in line with the removal direction of the limb or flesh. Dogs have a remarkable ability to control the strength of their bite. Pups appear to learn bite inhibition and control in the litter, both from their dam and from their littermates during play. This attack shows either less inhibitory control over a Level 2 attack, as the skin is broken, or an intentionally more serious bite aimed at achieving escape from the situation. Reduced inhibitions may arise from inadequate socialisation or medication (Hetts, 1999), but a more serious bite may reflect a higher level of arousal or fear due to the circumstances, perhaps as a result of temperament, which is also affected by early experience. This dog may perceive the threat to be greater, or that earlier signals have been ignored. This is believed to be the most common type of dog bite encountered as related by animal control authorities. According to Dunbar, and many others with relevant experience, animals involved in a bite at Level 1, 2, or 3 are those with the best chance of being safely retained by their owners, provided appropriate training and behavioural guidance is obtained.

4. A Level 4 bite is a major bite incident. More than just the canine teeth engage, and deeply. There is likely tearing, grasping and shaking. It is believed that a dog involved in this level bite intended to inflict significant damage. This may be extreme defensive behaviour from a threatened animal or relate to predatory behaviour that might ultimately lead to a kill. Although a dog that inflicts this type of injury may never bite again, if it does, it is believed that there is a high likelihood that it will be another major bite.

5. Multiple Level 4 bites are inflicted in a series of full force engagements. This dog is not expressing any socially related inhibition of the biting. This is the proverbial

'chainsaw with feet'. The animal in this type of incident is attacking with full intent to do massive damage to its intended target. An animal engaged in this sort of attack, (unless it is a trained police dog that is apprehending a combative suspect, which is a completely separate subject), is clearly a danger to the public, and to its owners. Prognosis for any sort of meaningful recovery for this dog is extremely poor, and if considering possible treatment of this dog, first consideration must be given to public safety and for the safety of owners or caretakers. Quality of life issues should also be a consideration in this case.

6.  When we consider a Level 6 bite we divert from quantifiable measurements of the bite itself to the outcome of the incident. This level is not necessarily composed of those Level 5 attacks that go on, unabated, until the human dies. These attacks are simply those that directly result in the death of a human.

    There are those that would argue, possibly from a biological perspective, against grouping all fatal incidents together. A single bite by a dog that happens to nick a major blood vessel could conceivably directly result in that person's death. Yet legally, and societally, we must consider these bites separately due to the extreme nature of their results.

    In almost all Level 6 cases in the United States the dogs are, by law, destroyed. A few cases exist wherein the dogs were allowed to be relocated to secure sanctuary, but those are extremely rare. In one case, when a dog named Onion killed one-year old Jeremiah Eskew-Shahan in the western US, the incident was thought to be due to many factors. Converging circumstances projected to be involved included time of day, lighting and the stress of the events prior to the bite. The fact that it was a single bite with immediate release differentiated this attack from those with multiple engagements, shaking, and tearing. Onion was relocated after a protracted legal battle (Keller v City of Henderson), but will never be permitted to live in a private home.

    Even though these dogs are destroyed it is essential that the incidents are investigated thoroughly, in order that we may learn from them. This may mean keeping the animal alive for a while after the incident to allow a professional behavioural evaluation of the animal first to see if there are any outstanding biological or psychological factors relating to the animal's behaviour that might help prevent a similar incident in future with another dog.

## 16.4 Documentation and collection of evidence

Bite marks can be documented by detailed photos that include a reference scale. A common reference tool is the ABFO (American Board of Forensic Odontology) photomacrographic scale (Hyzer and Krause, 1988). This tool is commonly available and provides a reference that, when included in evidentiary photographs, allows proper measurement and alignment of the target that can be supported in court testimony. Measurement can be conducted on a live dog, post-necropsy pre–defleshing, or may be conducted post-necropsy and after defleshing the skull. Figure 16.3 shows initial measurement of a defleshed skull. The scale used should be in the same plane as the plane of the bite, level with the base of the teeth, and parallel to the camera sensor plane. Caution is needed to make sure that during defleshing the teeth are not lost or displaced.

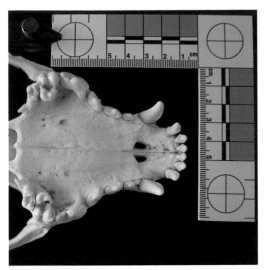

**Figure 16.3** Bite measurement of a canine jaw, ventral view of maxilla, post-defleshing using an ABFO #2 bite scale.

Bite marks can also be documented by using the techniques of tool mark casting. Flesh can retain the patterns of bite engagement, as can underlying bone if the bite is deep enough. Dams of malleable material can be placed surrounding a bite on a cadaver and casting material then poured to capture the detail. Casting material, whether to capture the profile of the bite or to document the subject dog's dentition, should be material that sets to a solid, inflexible state to maintain proper alignment and size measurement. Many orthodontic and regular dental casting materials are suitable.

We must keep several points in mind as we examine bite mark evidence. There are two classes of evidence when it comes to items such as bite marks: class characteristics and individual characteristics:

- Class characteristics are those that allow the assignment of evidentiary items into rough groups with characteristic common traits.
- Individual characteristics allow a piece of evidence to be attributed to a particular individual.

For instance, the morphology shown in a bite mark can establish whether a bite was inflicted by a dog or, for instance, a fox, a class of animal. DNA recovered from tissue at the scene may allow the identification of exactly which dog – or fox – was involved.

The collection of class characteristics and individual characteristics lead to the production of *identifying* evidence or *exclusionary* evidence. Identifying evidence is evidence that is identifiable to a single individual or item. Identifying characteristics must be permanent and unique. Examples of types of evidence that are considered identifying are fingerprints and DNA. In human cases, it is strongly suggested that bite mark comparison only be used as exculpatory evidence (Pretty, 2005). Serious debate exists as to whether a human's jaws, although they accumulate individual characteristics over a lifetime, are considered to be unique. Differences in jaw and dental morphology are not permanent; these details can change over time through a number of natural processes such as aging and natural wear. Although there are many potential points of comparison between dentition and bite marks, the question is if there are enough unique, permanent characteristics in a jaw, or a bite, that limit the marks produced to only a single, unique source for individual identification. Due caution would indicate that the potential uniqueness of a dog's dentition be subject to the same consideration.

Bite marks are, instead, best considered as exclusionary evidence. Individual characteristics can, depending on the potential pool of possible candidates, serve to include, or exclude, individual members of that pool if the size of the pool of candidates is sufficiently small. This means that, given a limited pool of potential suspects, if there are sufficient distinct markers, we may be able to exclude particular suspects from the ability to have produced those particular marks. Bites are either consistent with, or not consistent with, the physical characteristics of a particular dog.

As an example, in 2012 a Siberian Husky named Nikko was accused of killing three day old Howard Nicholson in his home in McKeesport, Pennsylvania. Although there were four dogs in the home at the time, Nikko was the only dog seized and accused. This author was called in to investigate the case. After examining the physical evidence, including details of Nikko's dentition and the autopsy documentation, Nikko was excluded from having inflicted the bite wounds on the infant based on significant differences in measurement and morphology of the bite wounds versus Nikko's jaws. The other three dogs were 'lost' by the local authorities and no further examination was possible. The court, after hearing arguments and examining the expert findings, ruled that Nikko was not the dog responsible and allowed Nikko to be removed from the jurisdiction and placed in safe sanctuary.

Dog bites have several parameters that can be examined, quantified, and compared. These are described below, but this topic is revisited within the broader context of the forensic process in Chapter 14.

* The number and positioning of teeth. Spacing of teeth varies based on age, physical size, breed, and individual differences. Irregular dentition in an older dog is illustrated in Figure 16.4.
* The breadth of the bite, the depth, and spacing of tooth marks are all bite characteristics based on dimension. Obviously, while keeping concerns such as tissue deformation in mind, simple dimensions are solid elimination criteria. A dog with an inter-canine distance of 2cm simply cannot make a pair of holes that are 5cm apart.

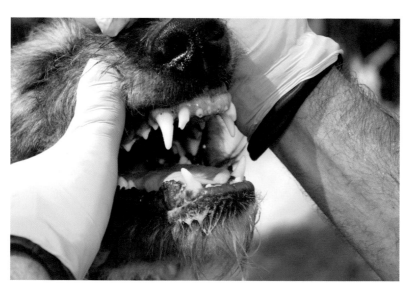

**Figure 16.4** Irregular canine dentition. This dog was excluded in a human fatality investigation based on the highly worn bite. DNA later confirmed the exclusion of this dog.

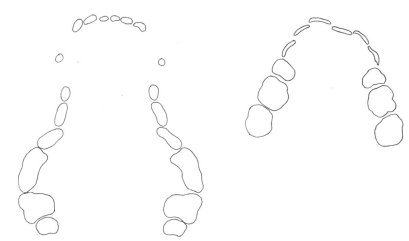

**Figure 16.5** Human and canine bite arch canine (left) v human (right) bite illustrated, approximately to scale. Note the size, shape, and orientation of the teeth. A key identifier is the presence of four incisors (human) v six incisors (canine).

4

- Overall morphology establishes more class characteristics. The hourglass shape of a generalised dog bite is clearly different from the typical bow shape of a human bite. When comparing them side by side, the rounder arc of a human bite is clear.
- In addition, if the bite is clear enough to distinguish, a simple count of incisors can easily differentiate human and canine bite as the typical human jaw has four incisors, whereas a dog has six. This simple difference has been a clarifying characteristic in a number of alleged dog bites over time, including the case of a dog named Phineas accused of biting a child in Missouri, USA, in 2013 (Patrick and Amber Sanders v City of Salem, Missouri). Examination of clear documentary photographs of that bite was sufficient to eliminate Phineas from the pool of possible candidates, and the morphology of the bite indicated strongly that the bite mark introduced as evidence in the case was human caused.
- Positioning of maxilla and mandibles, and gross alignment of the teeth engaged in a bite involving both upper and lower teeth engagement can assist in inclusion or elimination, since some dogs have teeth that are heavily misaligned, such as the English and French Bulldogs. Individual defects are more specific: these characteristics result from wear, damage, and injury. These include height above the gum line, broken edges and tips, missing or extremely worn teeth, and teeth that have broken longitudinally but remain in place. Alignment of individual teeth may also be influenced by injury or damage as they get twisted, pushed to one side, or shoved forwards or rearwards in relation to the surrounding teeth. Height, misalignment and angle of attack may reduce or obscure the engagement of observed oral dentition (Dorion, 2005). As stated in Lessig et al., (2006), 'The state of the dentition, the degree of breakdown and/or repair of the teeth may create a bite mark with a high level of individuality.' Note that Lessig reports that the bite may create a 'high level of individuality': individuality, based on the individual characteristics of wear, damage, or developmental differences, are less than the standard imposed upon fingerprints as identifying characteristics. As discussed previously, identifying characteristics are required to be unique and permanent.

Examination and evaluation of a bitemark must also consider the possibility of stretching or deformity of the substrate, in most cases skin and underlying tissue:

- Stress from the force of the bite may compress or distort the bite pattern. In a subject that survives the bite, swelling and treatment may distort the pattern.
- If the victim is fatally wounded there may be post-mortem changes due to decomposition and degradation of the tissue.
- Likewise, underlying decomposition may produce swelling and deformation of the surface skin, e.g. prior to the release of built up subcutaneous gasses. After dissipation of decomposition gasses the surface skin may retreat with drying, further complicating measurement and comparison.

Recovery of photographic images of a bite as soon as possible, and before treatment of the wound, are preferable. Bernstein states that even patterned impressions that do not pierce the skin can be recovered for up to approximately twenty minutes. Those injuries that cause skin breach and tearing, especially with underlying tissue damage, are easier to recover over a more extended time course, but recovery sooner than later is usually better.

Investigation of bite marks in alleged canine caused fatalities must also consider the difference between bites inflicted as part of an attack on a living victim, and those that may be the result of post-mortem scavenging. Domestic dogs are opportunistic scavengers. In cases where human victims die by other means but are accompanied by dogs, particularly in cases where the dog(s) and victim are closed up in a home or other structure, significant scavenging may occur. The dogs may use the deceased human as a food source if denied other options (Steadman and Worne, 2007). This may also occur in cases where humans in rural or open areas die and are undiscovered for a period of time.

## 16.5 Conclusion

Unlike the established system of identification of fingerprints by specific 'points', and a quantification of concurrence of points required to include or exclude a fingerprint as consistent with a particular subject, bite mark identification science is still evolving. Reliability in human cases is under examination (Pretty, 2005). Hard statistical agreement on consistency is not present, so each evaluator will have to make the best argument in each case. As case law develops, and examination science progresses, we can hope that standards will be established and accepted. Until then a forensic bite evaluator can best develop his or her opinion based on whether the bite mark in question is consistent or inconsistent with the pool of potential subjects established by other means. This opinion should be influenced heavily by supportive, hard evidence such as DNA, physical observation, blood, tissue recovered from the gastrointestinal tract, and other factors (See Chapters 14 and 15).

## 16.6 References

Bernstein, M. L. (2005). Nature of Bitemarks, In: Dorion, R. B. J. (ed) *Bitemark Evidence,* Marcel Dekker Pub, New York, pp.59–79.

Dorion, R. B. J., (2005). Dog Bitemarks, In: Dorion, R. B. J. (ed) *Bitemark Evidence*, Marcel Dekker Pub, New York, pp.293–321.

Dunbar, I. Dunbar dog bite assessment scale-official. Available at: www.dogtalk.com/BiteAssessmentScalesDunbarDTMRoss.pdf (accessed 10 March 2015).

Hetts, S. (1999). Pet Behavior Protocols, American Animal Hospital Association Press, Lakewood, Colorado, USA.

Hyzer, W. G., Krauss, T. C. (1988). The Bite Mark Standard Reference Scale, ABFO No. 2. *Journal of Forensic Sciences* 33(2):498–506.

Lapan, T. (2014). *The Las Vegas Sun*, Las Vegas, Nevada, USA, 29 January 2014. Web at lasvegas-sun.com/news/2014/jan/29/what-lessons-did-we-learn-onion-saga/ (accessed 17 July 2015).

Lessig R., Wenzel V., Weber M., (2006). Bite mark analysis in forensic routine case work, *EXCLI Journal* 2006; 5:93–102.

Pretty, I. A. (2005). Reliability of Bitemark Evidence In: Dorion, R. B. J. (ed) *Bitemark Evidence*, Marcel Dekker Pub, New York.

Steadman, D. W., Worne, H. (2007). Canine scavenging of human remains in an indoor setting. *Forensic Science International.* 173, 78–82.

## Legal citations

Nikko the Dog a/k/a Helo, Miscellaneous Docket #836-2012, Allegheny County Court of Common Pleas, Criminal Division.

Sanders, Patrick and Amber v City of Salem, Cause #12DE-CC00053, Circuit Court of Dent County, State of Missouri.

4

# CHAPTER 17

# Choosing a Dog Bite Expert

## *Tina Wagon*

## 17.1 Introduction

In court proceedings involving dog bite incidents there may be a requirement for expert testimony. This represents opinion evidence, as opposed to factual evidence (which is the normal evidence admissible by a lay person) and its purpose is to help the court understand and interpret technical matters based on technical expertise given the facts presented; this may include an opinion of expert consensus when factual evidence is lacking. To serve the court effectively the expert must explain clearly the basis for the opinion to show they are well-founded and logical. Although an expert may be approached and paid by one side of a dispute, his or her duty is to the court, which demands that they be objective, independent and unbiased, and they are liable for inexpert testimony. In this chapter we will look at the role of the dog expert largely in UK court proceedings and what the court requires of an expert witness in relation to dog bite incidents.

## 17.2 Who will the court accept as an expert?

The *Oxford English Dictionary* defines an expert witness as:

> '*A person whose level of specialised knowledge or skill in a particular field qualifies them to present their opinion about the facts of a case during legal proceedings.*'

Expert evidence is an exception to the general rule that a witness in criminal proceedings may only give evidence as to fact rather than opinion. A person may qualify as an expert by virtue of his or her experience rather than as a result of academic qualifications, but an expert must only give evidence within his/her area of expertise[1] and the issue of whether someone

---

1   Criminal Procedure Rules 2005, rule 33.1.

is competent to give expert evidence is decided not on a generalised basis but by reference to the specific issues to which the evidence relates.[2] Each time an expert appears in court he or she will need to have the relevant expertise recognised by the court and this is achieved by providing a detailed curriculum vitae upon which the expert may be cross-examined.

## 17.3  Duties of an expert witness

An expert witness has a duty to give 'objective, unbiased opinion on matters within his expertise'[3] both in the writing of reports and in giving oral evidence. He or she owes no allegiance to the party by whom the expert is engaged/instructed and may not enter into any arrangement where the amount or payment of fees is in any way dependent upon the outcome of the case.[4] Should the expert's opinion change from that given in a report, he or she is under a duty to inform all parties and the court.[5] An expert is not immune from negligence suits, so any evidence given either orally in court or in the form of a report prepared for the court proceedings, must be considered carefully.[6] Where both sides are calling an expert and the experts' opinions differ, they will usually be required to discuss the case and reduce the issues for trial by identifying areas of agreement and disagreement, and the court may ask for a joint statement setting out the points in dispute.[7] The experts prepare their reports, and may, after reviewing the other side's report, add dissenting opinion, but the experts do not come to any agreement, and they are both required to be in court. They are then examined and cross-examined and the court or jury makes up their minds on the basis of the court proceedings. By contrast, in the US, experts do not confer.

## 17.4  Why have a dog expert?

An expert is appointed to assist a court by explaining matters within his or her range of expertise in such a way that the court can understand them and therefore allow them to make informed decisions. They may be used both pre- and post-conviction. In the US, there may be a limitation on the use of an expert if an appeal is made against a conviction, unless a retrial is taking place, so it is essential that the need for expert testimony is recognised early in the process.

### *17.4.1  Pre-conviction:*

In the UK, section 5(5) of the Dangerous Dogs Act 1991 states that, where a dog is said to be a prohibited dog there is, unusually, a reverse burden of proof. Thus, once the police state that a dog is a prohibited type of dog, the onus is on the defendant to prove, on the

---

2   (R (on the application of Doughty) v Ely Magistrates Court, CPS interested party) WEHA 522 (Admin), (2008) 172 JPO.

3   Criminal Procedure Rules 2005, rule 33.1.

4   Criminal Procedure Rules 2005, rule 33.2.

5   Criminal Procedure Rules 2005, rule 33.3.

6   (Jones v Kaney [2011] UKSC 13, [2011] AC 398, [2011] All ER 671, [2011] 2 FLR 312).

7   Stones Justices Manual 2015 and Criminal Procedure Rules 2005, Part 24.

balance of probabilities that it is not. The court will require expert evidence to discharge this evidential burden, in which case it will be necessary for an expert to carry out a detailed assessment of the dog's conformation against the appropriate breed standard. As the courts are concerned with a dog's *type*, rather than its breed, it is not sufficient in the UK to adduce evidence of the dog's breed (for example Kennel Club certificates or DNA evidence). By contrast, in the US genetic evidence may be permissible, but this varies according to the jurisdiction.

Under section 3 of the Dangerous Dogs Act 1991, an offence is also committed if a person is caused to reasonably apprehend that they will be injured by the defendant's dog. If they are injured a more serious 'aggravated' offence is committed. The injury does not have to be a bite, a scratch or bruise will suffice. There are occasions where a defendant will accept that his or her dog has injured someone but disputes that the injury is a bite. Although this would not affect the verdict, it would have an impact on sentence as a dog that has accidentally caused an injury will be viewed as less dangerous than one that has bitten. There are also occasions where a defendant will dispute that his or her dog was responsible for the bite or injury, and this may be possible to prove from dental impressions (see Chapter 15). In an ideal world, during initial police investigations swabs would be taken from the wound and from the mouth of the alleged offending dog, but in practice this does not currently happen often (Chapter 14). It may be possible to instruct a forensic odontologist to consider the injuries but, the police rarely photograph the injuries against a scale rule so it may not be possible for an expert to reach any meaningful conclusions unless the dog has a particularly unusual dental pattern, or unless the images include an item for which an accurate measurement can be obtained in order to give a point of reference.

## 17.4.2 Post-conviction

In the UK, Section 4(1A)(a) Dangerous Dogs (Amendment) Act 1997 states that before placing a dog of one of the prohibited breeds on the Index of Exempted Dogs; or where a dog has injured someone, the court is required to order the destruction of the dog unless it is satisfied that the dog would not pose a danger to public safety. The court must consider the temperament of the dog and its past behaviour (Chapters 18 and 27). Since the introduction of the Anti-Social Behaviour Crime and Policing Act 2014 the court must now also consider the character of the defendant and whether he or she is a suitable person to own a dog of that type. It is now commonplace for police to object to a defendant being allowed to keep a dog if he or she has convictions on their record for drug-related offences or violence, or, more recently, if they have children in the house.

If no destruction order is made then the court must make a contingent destruction order.[8] This means that the dog will not be destroyed provided the owner adheres to the conditions of exemption for prohibited dogs or to whatever conditions the court deems appropriate for cases where injury has been caused. In cases where no injury is caused to a person the court has the discretion to make a destruction order or may alternatively make an order specifying conditions for its future control such as muzzling and/or keeping the

---

8    Dangerous Dogs Act 1991,section 4(1)(a) & s4(1A).

dog on a lead in public.[9] Such conditions are also imposed in many other countries, e.g. Germany (Chapter 27).

Expert evidence can assist the court in deciding what conditions would be appropriate to attach to a court order. It may also be necessary for the court to understand the welfare implications of such orders and the expert can assist with this.

Similarly, if a civil complaint under UK s2 Dogs Act 1871 is brought for owning a dog that is dangerous and not kept under proper control, the court may benefit from having a behavioural assessment to assist it in deciding whether the dog should be destroyed or whether conditions for its future control would be appropriate (Chapters 18 and 23).

Not all cases will require expert evidence as to the dog's temperament and behaviour. If the dog has never behaved aggressively or injured anyone before it may be sufficient for the defendant to produce character references for him or herself and the dog. If the dog has bitten previously, has caused serious injury to someone or has killed or seriously injured another animal, the prosecution will usually ask the court to make a destruction order. In such cases the court is likely to require favourable expert evidence if a destruction order is to be avoided.

## 17.5  Choosing a dog behaviour expert

Despite an increase in dangerous dogs prosecutions, many solicitors/attorneys will not have a great deal of experience in defending cases of this type and may not know of a suitable expert witness. In such cases an expert is often recommended by another solicitor, or one is found by consulting lists of vetted experts (e.g. UK Register of Expert Witnesses).

There can be an advantage in instructing a local expert if the dog is going to need some sort of remedial training or behavioural work after the court proceedings have concluded. Sometimes the client may have someone they wish to use, perhaps a dog trainer they have worked with but, extreme caution is urged here as such contacts rarely have the required qualifications or experience and are unlikely to be familiar with writing court reports, giving evidence in court or withstanding cross-examination (Chapter 18).

Cost can also be a factor as not all defendants will qualify for legal aid and obtaining a report from an expert, as well as funding his or her attendance at court, will usually cost in excess of £1,000, which may be beyond the reach of some defendants. Even if a defendant is funded publicly, there are strict limitations on the hourly rates that the Legal Aid Agency will pay, which could restrict the choice of expert.

### 17.5.1  Qualifications and experience

In an ideal world any expert witness would have a relevant degree, a number of years' experience working in the relevant field and would have kept his or her knowledge up to date by undergoing continual professional development training. However, as there is no statutory regulatory body for companion animal behaviour experts, assessing the calibre of an expert can be difficult. A witness can be deemed to be an expert by virtue of experience

---

9   Dangerous Dogs Act 1991, s4(1)(a).

rather than any formal academic qualification. Some experts belong to organisations whose criteria and codes of practice are defined clearly but, it is also possible to obtain qualifications from distance learning and from bodies whose qualifications are not verified externally.

There are now a number of organisations offering courses and training workshops in how to be an expert witness, covering such topics as report writing, preparing for and giving oral evidence and criminal law and procedure. Attending such a course may benefit a witness whose expertise is based upon experience rather that academic qualification (see www.cawc.org.uk/080603.pdf for a review of the situation in the UK).

## 17.5.2  The use of police officers as expert witnesses

It is common for the prosecution to rely on police officers to appear as expert witnesses to give evidence on whether a dog is a prohibited type of dog, and also to give evidence as to a dog's temperament and behaviour. This can give rise to a number of issues:

1.  *Can a police officer be said to be independent?* Most police forces now have dog legislation officers, who are usually specially trained officers usually drawn from the dog section. However, wildlife crime officers sometimes undertake the role. These officers will usually be independent of the investigation, which in theory gives them sufficient independence. However, it is questionable to what extent these officers can be truly independent given that they are salaried police officers.
2.  *Does a police officer have the right extent and relevance of expertise?* To work as a dog legislation officer in the UK, one must have completed a two-week course run by the Association of Chief Police Officers and now accredited by the College of Policing. The majority of this course is aimed at teaching police officers the legislation, with minimal time being spent on the conformation and history of the Pit Bull-type dog and even less time being devoted to canine behaviour and understanding aggression in dogs. Some police officers may be experienced and qualified police dog trainers but, depending on how long ago they learned their craft, not all of them will have an up to date scientific understanding of canine behaviour and few of them will have any sort of qualification in the field. They may be very skilled in handling a working dog, but this does not mean they have wider expertise in the science of dog behaviour. Other dog legislation officers will have had little or no professional experience with dogs prior to attending the course. They will often describe dogs as being aggressive and dangerous without any investigation and so may not be qualified to comment upon factors that may be the source of that aggression.

Once a police officer has recommended a destruction order for a dog he or she deems to be aggressive/dangerous, the court will require some very persuasive evidence that the dog does not pose a risk to the public.

## 17.5.3  Timescale of expert instruction

There is always a delay of several weeks, sometimes months, between a dog being seized and the matter coming to court. If a defendant is reliant upon legal aid to fund his or her case it is not possible to apply for legal aid until the date of the court hearing is known. Legal aid applications can take several weeks to process and, once granted, it is then necessary to apply to the Legal Aid Agency for funding for an expert assessment, which can take several more days. Once authority is granted the expert can be formally instructed and a date for the assessment can be arranged with the police. By the time the expert gets to see the dog it may well have been in kennels for several months, which could have an effect on the dog's physical condition and behaviour.

If a defendant pleads not guilty the case will be adjourned for a trial, which will take place several months ahead. As the courts double and treble list trials it is common for a trial not to go ahead on the planned date and it is not uncommon for a dog to remain in kennels for eighteen months or more waiting for the case to be heard. When the case is one of domestic violence or where a defendant is in custody, the case will be given priority over others but no priority is given to dog cases, despite the obvious welfare issues and the cost to the public purse of keeping a dog in kennels.

## 17.6  The expert's report (see also Chapter 18)

An expert report will usually set out the details of the offence, a certificate verifying that the expert understands his or her responsibilities under the Criminal Procedure Rules, the defendant's instructions, the background and history of the case and then the findings of the assessment and the expert's conclusions.

The report should outline the behaviour of the dog and the consequences of its actions in an objective manner. Rather than relying on the statements of witnesses who describe bites as 'nasty' or 'severe', use should be made of more objective descriptions (Chapters 14, 15, 16 and 21). Where possible, a diagnosis of the causes of the behaviour should be included.

Details of any home visit should be given as well as a full description of the dog's behaviour during the assessment. The expert should make clear where his findings are based on his own observations and assessment and where he is relying upon information provided to him by the owner. The report should state whether or not, in the expert's opinion, the dog poses a risk to the public and set out any recommendations the expert may have to protect the public in future. These may include both physical management and behaviour modification plans.

Details of the behavioural assessment and report are described in Chapters 18 and 27, with a different emphasis given to the type of assessment depending on local legislative requirements.

In the UK, once the expert has provided a report it must be approved by the defendant before it can be served on the court or the prosecution. If the report is unfavourable there is no requirement on the defence to disclose it to the court or the prosecution and there is nothing (other than funding issues) to stop it from instructing an alternative expert if it does not like the findings of the first expert. The prosecution must, however, disclose the existence of any report it has commissioned.[10]

In the UK, the prosecution can reasonably expect to have a copy of the defence report no less than two weeks before the trial and may then ask its own expert to carry out a

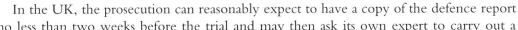

10   The Criminal Procedure & Investigations Act 1996, Part 1, ss 1–21.

further assessment of the dog. If the expert's findings are not disputed then the experts will not usually need to attend court and the court will simply use their reports to assist them in reaching a decision. In the US, both sides may stipulate that they accept the report(s) as they stand, especially if they substantially agree.

## 17.7 Conclusion

There is a need for good quality expert witness testimony in many cases, and it is important that this need is identified early in the legal proceedings so that an appropriately qualified and independent expert can be instructed. This may require that they have expertise in the growing science of analysis of dog bites and/or dog behaviour. Indeed, in some situations different experts may be indicated to cover each aspect of the dispute. Given the increasing scientific knowledge base surrounding dogs, the value of a 'general dog expert', or simply someone with a history of experience with dogs in a range of potentially irrelevant settings, is questionable.

# CHAPTER 18

# The Assessment of Dogs for Legal Cases – a UK Perspective

### *Kendal Shepherd*

## 18.1 Background

Dangerous dogs legislation in England and Wales is at present divided into two parts – those dogs that by their appearance only, are assumed to be dangerous (Dangerous Dogs Act 1991 Section 1) and those dogs that are thought to have behaved in a dangerous manner, with or without injurious consequences (Dangerous Dogs Act 1991 Section 3). Offences under this Act are criminal in nature. Civil offences may also be charged under the Dog Act 1871 or the Animals Act 1971, although this is far less common. For more information see Chapter 13.

## 18.2 The Dangerous Dogs Act Section 1

As enacted in 1991, Section 1 applies to four specific breeds of dog, namely the Japanese Tosa, the Dogo Argentino, the Fila Brasileiro and the American Pit Bull Terrier. Contrary to almost all UK law, the offence of owning such a dog carries a reverse burden of proof, so that it is incumbent on a defendant to show his or her dog is not a certain breed/type, and therefore innocent, rather than the prosecution to prove guilt. The only breed to which this has realistically applied over the years in the UK is the Pit Bull Terrier, there being only a handful of cases involving the other breeds/types.

- Subsequent to a High Court ruling in 1993 (Dunne and Brock, Knightsbridge Crown Court), the definition of a Pit Bull breed was extended to the notion of 'type' – in other words, a dog of any breeding that substantially conformed to the appearance of the pure-bred dog fell under the legislation. The standard that was to be applied in order to determine conformity was as defined by Ralph Greenwood of the American Dog Breeders Association (ADBA) in 1977 (*The Pitbull Gazette*, Vol 3, Issue 1, 1977). Since then, any dog fitting this description may be deemed to be *prima facie* 'dangerous' by its appearance and conformation, and falls under Section 1 of the Act, regardless of breed.

- The 1993 High Court ruling also decreed that the behaviour of a dog was not irrelevant, thus allowing for behavioural traits to be included in any assessment. As human-directed aggression in any form is deemed a fault in the Pit Bull Terrier, the paradox now exists that a human-friendly dog therefore conforms more highly to the ADBA standard in terms of behaviour, thus is more likely to be deemed 'dangerous' under this law as a Pit Bull type, than a similar looking dog that actually shows aggression.
- Initially all dogs thought to comply with either breed or type were compulsorily destroyed. In 1997, the Dangerous Dogs Amendment Act was passed, allowing dogs deemed of type but thought not to present a danger to the public to be entered on to a Register of Exempt Breeds, which is currently administrated by the Department for the Environment, Food and Rural Affairs. However, there has been no standard means whereby behaviour, and hence potential 'dangerousness', has been assessed. Indeed, in my experience, the majority of dogs on the Exempt Register appear to have had no behavioural assessment, other than acceptably tolerating handling for a conformational examination by a police officer, and few dogs in total have had any second opinion as to their type and behaviour.
- It is relatively uncommon for dogs deemed by appearance to be Pit Bull types to have also behaved in a dangerous manner and their owners also have a charge under Section 3 of the Act; from the author's own records, of 120 dogs charged with being Pit Bull types that she has examined from November 2008 to the time of writing (early 2015), only sixteen dogs also carried a Section 3 charge, not all of which were substantiated in court. This calls into question the legitimacy of deeming dogs dangerous simply by their appearance.

## 18.3  Section 3 of the Dangerous Dogs Act

Section 3 applies to those dogs deemed to have been 'dangerously out of control' of their owner or handler, which is defined as having given a person 'reasonable apprehension' that an injury might occur.

- An aggravated offence under Section 3 is committed if an alleged injury (of any kind) does actually occur. This offence carries a strict liability, so that an owner is obliged to plead guilty if they accept that their dog caused injury (which may be by biting but also by scratching or knocking a person over).
- Contrary to most owners' beliefs, being on lead, or even having obeyed a command to sit just prior to the incident, is not evidence of a dog being sufficiently under control. The legal view is that, if a dog caused injury or fear of injury, then however well-behaved immediately before or immediately afterwards and regardless of circumstance, an offence has been committed.

Under UK law, a court is obliged to consider a destruction order as a starting point for dogs whose owners are found guilty under either section of the Act and indeed are frequently urged to do so by the prosecution, based in some cases more on the nature of the owner of a dog, rather than that of the dog itself. It is now a requirement for an owner to be shown to be a fit and proper person to take care of a dog, as well as providing evidence that his or her dog does not generally present a danger. If the court is persuaded that a dog, as well as an owner, does not present a danger to the general public, then an animal deemed to be of the Pit Bull type may be entered under stringent conditions on to the Exempt Register. Similarly, a dog that has frightened or injured a person can be subject to a Contingent Destruction Order (or 'stay of execution'), again under usually stringent conditions.

On relatively rare, but significant, occasions in the past, a court may find the owner not guilty or, if guilty, that no control conditions are required, accepting that the incident was purely the result of human, rather than canine, failing. This decision is now supported by recent case law (R. v. Pierre-Robinson 2013) where the victims of a dog 'attack', namely police officers, were deemed to be the orchestrators of their own demise, since the dog was expressing in behavioural terms, an evolutionarily adaptive defensive action towards a threat to itself and its territory. In this case, the owner was found not to have contributed to the incident either by act of commission or omission. Inappropriate means of dealing with incidents by the authorities involving people accompanied by their dogs, may often contribute to the eliciting of aggressive, and therefore 'dangerous', behaviour – the following is taken from a report on a dog seized from a taxi in which his owner was behaving in a 'drunk and disorderly' manner:

*'It is to me an irony that the reason for K being seized was not because he had injured anyone but simply because he was very frightened and doing the job for which dogs have been selected – that of defending himself and his owner. The fact that he has now, rightly or wrongly, been identified as a Pit Bull is immaterial to this fear-based aggressive behaviour, which from a behavioural stand-point, makes it less likely that he is of the type.'*

(written by the author regarding a dog assessed by her in 2009)

## 18.4 Information required by the courts

It is upon this background that assessments of dogs for legal purposes, both as regards their conformation and their behaviour, is carried out. One's brief as an expert is to help a court make as informed a decision as possible regarding a dog's future. This must entail a prognosis, using all available information and factors upon which a prognosis, for better or worse, depends. In order to do this, the author, as a veterinary surgeon, treats the exercise as she would any clinical veterinary case where – by taking into account history, present examination, investigation and tests, required treatment and owner potential for compliance – a realistic prognosis is created as to the future of the dog, in terms of behavioural, rather than purely physical, health. The importance of veterinary behaviourists (as opposed to simply veterinary surgeons or behaviourists) has now been recognised by the Legal Aid Agency as a distinct amalgam of skills in this regard, and is to be listed in the 2015 revised list of expert witnesses eligible for public funding.

Crucial to producing a report for court and giving evidence is the maintenance of complete independence in giving one's opinion, regardless of whom one is instructed by and any potential outcome of a case. It may appear that, in having a duty of care to an animal being assessed, and through communication with the owner, such independence is compromised. However, if one has the requisite skills and knowledge and uses these to follow the same investigative, diagnostic and prognostic model for a legal case as for a clinical case, then one ought to be no more likely to pronounce potentially dangerous behavioural tendencies as benign, than to give a misdiagnosis for any serious disease condition.

All dogs considered to be of a banned breed or type are mandatorily seized, whereas owners charged only under Section 3 of the Act, may or may not be allowed to keep their dog at home, at the discretion of police officers in charge of the case. In an ideal world, a dog should always be assessed in the presence of its owner, as the behaviour and demeanour of human companions affects that of their dogs. However, this is not possible in dogs that have been seized by the police; in contrast to other countries, UK owners are not allowed to visit their dogs, or to take part in any behavioural assessment. In these instances allowances have to be made for the many months a dog will frequently have spent kennelled in social isolation since seizure, where the quality of care is unknown. Even if a dog is unable to be assessed in its home situation, information regarding the home environment is strongly recommended to be sought and included in the report.

## 18.5  The purpose of an assessment

The purpose of any assessment is to inform the judgement as to whether the dog is deemed 'dangerous' and what 'being dangerous' entails. If there is incontrovertible evidence that a dog has indeed injured, then rational and informed explanation of why this happened is required. Prior to any assessment, it is therefore imperative to obtain all available evidence regarding the context of an alleged incident, including 'victim' statements and their own actions, those of the attending police officers, any medical evidence and the extent of treatment required, as well as the version of events from the perspective of the dog owner or handler at the time. Any practical behavioural assessment must be carried out and interpreted in light of such statements.

In a multi-dog incident, the identity of the culprit may be in dispute. In which case, it is possible, providing rigorous information is provided by the statements and medical evidence, as well as the behavioural assessments, to help confirm or refute the identity of the offending dog. If there is no dispute, then a rationale should be provided for the dog's behaviour during the alleged incident.

In addition, the likelihood of recurrence ought to be gauged. It is this 'likelihood of recurrence', and how likely it is that a specific triggering circumstance can be avoided in the future, that determines 'dangerousness'.

- If the likelihood that a dog will bite again is so high as to make even thoroughly informed human action to obviate risk unlikely to succeed, then in the author's experience euthanasia must be recommended.
- In others, control measures may well be necessary to ensure public safety (ranging from simple common sense precautions such as repairing a garden fence, to muzzle and lead control in public places). It is the decision of the court as to whether an owner is likely to abide by such measures.

There is a concern in the author's experience that the welfare implications for the dog of such control measures have not been taken into account, nor has the essential need for counselling and behavioural advice to be given to the owner of such dogs. If muzzles and leads are placed on dogs with impunity simply to prevent biting, without any attention to the frustration and social deprivation that may result, then further potentially dangerous behaviour may be created – the opposite to what the law intends.

## 18.6  The importance of a behavioural history

In a legal context, history is at risk of being relegated to the realms of hearsay (in that it relates to events not actually observed oneself) and therefore deemed inadmissible. However, in the medical/veterinary context, information regarding past events is intrinsic and essential to a thorough diagnostic and prognostic process. In other words, when determining what one needs to investigate and ultimately what the prognosis might be, it is just as important to know how often a dog looks frightened or growls, as how often it may scratch, limp or have diarrhoea. In addition, past and present health problems, particularly painful ones, will have a bearing upon how a dog views its environment and its behavioural responses.

Therefore, a full behavioural and medical history should be obtained from the owner for any dog to be examined, whether or not it is alleged to have bitten or injured a person. Under current legislation, which is concerned only with whether or not a dog is likely to or has injured a person, a dog's ongoing apprehension of or antipathy towards other dogs is often overlooked. Yet in the author's experience, intervention in a dog fight is a frequent cause of inadvertent human injury, despite no intent on the part of a dog. Although the Dangerous Dogs Act was never intended to apply to aggression directed towards other dogs, case law exists under the civil Dogs Act 1871 (Briscoe v. Shattock 1998) that has confirmed that if a dog has been shown to be dangerous towards other dogs, this may be used to imply that it is also a danger to people. The dog must therefore be assessed and treated as a whole if all future eventualities are to be addressed.

In particular for dogs perceived by their owners as likely to misbehave in public, it is highly likely that the dog has experienced reprimands and punishment for its real or threatened behaviour. The use of coercive 'dominance' and threat-based training techniques is associated with aggressive behaviour problems (Casey et al., 2014) and it is plausible that the fear produced by them may lead to or exacerbate the aggressive behaviour. Therefore the eliciting of non-judgmental information regarding previous training attempts is essential to analyse a dog's alleged or current emotions and actions.

Finally, the history given by an owner is a means of assessing his or her own accuracy. Just as a clinical examination may belie a history that suggests a much shorter time-span for an illness than is obviously the case, the behavioural assessment may confirm or refute assertions and history, such as which commands a dog knows, what it likes playing with, and how much it enjoys being cuddled. In this way, the reliability of the owner can be gleaned. In the author's experience, the behaviour of the dog is often generally as described by its owner, even taking into account often many months of confinement.

## 18.7 Procedure for assessment

If a dog is in police custody, it is rare for an expert instructed by the defence to be allowed into the kennels in which the dog is being held. This may vary between police forces in the UK and is due to the perceived risk in transporting a dog behaving aggressively in confinement. Most commonly, however, the dog is delivered to a police-designated venue in order for an assessment to be carried out. There is no standard provision of assessment facilities but attempts should be made in advance to ascertain what will be available (secure area, surface, e.g. concrete or grass, whether under cover, etc). Unfortunately in the UK, as mentioned above, almost without exception the police do not permit owners to be present during the assessment of their seized animal.

If the dog has been left at home, then contact will be made directly with the owners, and a full explanation should be given at this time regarding the purpose of the assessment, how it will be carried out and who will be attending. Owners may feel very defensive at such times and need reassurance that the assessor is not there to unduly stress their pet. The purpose is to interpret any behavioural allegations, diagnose causes and create a prognosis in the light of the assessment; thus the more truthful an owner is, the more likely it is that the diagnosis and prognosis will be accurate.

It is imperative that every assessment, wherever it is carried out, is fully video-recorded, with a copy of the recording made available to all relevant parties. This is not only to ensure transparency and review of one's actions and interpretation by other parties, but also to enable one's own later review of the behaviour of the dog, as well as that of any assistants and bystanders. Much may be seen later that is not necessarily seen at the time.

## 18.8 Real-life events that may trigger aggressive behaviour

In order to ascertain whether or not potential 'danger' exists with a dog that has been seized, then day-to-day events commonly known to elicit defensive aggression should be enacted in order to test the dog's tolerance.

The assessment of seized dogs most commonly involves van transport in a small cage, to be greeted at the end of the journey by the assessor, a complete stranger. In some cases, as a result of the perceptions of 'danger' by the dog's keepers the animal may have been forced into the van on a dog 'catch' pole/'long arm'. Dogs are also generally presented without a collar. Therefore, the first test of their tolerance of interaction with a person is, of necessity, one's approach to the transport van to open the cage door of a possibly already very stressed dog, and to reach in and place a slip lead over the head in order to let the animal safely exit the cage (Figure 18.1).

The assessor should then proceed to behave as far as is possible and safe as a pet owner, as opposed to a behaviourist, might do, although this might mean that the dog is handled and petted, in what might be considered to be ill-advised ways. Important contexts to assess are:

- Handling while eating and removal of food in order to test for any guarding propensities
- Grooming
- Exposure to simulated human argument and fighting

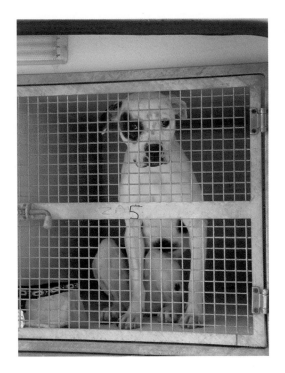

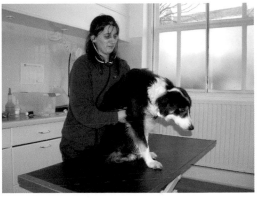

**Figure 18.2** Veterinary examination is a common trigger for defensive aggression.

**Figure 18.1** Dog in transport cage.

4

- Response to verbal and physical reprimand
- Reaction to physical restraint and coercion to 'obey'
- A mock veterinary examination, with restraint if required (Figure 18.2) as this is a common cause of alarm and defensive action
- Walking on lead with and without a baby buggy, particularly if the dog lives with small children
- Exposure to other dogs, as far as is safely possible, to observe the response.

At all times, it is essential for the assessment itself not to cause any behavioural deterioration and assessors must accept responsibility for the risks they take in order to gain a thorough assessment that is useful to the court. The various tests are therefore interspersed with relaxed interaction, including the giving of toy or food rewards for compliance (Figure 18.3).

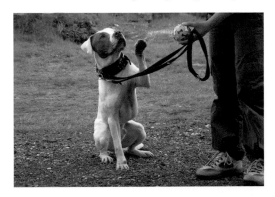

**Figure 18.3** A behavioural assessment must include opportunities for relaxation and compliance.

## 18.9 Behaviour of dogs that may result in accidental injury

Many dogs are inclined to jump up in greeting and it is a behaviour that commonly results in inadvertent reward in the form of petting and pleasant attention (Figure 18.4). Pawing and mouthing of clothes and hands may also be involved. Although intended by the dog and understood by an owner as a friendly overture, such behaviour may be sufficient to cause alarm among those unfamiliar with normal dog behaviour. Behaviour that is entirely playful in intent may also have damaging consequences if dogs have never learned to be gentle, or have ill-advisedly been encouraged to be very vigorous and rough in play. Lack of bite inhibition may result in playful mouthing or nipping causing actual damage, as may rough contact with fingers instead of the held toy. 'Tug of war' type play misdirected on to pigtails or scarves around a child's neck can have very traumatic consequences. It is therefore useful to assess:

- Is the dog gentle in taking a food reward from the hand or does it snatch with no self-control? Although not evidence of aggression by any definition, such actions may deem a dog dangerously out of control under the law.
- The dog's response to provocation and teasing in play to determine its tenacity and the ability for vigorous play to be successfully interrupted with commands, for example to sit.

Although muzzling in public may be perceived to be the solution to inappropriate play, more awareness is needed of the frustration caused by being unable to play again on walks in dogs with a high play drive that are accustomed to playing, and how such frustration may exacerbate aggression.

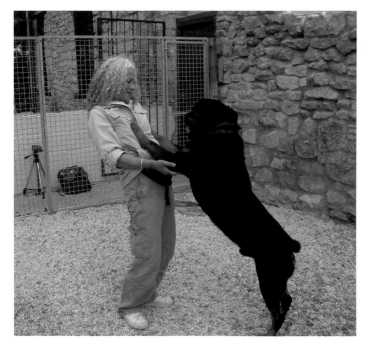

**Figure 18.4** Jumping up is a normal behaviour, potentially deemed dangerous.

## 18.10 Reconstruction of alleged episode

Where possible, the site of the incident itself should be examined, and the assessment of this taken into account in one's analysis of any alleged incident. Insecure properties that allow a dog to become free without supervision feature in many legal cases, so the simple expedient of ensuring security, for example by the provision of double barriers to the outside, may be sufficient to prevent recurrence.

Much information can be gained from a site visit in determining the veracity of statements, as well as allowing (if safe) an *in situ* reconstruction of alleged events. In the case of a seized dog, aspects of the alleged incident are recreated as far as possible in the facilities provided, with the dog muzzled if necessary. Placement of a muzzle itself may alter a dog's immediate response, so this must also be taken into consideration in interpretation. Common scenarios include:

- human intervention in a dog-on-dog-incident, for example by lifting a small dog up or by pushing or pulling a dog away
- chasing and jumping up at running and/or screaming children
- being petted or hugged
- jumping up at a passer-by
- chasing passing cyclists or joggers
- lack of guidance and subsequent intervention in human argument or dispute
- owner or victim being drunk or drugged
- owner or others being arrested.

## 18.11 Trainability/responsiveness

Regardless of what a dog has done in the past, it is essential to determine the ability of an animal to change for the better either within an existing relationship or, if the owner is deemed by the court unsuitable, in the care of another person. Throughout all features of the assessment, therefore, the dog's responsiveness to human guidance and its learning capabilities should be determined:

- Has it remained as unresponsive to a sit command, for example, or similar behaviour at the end of the assessment as at the beginning?
- If an owner is present, has he or she shown a willingness to take advice for the future and understand that simply shouting at the dog is not the answer?
- Is the dog already very well-trained, but paradoxically all the more uncertain what to do when momentarily left without essential information normally given by the owner and upon which it relies? (Many police dogs that bite at the wrong time fall into this category).

In the vast majority of dogs, great learning capacity is shown, regardless of age, and an extreme willingness to comply with human requirements once they are clearly shown those requirements.

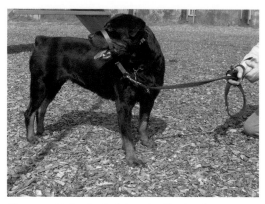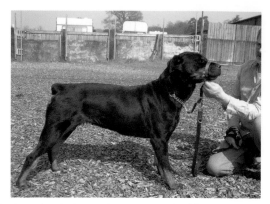

**Figures 18.5a–b** a) A head collar is a humane and educational alternative to a muzzle. b) A head collar allows the mouth to be held shut if needed.

## 18.12 Tolerance of muzzle/head collar

The prognosis for owner compliance and the risk of reoffence (either by biting or by contravening the requirements of the Exempt Register) are largely dependent on an individual dog's tolerance of the physical restrictions placed upon it. For any dog agreed to be of a Pit Bull type, it is mandatory for it to be muzzled and on a lead at all times in public. However, owner instruction as to how to humanely accustom the dog to wearing a muzzle and to perpetual restraint on lead, has generally been lacking in control orders, as has information as to how to replace the reward of play with food and owner attention. In dogs for whom the court has discretion as to whether a muzzle or other forms of head control are more appropriate, courts may be persuaded by the humane and educational features of some head collars, (Figures 18.5a and 18.5b), which allow head control and toy-directed play, but also have a semi-muzzling action should the need arise.

## 18.13 Behavioural and management advice

In all cases however, it is essential to have as a goal that a dog does not perceive the need to bite again. An assessment ought therefore to include preventative advice directly to the owner if possible, or included in a written report. Therefore behaviour modification and training should be included in all control orders, not only to alter the behaviour of dogs that have injured, but also to avoid ill-effects of measures imposed upon dogs deemed to be dangerous by their conformation, e.g. by increasing frustration.

In summary, an assessment report should ideally be based on the following, as well as information gleaned from practical assessment:

- The complete history of a dog with its owner or family, both medical and behavioural, e.g. training methods.
- How it is said or assumed to have behaved during an incident from any statements.
- Comprehensive medical evidence regarding any injuries to a 'victim' and treatment required.

- If seized, information from the housing kennels since seizure, regarding both veterinary attention and behaviour.
- The attitude and capabilities of an owner in following advice and ensuring safety in the future.
- Security of the home and measures taken to prevent escape from premises.

## 18.14 Conclusions of assessment and report writing

The purpose and conclusions of any assessment and report (see Box 1) must be borne in mind from the point of instruction onwards and must concentrate on what the court will need to know from an expert. The facts of the case will be decided largely upon evidence and the relative credibility of witnesses, although it may be that expert opinion will sway a bench in favour of one version of events compared to another. However, in the majority of cases, one's analysis and opinion on canine behaviour should focus on prognosis for the future and the relative importance of the dog itself; the owner; control measures; and the potential for training measures in creating this prognosis (See Box 18.1).

Ultimately, the questions to be answered are:

- Does the dog need to be put to sleep (as this is the starting point assumption in any DDA case)?
- Are the current owners able to ensure safety in the future?
- Can the dog be rehabilitated if necessary or is secure management sufficient?
- Can the dog be rehomed if an owner deemed to be unfit to have a dog returned?

## 18.15 Further Reading

*The Pitbull Gazette*, Vol 1, Issue 3 (1977). Reproduced in Stevens, Bob (1983) Chapter 2 'History' in 'Dogs of Velvet and Steel', Herb Eaton Historical Publications, North Carolina pp.68–73.
Sweeney, N. 'Dogs of law' (2015). Alibi, imprint of Veritas Chambers, Bristol.

## Useful links

Specialist dog-related legislation advice www.doglaw.org.uk
'Dealing with dangerous dogs' www.acpo.police.uk/documents/uniformed/2009/200903UNGDD01.pdf
Defra 'Dangerous Dogs Law guidance for enforcers' https://www.gov.uk/government/uploads/system/uploads/attachment_data/file/69263/dogs-guide-enforcers.pdf
Defra http://archive.Defra.gov.uk/wildlife-pets/pets/dangerous
Royal College of Veterinary Surgeons guidance on 'Giving evidence for court' https://www.rcvs.org.uk/advice-and-guidance/code-of-professional-conduct-for-veterinary-surgeons/supporting-guidance/giving-evidence-for-court
The Academy of Experts, 3 Gray's Inn Square, London WC1R 5AH, www.academyofexperts.org/

## Box 18.1  What should be in the report?

<u>Instructions from solicitor</u>
What exactly have you been asked to do and give an opinion on?
Is there anything else that you feel needs to be included in your report apart from your brief?
Look at the brief and what you need from all sides regardless of who is instructing you. Solicitors don't know about dogs and don't think of everything!

<u>The documentation received – listed and dated</u>
All statements so far disclosed to your instructing solicitor
Ask for anything that ought to be there but is not – veterinary records of injured dogs, medical records of injured people, how a dog has behaved in kennels if seized. Solicitors may not ask for information that may be detrimental to their case but very important for your assessment.

<u>History of the offending dog</u> – medical and behavioural, family details, socialisation history, training methods.

<u>Details of the behaviour assessment – all video recorded and photographed</u>
Exactly what you did and why – relevance to incident?
What information could be gleaned from it?

<u>Comments upon the incident with reference to the results of assessment</u>
Has the assessment shed light on what happened?
Has the assessment cast doubt on what is alleged to have happened?
Do the statements conflict with each other?
In the light of the assessment, do you prefer one view to another?

<u>Conclusions reached regarding the nature of the dog</u>
Does the dog present a risk to the general public under normal circumstances?
Were the circumstances unusual?
How many and what kind of provocations does the dog need to become aggressive?
How likely is it that these circumstances will combine again?
What can be done to prevent such a circumstance happening again?

Addenda

* A full Curriculum Vitae relevant to your expertise in this field
* Declaration of Independence as An Expert Witness
* Any references or other material supporting the opinion given.

## Relevant legislation and case law

Animals Act 1971 www.legislation.gov.uk/ukpga/1971/22

Dangerous Dogs Act 1991 www.legislation.gov.uk/ukpga/1991/65/contents

Dangerous Dogs Amendment Act 1997 www.legislation.gov.uk/ukpga/1997/53/contents

Dogs Act 1871 www.legislation.gov.uk/ukpga/Vict/34-35/56

Briscoe v. Shattock October 1998 Queen's Bench Division (Dogs Act 1871 case).

R. v. Knightsbridge Crown Court, ex parte Dunne, Brock v. Director of Public Prosecutions, Queens Bench Division July 1993.

R.v. Robinson-Pierre December 2013 CA, Criminal Division (Dangerous Dogs Act 1991 Section 3 case)

## References

Hilby, E. F., Rooney, N. J., Bradshaw, J. W. S. (2004). Dog training methods: their use, effectiveness and interactions with behaviour and welfare. Animal Welfare 13, 63–69.

Casey, R. A., Loftus, B., Bolster, C., Richards, G. J., Blackwell, E. J. (2014). Human-directed aggression in domestic dogs: occurrence in different contexts and risk factors. Applied Animal Behaviour Science 152, 52–63.

# Section 5
# Health Issues

In Section 5, we consider the wider human health impact of dog bites. While many bites may be relatively innocuous, it is important to differentiate these from those requiring greater medical attention. In the first chapter of this section, Chapter 19, Matthew Burgess provides an essential overview of first line assessment necessary for dog bite cases and the medical priorities for anyone encountering the victim of a bite. This theme is developed further in the subsequent chapters of this section. In Chapter 20, Lorna Lancaster reviews the infectious risks from dog bites and the microbiology of these injuries. Different bacteria may be associated with different types of wound, and while some of the infectious agents may come from the dog, others may come from the resident human flora. As in both the preceding and subsequent chapter, the importance of cleaning the wound effectively early on is emphasised. The routine use of antibiotics at a time of rising concern over the development of resistance is unwise, although there are special groups that fall outside this generalisation.

Only once the issues of potential infection have been addressed can surgical intervention be considered and in Chapter 21 Chris Mannion emphasises the importance of carefully evaluating both the patient and the wound to maximise the benefit of any surgical intervention. This is something that his own data illustrate is not routinely done very well, and this chapter is a timely reminder of best practice. Reconstructive surgery is not just cosmetic, but it may play an important role in the mental rehabilitation of the patient. The special case of the risk of rabies is considered in Chapter 22 by Lorraine McElhinney. Rabies is a disease that strikes fear into many bitten by a dog where the disease is endemic. This is a global disease problem, but one which, she argues, need not cause high mortality in humans if the right measures are put in place by government for the management of dogs and bite victims. Indeed, if we understood dog bites as well as we understood rabies, then clearly the risks to society would be greatly reduced. Finally, Carri Westgarth and Francine Watkins highlight a much overlooked health consequence of dog bites: its psychological impact. Drawing on new data, they show how great this can be even for minor incidents. At the severe end of the scale is the potential for further complications such as post-traumatic stress disorder. Like all the authors in this section, they argue strongly for a much more joined up process to the management of victims, in order to minimise the risks involved.

# CHAPTER 19

# First Aid and Practical Medical Management for Dog Bites

## Matthew Burgess

## Disclaimer

The views expressed herein are those of the author and do not necessarily reflect the official policy or position of the Department of the Navy, Department of Defense, or the United States Government.

## 19.1 Introduction

Animal bites are a common occurrence around the world, with dog bites representing up to 90% of all mammalian bites (Endom et al., 2015). Owing to its common occurrence, it is important to know what to do if a dog bite occurs, when to seek medical care, and what the primary concerns are following a bite.

For the purposes of this chapter, a dog bite will describe any incident where a dog has its jaws on/around a person. With this broad definition, one can see that many 'dog bites' are bound to occur, especially when playing or when a dog attempts to protect itself with a simple nip. Oftentimes, nothing is needed to be done for these simple, sometimes playful, 'bites', but if these accidental bites become more harmful, then they should be handled the same way that an intentional attack is handled (see subsequent chapters in this section for more detail on the wider health issues). As described elsewhere in the text, an important aspect of treating dog bites is preventing them in the first place (see Chapters 29, 30 and 31).

## 19.2 Initial priorities

Once a dog bite has occurred, the first and most important thing to do is to separate the victim from the attacking animal. This can be via escape to another room, restraining the animal, or a number of other ways (see Chapters 24 and 25). This will prevent continued attacks and allow an opportunity to fully assess the injury.

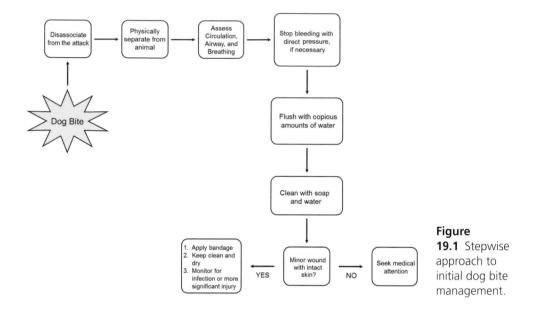

**Figure 19.1** Stepwise approach to initial dog bite management.

As with most first responder situations, the primary survey or Basic Life Support (BLS) principles then take priority (Field et al., 2010). These are, in order, assessment of:

1. Circulation
2. Airway
3. Breathing.

Even seemingly innocuous incidents can result in more significant injuries, such as an elderly person suffering a heart attack or a bite on the extremity that severs an artery and causes exsanguination (Chapter 11).

If a victim is conscious and talking, then airway and breathing are accounted for at that time. The primary concern at such point will be assessing the extent of bleeding. **Significant bleeding** can be controlled and eventually stopped with **continuous direct pressure** (Endom et al., 2015). It is important to avoid the common mistake of applying pressure and then checking after a short amount of time to see if the bleeding has stopped because the bleeding will often resume with the reduction in pressure.

Figure 19.1 provides a simple overview of the process involved in assessment and initial management.

## 19.3 Whether or not to seek medical attention

Large or deep wounds, injuries to vital organs, or involvement of the head and/or neck will surely lead nearly every victim to seek medical attention. Minor injuries that do not break the skin can easily be treated at home and likely pose little risk of more significant injuries. It is the intermediate wound that may be small or seemingly minor that will likely have individuals questioning whether to seek medical attention. In the author's opinion, the safest and easiest approach is to seek medical attention whenever a bite breaks the skin, if only to get professional assessment of the immediate or delayed health risks.

While ultimately the decision to seek medical attention is an individual choice, the following are what physicians are concerned about in regards to managing dog bites:

- Wound care (Chapter 20)
- Damage to underlying structures such as nerves, blood vessels, muscles, tendons, bones, and vital organs
- Retained foreign bodies such as teeth
- The need for antibiotics or sutures (stitches) (Chapter 21)
- The chance of rabies or needing a tetanus vaccination (Chapter 22).

If the individual can satisfactorily address each of these concerns then perhaps the wound is minor enough and does not need medical attention. However, the wound should be monitored for signs of infection (fever, redness, swelling, pus, etc) and more significant injury (e.g. numbness, loss of movement or strength). Regardless, the most important step in treating a dog bite is wound care, which includes flushing the wound with a copious amount of water and washing it with soap and water (Endom et al., 2015; Melton, 2004). These two steps alone will greatly reduce more significant injury due to infection or retained debris.

## 19.4  General medical assessment

As with any patient presenting to the accident and emergency department, it is important for the attending clinician to obtain a thorough history and physical exam. Important aspects to consider are:

- Patient age and comorbidities
- When the injury occurred
- What has been done to the wound since the bite occurred
- Vaccination status of the patient
- Any information about the dog such as size, breed, familiarity (family pet, stray), and vaccination status (along with evidence of the reliability of this information).

Assessment of the wound should include:

- Where the wound is located
- The type of wound
- The extent of damage.

Particular attention should be paid to the neurovascular exam and damage to underlying structures. Deep wounds to vital organs should be treated as major penetrating trauma (Endom et al., 2015).

## 19.5  Bite wound treatment

Once it has been determined that the patient is stable, the focus should be on wound care. This is the most important aspect of treating a laceration from a dog bite.

1.  The first step is *irrigation*. The wound needs to be flushed with an appropriate amount of water or saline for the size of the wound. High pressure washing, especially with puncture wounds, can be counterproductive as it runs the risk of powering infectious organisms and millieu deeper into the wound (Endom et al., 2015). It may be appropriate to anesthetise the area in order to appropriately clean and explore the wound.
2.  Devitalised tissue should be *debrided* after irrigating the wound sufficiently, and the wound can again be explored to identify damage to underlying structures and the presence of foreign bodies such as a retained canine tooth.
3.  The next decisions relate to the needs of *suturing* the wound closed and prescribing *antibiotics*, which are related and so dealt with together here. Chapter 21 deals with the specifics relating to the decision to suture the wound, and the outcome of this may affect the decision to use antibiotics. Prophylactic antibiotics, such as amoxicillin-clavulanate, clindamycin plus ciprofloxacin, or clindamycin plus trimethoprim-sulfamethoxazole, for dog bites continues to be a controversial subject (Chapter 20, Fleisher, 1999). In general, antibiotics are not recommended routinely except for high risk or complicated wounds such as puncture wounds, those involving the hands, those requiring surgical repair, or those with delayed initial treatment (Endom et al., 2015; Melton, 2004). Additionally, high-risk patients such as the elderly, diabetics, and the immunocompromised likely benefit from prophylactic antibiotics. Wounds that are obviously already infected need to be treated with broad-spectrum antibiotics, and significant infections may require admission and parenteral antibiotics (Melton, 2004). Culturing bite wounds are of little value except perhaps in wounds that are already infected (Endom et al., 2015).
4.  Another consideration is whether to obtain radiographs or other forms of *diagnostic imaging*. If there is concern for retained foreign body, underlying fracture, or evidence of infection then radiographs are reasonable. Additionally, deep bites to the scalp or head, especially in small children, may necessitate head computed tomography (CT) scans to assess for depressed skull fractures or intracranial involvement. Ultrasound may be helpful to assess abscess formation or retained radiolucent foreign body (Endom et al., 2015).
5.  Lastly, *tetanus and rabies* must be considered. Dog bites are considered 'dirty' wounds and thus prone to tetanus infections.

    *   Patients with two or fewer tetanus toxoid vaccinations should receive both tetanus toxoid vaccination and human tetanus immune globulin at initial presentation. The two injections should be administered at different sites and the tetanus vaccination should be continued through to completion as necessary (Endom et al., 2015).
    *   For patients that have already received three or more tetanus toxoid vaccinations, they should receive a vaccine booster if their last tetanus dose was five or more years ago. One should also refer to one's regional tetanus guidelines.

Rabies is a concern from dog bites, especially in the non-industrialised world (See Chapter 20). Unprovoked attacks, attacks from wild/stray dogs, or attacks from dogs that appear ill or behave erratically necessitate post-exposure prophylaxis unless the animal is killed and its brain tests negative for rabies (Fulton and Salata, 2007). Treatment consists of a series of four to five doses of rabies vaccinations and one injection of rabies immune globulin (CDC, 2011), if the patient has not previously been vaccinated. Healthy-appearing dogs can be quarantined for ten days and killed if signs of illness appear (Corrall, 2004; Fulton and Salata, 2007). If they remain normal and/or are appropriately vaccinated, then rabies treatment for the dog bite victim is not necessary. Again, there are local geographic guidelines in regards to managing potential rabies exposed victims.

## 19.6 Conclusion

Dog bites are common occurrences in domestic life. It is important to remember the basics when a dog bite does occur and Figure 19.1 provides a guide for initial management. Ending the attack, assessing the victim in a safe environment, and ensuring circulation, airway, and breathing are the initial priorities. Wound care and irrigation are crucial once the victim is stabilised. Lastly, the decision to seek medical care can be challenging but when in doubt, it is reasonable to ensure no additional management is needed by having a medical professional examine the wound(s).

## 19.7 References

CDC (2011) Rabies. Available at: www.cdc.gov/rabies/exposure/index.html (accessed 13 September 2015).

Corrall, C. J. (2004). Tetanus and rabies. In: Ma, O. J., Cline, D. M. (eds.) *Emergency Medicine Manual*, 6th edn. The McGraw-Hill Companies, Inc., United States of America, pp.423–425.

Endom, E. E., Danzl, D. D., Wiley II, J. F. (2015). Initial management of animal and human bites. Available at: www.uptodate.com/contents/initial-management-of-animal-and-human-bites (accessed 29 August 2015).

Field, J. M., Hazinski, M. F., Sayre, M. R., Chameides, L., Schexnayder, S. M., Hemphill, R., Samson, R. A., Kattwinkel, J., Berg, R. A., Bhanji, F., Cave, D. M., Jauch, E. C., Kudenchuk, P. J., Neumar, R. W., Peberdy, M. A., Perlman, J. M., Sinz, E., Travers, A. H., Berg, M. D., Billi, J. E., Eigel, B., Hickey, R. W., Kleinman, M. E., Link, M. S., Morrison, L. J., O'Connor, R. E., Shuster, M., Callaway, C. W., Cucchiara, B., Ferguson, J. D., Rea, T .D., Vanden Hoek, T. L. (2010). Part 1: Executive Summary: 2010 American Heart Association Guidelines for Cardiopulmonary Resuscitation and Emergency Cardiovascular Care. *Circulation* 122(18 Suppl 3), S640–656.

Fleisher, G. R. (1999). The management of bite wounds. *The New England Journal of Medicine* 340(2), 138–140.

Fulton, S. A., Salata, R. A. (2007). Infections of the nervous system. In: Andreoli, T. E. (ed.) *Andreoli and Carpenter's Cecil Essentials of Medicine*, 7th edn. Saunders Elsevier, Philadelphia, PA, pp.917–918.

Melton, C. (2004) Puncture wounds and mammalian bites. In: Ma, O. J. and Cline, D. M. (eds.) *Emergency Medicine Manual*, 6th edn. The McGraw-Hill Companies, Inc., United States of America, pp.115–116.

5

CHAPTER 20

# The Microbiology of Dog Bite Wounds

*Lorna Lancaster*

## 20.1 Introduction

There were reported to be nearly 7,000 admissions to hospital in England in 2013 due to dog strikes and bites (HSCIC, 2014) and in USA there are on average more than 350,000 people treated for bites in emergency departments with a calculated cost of $164 million annually (Centers for Disease Control and Prevention, 2003; Quinlan and Sacks, 1999; Benson et al., 2006). It is reported that perhaps 50% of bites require medical treatment (Beck and Jones, 1985) with the most frequent complication being infection (Centers for Disease Control and Prevention, 2003). Children are the most likely to be hospitalised for dog bites. There were 12,777 mammalian bites reported in USA between 1990 and 1992 with 25% of these involving children under six years old and 34% involving children aged between six and seventeen years old (Litovitz et al., 2001).

Dog bites can result in severe injuries but complications caused by infection can increase the severity of the injury and have been estimated to occur in 3–25% of cases (Talan et al., 1999). The impact of infection of the wound can range from minor afflictions to more serious conditions, such as fever, lymphangitis (swelling of the lymph nodes) and abscesses. In some cases, the infection can cause severe systemic diseases, such as bacteraemia (infection of the blood stream), endocarditis (infection of the heart), septic arthritis (infection of joint tissue), meningitis and septic shock. These diseases often cause severe long–lasting side effects that can impede the life of the victim (Hloch et al., 2014; Wareham et al., 2007; Monrad and Hansen, 2012). The risk of infection can depend on the location and the type of injury caused by the bite, with puncture wounds more likely to cause infection (Talan et al., 1999). The infections themselves can be caused by a variety of bacteria that are found in the mouths of dogs or on the skin of the victim (Thomas and Brook, 2011). Wounds can be infected with more than one species of bacteria and often up to sixteen different bacterial species are involved (Talan et al., 1999).

Treatment of dog bite wounds should be performed quickly to avoid risk of infection and should be treated as any other contaminated wound (Chapter 19, Esposito et al., 2013;

Looke and Dendle, 2010). There is still some debate as to whether the wound should be closed immediately or left for twenty-four hours to determine the possibility of an infection (Chapter 21). There also needs to be some consideration about the use of antibiotics in order to prevent infection developing. With the large range of bacterial contamination within a wound making it very difficult of being confident that the correct antibiotic has been selected and with increasing levels of antibiotic resistance in the community, antibiotic usage should be focused on where there are clear indications. This chapter discusses the bacteria that have been found in infections from dog bite wounds and the possible bacterial species found in dogs' mouths and on the human skin that are likely to cause infection. The treatment of dog bites is discussed briefly with a focus on prevention of infection and the recommended antibiotics to use either in preventing infection or to treat the most common occurring infections.

## 20.2 Origin of dog bite wound infections

With up to 25% of dog bite wounds becoming infected, it is important to understand the infection and where the bacteria causing the infection have come from. For most dog bite wounds, the infection develops from bacteria that originated in the mouth of the dog, the skin of the victim or the environment (Thomas and Brook, 2011). It is, therefore, important to understand the microbiology of these sources.

### 20.2.1 Microbiology of dogs' mouths

The mouths of animals contain a diverse range of ecological areas that are perfect for the growth of a large number of different micro-organisms, especially bacteria (Keijser et al., 2008; Zaura et al., 2009; Xie et al., 2010). The microbiology of the mouth of a dog has been studied by a variety of methods. Until recently, bacterial species were identified by culturing methods within the laboratory and identified by similarities to other bacteria already categorised from the human mouth. About 300 different species were identified by this method. Recently, new technology in genetics and molecular biology, such as high throughput pyrosequencing of the 16S rRNA gene, have made it possible to identify bacterial species that we are unable to cultivate in the laboratory.

When analysing the microbiology of dogs' mouths it was found that there were 181 different genera of bacteria, with many different species in each genera. Many of these genera and species were found in all dogs tested, indicating that there is a stable core of bacteria that inhabit dogs' mouths (Sturgeon et al., 2013). The most common genera of bacteria found within dogs' mouths include *Porphyromonas, Fusobacterium, Capnocytophaga, Derxia, Moraxella, Bergeyella,* and *Clostridia* (Sturgeon et al., 2013; Dewhirst et al., 2012; Davis et al., 2013). The genera *Peptostroptococcus, Actinomyces,* and *Peptostreptococcaceae* should also be noted as they are found commonly in dogs with tooth decay and may be more likely to cause infection if the dog is suffering from this condition (Davis et al., 2013). It is interesting to note that the species of bacteria found within dogs' mouths share only 16.5% similarity with the bacterial species found in the human mouth and therefore, comparisons should not be made between the two.

One of the genera found within the dog's mouth, *Capnocytophaga,* has recently been discovered to be a significant infecting bacteria, especially in immuno-compromised patients (Wareham et al., 2007; Hloch et al., 2014). This species is normally identified by culture-based methods within hospitals, but this genus of bacteria is often slow growing and can sometimes be missed in analysis. Two studies have examined the carriage of *Capnocytophaga canimorsus* species within dog mouths (Dilegge et al., 2011; Suzuki et al., 2010). One study used traditional culture methods (Dilegge et al., 2011) and identified that 22% of dogs carried this bacteria within their mouths. By contrast, Suzuki et al. (2010) found the bacteria in 74% of dogs' mouths when using a specific polymerase chain reaction to identify the 16S rRNA. The difference in carriage rates found by these two studies indicates the issues of identification methods for bacterial species that may cause infection, so there may be an underestimation of the carriage of this bacterial species and the infections caused by it.

Viruses have not been found to be part of the normal microbiome of the dog mouth, however, dogs may be infected with viruses that can be present within the mouth, including parvovirus, canine oral papillomavirus and rabies (McKnight et al., 2007; Sundberg et al., 1986; Wacharapluesadee et al., 2012). Parvovirus and canine oral papillomavirus do not infect humans so do not need to be considered as a possible infection when dog bites occur. Rabies is a serious infection and preventative treatment should be administered in areas where rabies is endemic or if the vaccination background of the dog cannot be obtained (Chapter 22).

### 20.2.2 Microbiology of human skin

Human skin can harbour a wide array of microbes and has been studied in great detail. The skin consists of a range of micro-environments that are diverse in their temperature, pH, moisture content and topography. This diverse range of environments can influence the variety of microbial content. The changes in microbial growth on the skin in different regions may affect the type of infection acquired depending on the site of the wound and can be described as a site-specific infection. Many of the microbes found on the skin and, therefore possibly in wound infections, can be host specific (Oh et al., 2014) where an individual's skin can have very different pH, moisture content and topography compared with other individuals that will influence the growth of certain microbial species compared with others (Oh et al., 2014).

Oh et al., (2014) found that bacterial species are the most abundant micro-organisms on the skin but DNA viruses and species of fungi are also found; this is unique to the skin compared to other body organs (Oh et al., 2014). Bacterial genera most commonly observed were *Corynebacterium*, *Propionibacterium* and *Staphylococcus*. The most common species found were *Propionibacterium acnes*, which was predominantly host specific, and *Staphylococcus epidermidis*, which was predominantly site specific (Oh et al., 2014). It was also determined that there was a variety of potential antibiotic resistant bacterial species (Oh et al., 2014), which may cause issues when trying to treat wound infections. Fungi were the least common organism found, with the main species observed being *Malassezia globosa* and *Malassezia restricta*. Fungal species were found to have a higher abundance around the head and ears (Oh et al., 2014). Sites of high viral content have also been observed mostly around the nose. These viruses were mostly harmless but some pathogens such as *human papillomavirus*, *Merkel cell polyomavirus* and *Molluscum contagiosum*, have been found (Oh et al., 2014).

## 20.2.3 Microbiology of the environment

The environment has a rich diversity of micro-organisms, which will depend on the geography of the land and are therefore too numerous to list here. However, one bacterial species of note that should be considered in all potentially dirty wounds is *Clostridium tetanii*, the cause of tetanus. As dog bite wounds are classed as a dirty wound, tetanus should be considered in the treatment plan (Chapter 19, Esposito et al., 2013).

## 20.3 Dog bite associated infections

Dog bites in adults generally occur around the hands and legs but in children often the face, head and neck are injured (Ostenello et al., 2005). Bites to the hand tend to have a higher risk of infection (Table 20.1), possibly because they tend to be more likely to involve crush injuries which increases the risk of infection as deeper wounds are involved (Ward, 2013; Rothe et al., 2002). With face, neck and head injuries, wound infection is rare but can lead to more severe complications, including fatal intracranial infection, parotid gland fistulas and nasolacrimal injury (Rui-feng et al., 2013). The age of the patient, the injury depth and secondary presentations at emergency departments are all risk factors for serious injury and infection (Table 20.1), leading to hospitalisation (Pfortmueller et al., 2013). The elderly are at an increased risk of infection, most likely due to decreased immune system function along with other medical compromises (Pfortmueller et al., 2013).

Dogs tend to cause either puncture or laceration injuries with an estimated 60% of dog bite injuries having punctures only, 10% lacerations only and 30% having both lacerations and punctures (Talan et al., 1999). Lacerations tend to be easier to clean and disinfect, so are less likely to develop infection compared with puncture wounds (Abrahamian, 2000).

**Table 20.1** Risk factors for developing an infection and the reasons for this risk.

| Risk Factor for infection | Reasons for risk | Reference |
|---|---|---|
| Bite to the hand | Hands have many small compartments and they do not have much soft tissue. Infection can penetrate joint tissue easily. | Rothe et al., 2002 |
| Depth of injury | Deeper wounds are difficult to clean. Anaerobic bacterial species can thrive in this environment. | Talan et al., 1999 |
| Age of wound | The bacteria are given time to establish before adequate cleaning may take place. Often the wound is not seen in the hospital until the wound is infected. | Pfortmueller et al., 2013 |
| Age of the patient | Elderly or very young are more prone to infection most likely due to reduced immune response. | Pfortmueller et al., 2013 |
| Immuno-compromised patients | Patients with a compromised immune system are unable to fight the infection effectively, leading to more severe infections. | Wald et al., 2008; Monrad and Hansen, 2012; Stiegler et al., 2010; Hloch et al., 2014 |

Infections occurring in dog bite wounds tend to be polymicrobial with variations on numbers and types of bacteria depending on the infection caused (Talan et al., 1999). Wound infections can be characterised into three groups:

1.   Presence of an abscess
2.   Purulent (presence of pus)
3.   Non-purulent (no pus produced) with lymphangitis or cellulitis.

Talan et al. (1999) found that 48% of infection cases had purulent infections, 36% non-purulent infections with lymphangitis and 16% abscesses. It was also found that 48% of dog bites had infections with mixed aerobic and anaerobic bacteria, 42% with aerobes only but only 1% with anaerobes only. The number of isolates found in each wound type varied depending on the type of infection observed. The median of bacterial isolates observed in an abscess was higher at seven and a half compared with purulent wounds with a median of five and non-purulent wounds with a median of two. The highest bacterial number observed in this study was found in a purulent wound that contained sixteen different bacterial species (Talan et al., 1999).

Bacteria most commonly isolated from dog bite wounds include *Pasteurella canis*, *Capnocytophaga canimorsus*, *Streptococci* spp., *Staphylococci* spp., *Moraxella* spp., *Neisseria* spp., *Fusobacterium* spp., *Bacteriodes* spp., *Porphyromonas* spp. and *Prevotella* spp. (Talan et al., 1999; Abrahamian, 2000). Most of these bacteria are found commonly in the mouths of dogs except *Staphylococci* and *Streptococci*. These species were not commonly found in the mouth of dogs in more recent studies (Dewhirst et al., 2012; Davis et al., 2013; Sturgeon et al., 2013; Dilegge et al., 2011) but they are a normal part of the skin microflora of humans (Oh et al., 2014).

Anaerobes (*Bacteroides*, *Fusobacterium* and *Porphyromonas*) were found most commonly in abscesses compared with other types of infection and in puncture wounds compared with other injuries. Anaerobic bacteria can increase significantly the severity of infection because of their synergistic relationship with aerobic bacteria, making the infection harder to eliminate and selecting antibiotics that can kill both types of bacteria more complicated. *Streptococci* and *Staphylococci* were found more frequently in non-purulent wounds with lymphangitis.

*Pasteurella* spp. were common in both abscesses and nonpurulent wounds and most commonly isolated from puncture wounds from the arms (Talan et al., 1999). *Pasteurella multicoda* is often found in dog bite wounds and requires special mention as it is highly likely to spread and cause severe disease and side effects. Wounds infected by *P. multicoda* are often purulent and inflammation develops rapidly. In severe cases, the infection can progress rapidly to cause bacteraemia (infection of the blood), osteomyelitis (inflammation of the bone), endocarditis (inflammation of the heart) and meningitis (as reviewed in Wilson and Ho, 2013).

Another infection of note is *Capnocytophaga canimorsus*. It does not cause many infections but when it does it can be severe and cause death. The infection mostly occurs in patients with a compromised immune system caused by underlying conditions, such as alcohol addiction or spleen removal (Wald et al., 2008; Monrad and Hansen, 2012; Stiegler et al., 2010; Hloch et al., 2014). However, fatal infection has been observed in healthy individuals with no underlying conditions (Hantson et al., 1991). *C. canimorsus* can cause a number of severe infections including bacteraemia, endocarditis and meningitis (Hloch et al., 2014; Wareham et al., 2007; Monrad and Hansen, 2012) and has a high mortality rate if it causes septic shock or multi-organ failure (Lion et al., 1996). Hloch et al. (2014) described a case of a patient who had undergone a splenectomy and had become infected with *C. canimorsus* from a minor dog bite. The infection developed into septic shock and was treated with antibiotics (clindamycin). The patient started to recover from the initial infection but developed two secondary infections from the treatment – *Enterococcus faecalis* and *Candida albicans*. The patient survived but required 102 days in hospital and was severely ill. This case study indicates the need for quick treatment of dog bite infections, especially in patients with a compromised immune system.

## 20.4 Antibiotic resistance

Antibiotic resistance is an increasing problem that is making the treatment of infections more difficult. As more bacterial species become resistant to more of the antibiotics we use to fight infection, the more difficult it is to treat the infections. There is limited published research on the antibiotic resistance of bacterial infections from dog bites in humans. However, there is some evidence that the incidence of methicillin resistant *Staphylococcus aureus* (MRSA) and methicillin resistant *Staphylococcus pseudointermedius* (MRSP) is increasing (Looke and Dendle, 2010; Oehler et al., 2009; Ruscher et al., 2010; Weese and van Duijkeren, 2010).

Dogs tend to acquire MRSA from their owner (Oehler et al., 2009), therefore, if the prevalence of MRSA is high within the community, it has a higher possibility of infecting a bite wound. MRSP is commonly found as part of the normal microbiota of dogs and might be found on dogs eleven months or more after an infection within the dog has been diagnosed (Windahl et al., 2012). There has also been a study into the carriage of antibiotic resistant *E. coli* in dogs (Martins et al., 2013). Some 124 strains of *E. coli* were isolated and a large percentage of these were found to have antibiotic resistance. Although *E. coli* does not seem to be a major cause of dog bite wound infections, they may still need to be considered if treatment is not effective or *E. coli* has been identified as the infecting agent.

Once the infecting agent has been identified, antibiotic susceptibility testing should be performed to diagnose if an antibiotic resistant bacteria is present, then the correct antibiotic can be selected to treat the infection.

## 20.5 Management of dog bite wounds

Dog bite wounds should be treated as any other contaminated wound (Chapter 19). The management of dog bite wounds can to be broken down into several stages (Morgan, 2005; Ward, 2013) (Table 20.2). The wound will need to be treated but certain aspects of the wound and the circumstances surrounding the injury need to be considered, therefore a careful history should be taken so decisions can be made about the best method of treatment. The site of the wound should be analysed to determine any risk factors for infection (Table 20.1). The wound then needs to be cleaned thoroughly and the requirement for sutures determined. If there is evidence of an established infection, the wound needs to be

**Table 20.2** Stages of wound management of a dog bite.

| Stage of Management | Procedures |
| --- | --- |
| Clinical Assessment | Full history, was the attack provoked, time since injury, immunisation history. |
| Risk of Infection Assessment | Any underlying immune-compromising conditions, age of patient, depth of wound, site of wound. |
| Wound management | Irrigation and debridement of wound, closure of the wound dependent on site. |
| Wound infection management | Infected wounds are opened and drained, cultured as soon as possible, antibiotics when required or if risk factors are indicated. |

drained, cleaned and treated and should be swabbed and cultured to identify the infecting agents to allow the correct treatment to be used (Morgan, 2005).

## 20.5.1 Clinical history

A careful history should be taken to determine the risk factors of infection and the best method to proceed. If the attack from the dog appeared unprovoked or occurred in a rabies endemic area with no vaccine history of the dog there may be a risk of rabies infection (Ward, 2013) and this should be considered in the treatment plan. It will also need to be determined if any underlying immune compromising conditions are present in the patient, for example HIV, spleen removal, alcoholism, cirrhosis, or elderly, as this can lead to more severe infection conditions (Rothe et al., 2002; Pfortmueller et al., 2013; Wald et al., 2008; Monrad and Hansen, 2012; Steigler et al., 2010; Hloch et al., 2014). The vaccination status of the patient should be evaluated to determine the requirement for a tetanus booster (Ward, 2013).

A physical examination is also required in the assessment of the patient. The type, location and depth of wound should be analysed and the range of motion evaluated if the bite is in the area of a joint (Ward, 2013). If the wound is more than six hours old, it should be assessed for any signs of infection. If infection is present, there may be signs of wound discharge, lymphangitis and cellulitis (Ward, 2012; Morgan, 2005). If the wound is to the hand, special attention is required as severe injury may occur and there is a higher risk of infection (Rothe et al., 2009). Wounds to the face, neck and head also need special attention as they should be treated and closed quickly to prevent infection, deformity and scarring (Morgan, 2005; Rui-feng et al., 2013). The depth of wound should be examined as deeper examples cause more severe injury and have a higher risk of infection (Pfortmueller et al., 2013). It is also important to examine the type of wound as lacerations have a lower risk of infection compared to punctures and different bacterial species have a tendency to infect the different types of wound with anaerobic bacteria and *Pasteurella* spp. more commonly found in puncture wounds (Talan et al., 1999).

## 20.5.2 General wound management

In the first line of treatment, wounds should be cleansed and any foreign objects removed (see Chapter 19 for further details). Copious irrigation is required for all wound types, even if minor, to reduce risk of infection. The use of pressure for the irrigation should be done with care to avoid driving infection into the wound. Pressure can be applied by using an 18- or 19- gauge needle or catheter attached to a large syringe (Taplitz, 2004) and about 1 litre of solution used (Looke and Dendle, 2010). It is also important to remove any devitalised tissue surrounding the wound (Ward, 2013; Rui-feng et al., 2013). If infection occurs, signs of redness, swelling and purulent drainage are usually visible after twelve to forty-eight hours (Morgan, 2005).

## 20.5.3 Closure of wounds

Many dog bite wounds may require closure by suturing (see Chapter 21), but there is some controversy in the scientific literature whether suturing wounds as soon as possible or leaving them open for twenty-four hours to prevent infection is preferable. Traditionally, it has been recommended that dog bite wounds be left open to allow access for cleaning and bleeding to remove any infection (Morgan, 2005; Fleischer 1999; Goldstein, 1992; Griego et al., 1995). However, Maimaris and Quinton (1988) performed a randomised trial examining the primary closure of a wound from a dog bite and found that there was no increased risk of infection after primary closure. More recently, a randomised control trial (Paschos et al., 2014) also found that there was no increased risk of infection when the wound was closed immediately. The advantage of suturing immediately is that the cosmetic appearance is much improved after healing (Paschos et al., 2014). Face, head and neck wounds should be closed as soon as possible, after cleaning and debridement, as the risk of infection is lower at this site and results in a better cosmetic appearance (Rui-feng et al., 2012; Paschos et al., 2014).

If the wound is presented for treatment some time after the injury, the wound has a higher risk of infection. It is not clear whether closure of older wounds can prevent infection or within what time period the wound can be closed safely without increasing the chance of infection (Zehtabchi et al., 2012; Van den Baar et al., 2010; Berk et al., 1988).

## 20.5.4 Prophylactic antibiotics

The use of antibiotics to reduce the risk of an infection developing from a dog bite wound has advantages in some cases, however, the standard use of antibiotics in all cases of dog bite injury is controversial. There have been few controlled trials performed to analyse the effectiveness of the use of antibiotics to prevent serious infection. One meta-analysis indicated that prophylactic use of antibiotics reduces the incidence of infection but fourteen patients would need to be treated to prevent one infection (Cummings, 1994). Another, more recent trial found that there was no significant difference between infection rates in those treated with antibiotics to prevent infection compared with no preventive antibiotics prescribed (Medeiros and Saconato, 2001). With antibiotic resistance rates increasing from their overuse, it is worth considering restricting the use of prophylactic antibiotics to high-risk injuries or high-risk patients only (Looke and Dendle, 2010; Ward, 2013). Antibiotics are recommended if the patient is immunocompromised and at high risk of severe infection (Hloch et al., 2014; Wareham et al., 2007) or if the wound is a deep puncture, there is crushing of tendons with a lot of dead tissue, or particularly dirty wounds (Looke and Dendle, 2010; Rothe et al., 2002).

## 20.6 Treatment of infected wounds

If a wound becomes infected, the wound should be opened, cleaned thoroughly and drained. Swabs should be taken as soon as possible to identify the infecting bacteria to allow the correct selection of antibiotic (Morgan, 2005; Esposito et al., 2013). For treatment to start before identification of the infecting agent there must be some educated presumptions made. Penicillin and ampicillin have often been used as general therapy for infections as they were known to be effective against *Pasteurella* spp. which are common in dog bites. However, studies have shown that *Staphylococci* spp. and anaerobes may also be involved and these are resistant to these antibiotics (Brook, 2003; Talan et al., 1999). Studies into the best selection of antibiotic for dog bite wounds are limited but the literature suggests that amoxicillin/clavulanate, taken orally is effective against most of the bacterial species most likely to be involved in the infection (Ward, 2013; Esposito et al., 2013; Morgan, 2005). In the case of allergy to penicillin-based antibiotics, extended-spectrum cephalosporins or trimethroprim-sulfamethoxazole can be used, or metronidazole plus doxycycline, or metronidazole plus oxytetracycline. First generation cephalosporins, macrolides or lincosamides should be avoided as *Pasteurella* spp. are not susceptible to these (Looke and Dendle, 2010). In severe infection, the antibiotic ampicillin-sulbactam given intravenously is recommended (Ward, 2013). If the infection appears to be caused by *Staphylococcus* spp. and the community has a high rate of methicillin-resistant *Staphylococcus aureus* (MRSA), then the antibiotic selection will depend on the severity of the infection, the age of the patient and local susceptibility patterns. Potential recommendations include vancomycin, clindamycin, trimethropim-sulfamethoazole or a tetracycline (Ward, 2013).

## 20.7 Tetanus and rabies prophylaxis

The risk of a tetanus infection after a dog bite is rare but the risk should be considered as with any contaminated wound (Esposito et al., 2013). Tetanus toxoid along with tetanus human immunoglobulins are recommended in children who have not received the full schedule of the tetanus vaccine. A tetanus booster should also be considered if it has been longer than five years since the last tetanus vaccine or booster (Howdieshell et al., 2006). There is a small risk of this infection in any contaminated wound.

Rabies prophylaxis should also be considered if there is a risk that the dog may be infected. The requirement of rabies immunisation will depend on the epidemiology of the area where the patient was bitten and if the dog can be observed. Prophylaxis is effective if the wound is treated effectively and the vaccine and immunoglobulins are given promptly (Warrell, 2012).

## 20.8 Conclusion

Up to 25% of dog bites can result in infection taking hold. Sometimes these infections can lead to severe complications that require hospitalisation and treatment for long periods. To prevent infection, quick treatment is required, including cleaning and debridement of the wound and understanding of the risks of infection. Generally, antibiotics are not required but in cases where risk of severe infection is high, due to the patient or wound type, antibiotics should be given as a preventive measure. To reduce the usage of antibiotics for dog bite wounds, some research into improved, faster methods of diagnosis is required. If infection can be diagnosed quickly then antibiotics can be used only when necessary and not as a preventative measure. The selection of antibiotics will depend on the infecting bacteria, the type of wound and the antibiotic resistance pattern within the community. It is still unclear how many dog bite wounds are infected with antibiotic resistant bacteria and this needs to be studied further to ensure the correct use of antibiotics. With severe complications possible, it is better to prevent the wound in the first place by educating children and adults about the risks of dog bites, how to behave safely around dogs, alongside measures aimed at encouraging responsible dog ownership.

## 20.9 References

Abrahamian, F. M. (2000). *Dog bites: bacteriology management and prevention. Curr Infect Dis Rep.* 2, 446–453.

Beck, A. M., Jones, B. A., (1985). *Unreported dog bites in children. Public Health Rep.* 100, 315–321.

Benson L. S., Edwards, S. L., Schiff, A. P., Williams, C. S., Visotsky, J. L. (2006). *Dog and cat bites to the hand: treatment and cost assessment. J Hand Surg Am.* 31, 468–473.

Berk, W. A., Osbourne, D. D., Taylor, D. D. (1988). *Evaluation of the 'Golden Period' for wound repair: 204 cases from a third world emergency department. Annals Emerg Med.* 17, 496–500.

Brook, I. (2003). *Microbiology and management of human and animal bite wound infections. Prim care.* 30, 25–39.

Centers for Disease Control and Prevention (CDC) (2003). *Nonfatal dog bite-related injuries treated in hospital emergency departments – United States, 2001. MMWR Morb Mortal Wkly rep.* 52, 605–610.

Cummings, P. (1994). *Antibiotics to prevent infection in patients with dog bite wounds: a meta-analysis of randomized trials. Ann Emerg Med.* 23, (3) 535–540.

Davis, I. J., Wallis, C., Deusch, O., Colyer, A., Milella, L., Loman, N., Harris, S., (2013). *A Cross-Sectional Survey of Bacterial Species in Plaque from Client Owned Dogs with Healthy Gingiva, Gingivitis or Mild Periodontitis. PLoS One.* 8 (12) e83158.

Dewhirst, F. E., Klein, E. A., Thompson, E. C., Blanton, J. M., Chen, T., Milella, L., Buckley, C. M. F., Davis, I. J., Bennett, M-L., Marshall-Jones, Z. V., (2012). *The canine oral microbiome. PLoS One.* 7 (4) e36067.

Dilegge, S. K., Edgcomb, V. P., Leadbetter, E. R., (2011). *Presence of the oral bacterium Capnocytophaga canimorsus in the tooth plaque of canines. Vet Microbiol.* 149, 437–445.

Esposito, S., Picciollo, I., Semino, M., Principi, N. (2013). *Dog and cat bite-associated infections in children. Eur J Clin Microbiol Infect Dis.* 32, 971–976.

Fleisher, G. R. (1999). *The management of bite wounds. New Eng J Med.* 340, 138–140.

Goldstein, E. J. (1992). *Bite wounds and Infection. Clin Infect Dis.* 14, 633–638.

Griego, R. D., Rosen, T., Orengo, I. F., Wolf, J. E. (1995). *Dog, Cat and human bites: a review. J Am Acad Dermatol.* 33, 1019–1029.

Hantson, P., Gautier, P. E., Vekemans, M. C., Fievez, P., Evrard, P., Wauters, G., Mahieu, P. (1991). *Fatal Capnocytophaga canimorsus septicaemia in a previously healthy woman. Ann Emerg Med.* 20, 93–94.

Hloch, O., Mokra, D., Masopust, J., Hasa, J., Charvat, J. (2014). *Antibiotic treatment following a dog bite*

5

*in an immunocompromized patient in order to prevent Capnocytophaga canimorsus infection: a case report.* BMC Research Notes. 7, 432–435.

Howdieshell, T. R., Heffernan, D., Dipiro, J. T. (2006). *Surgical infection Society guidelines for vaccination after traumatic injury.* Surg Infect. 7, 275–303.

HSCIC (2014). Dog Bites: hospital admissions in most deprived areas three times as high as least deprived. www.hscic.gov.uk/article/4722

Keijser, B. J. F. B., Zaura, E. E., Huse, S. M. S., van der Vossen, J. M. B. M. J. M., Schuren, F. H. J. F., Montjin, R. C. R., ten Cate, J. M. J., Crielaard, W. W., (2008). *Pyrosequencing analysis of the oral microflora of healthy adults.* J. Dent. Res. 87, 1016–1020.

Lion, C., Escande, F., Burdin, J.C. (1996). *Capnocytophaga canimorsus infections in human: Review of the literature and case report.* Eur J Epidemiol. 12, 521–533.

Litovitz, T. L., Klein-Schwartz, W., White, S., Cobaugh, D. J., Youniss, J., Omslaer, J. C., Drab, A., Benson, B. E. (2001). *2000 annual report of the American Association of Poison Control centers Toxic Exposure Surveillance System.* Am J Emerg Med. 19, 337–395.

Looke, D., Dendle, C., (2010), *Bites (Mammalian).* BMJ Clin Evid. 07, 914.

Maimaris, C., Quinton, D. N., (1988) Dog bite lacerations: a controlled trial of primary wound closure. Arch Emerg Med. 5, 156–161.

Martins, L. R., Pina, S. M., Simoes, R, L., de Matos, A.j., Rodrigues, P., da Costa, P. M. (2013). *Common phenotypic and genotypic antimicrobial resistance patterns found in a case study of multiresistant E. coli from cohabitant pets, humans and household surfaces,* J Environ Health. 75 (6), 74–81.

McKnight, C. A., Maes, R. K., Wise, A. G., Kiupel, M. (2007). *Evaluation of Tongue as a complementary sample for the diagnosis of parvoviral infection in dogs and cats.* J Vet Diag Invest. 19 (4), 409–413.

Medeiros, I., Saconato, H. (2001). *Antibiotic prophylaxis for mammalian bites.* Cochrane Database Syst Rev. 2, CD001738.

Monrad, R. N., Hansen, D. S. (2012). *Three cases of Capnocytophaga canimorsus meningitis seen at a regional hospital in one year.* Scand J Infect Dis. 44, 320–324.

Morgan, M., (2005). *Hospital management of animal and human bites.* J Hosp Infect. 61, 1–10.

Oehler, R. L., Velez, A. P., Mizrachi, M., Lamarche, J., Gompf, S. (2009). *Bite-related and septic syndromes caused by cats and dogs.* Lancet Infect Dis. 9, 439–447.

Oh, J., Byrd, A. L., Deming, C., Conlan, S., NISC Comparative Sequencing Program, Kong, H.H., Segre, J. A. (2014). *Biogeography and individuality shape function in the human skin metagenome.* Nature. 514, 59–64.

Ostenello, F., Gherardi, A., Capriolo, A., La Placa, L., Passini, A., Prosperi, S. (2005). *Incidence of injuries caused by dogs and cats treated in emergency departments in a major Italian city.* Emerg Med J. 22, 260–262.

Paschos, N. K., Makris, E. A., Gantsos, A. (2014). *Primary closure versus non-closure of dog bite wounds. A randomised controlled trial.* Injury. 45, 237–240.

Pfortmueller, C. A., Efeoglou, A., Furrer, H., Exadaktylos, A. K. (2013). *Dog Bite Injuries: Primary and Secondary Emergency Department Presentations – A Retrospective Cohort Study.* Sci World J. 2013, 393176.

Quinlan, K. P., Sacks, J. J. (1999). *Hospitalizations for dog bite injuries.* JAMA. 281, 232–233.

Rothe, M., Rudy, T., Stankovic, P. (2002). *Treatment of bites to the hand and wrist – is the primary antibiotic prophylaxis necessary?* Handchirurgie, Mikochirurgie, Plastiche Chirurgie. 34, (1) 22–29.

Rui-feng, C., Li-song, H., Ji-bo, Z., Li-qui, W. (2013). *Emergency treatment on facial laceration of dog bite wounds with immediate closure: a prospective randomized trial study.* BMC Emergency Medicine. 13, (Suppl 1) S2.

Ruscher, C., Lubke–Becker, A., Semmler, T., Wleklinski, C. G., Paasch, A., Soba, A., Stamm, I., Kopp, P., Wieler, L. H., Walther, B. (2010). *Widespread rapid emergence of a distinct methicillin- and multidrug-resistant Staphylococcus pseudintermedius (MRSP) genetic lineage in Europe.* Vet Microbiol. 144, 340–346

Stiegler, D., Gilbert, J. D., Warner, M. S., Byard, R. W. (2010). *Fatal dog bite in the absence of significant trauma: Capnocytophaga canimorsus infection and unexpected death.* Am J Forensic Med Patol. 31, (2) 198–199.

Sturgeon, A., Stull, J. W., Costa, M. C., Weese, J. S., (2013). *Metagenomic analysis of the canine oral cavity as revealed by high-throughput pyrosequencing of the 16S rRNA gene.* Vet Microbiol. 162, 891–898.

Sundberg, J. P., O'Banion, M. K., Schmidt-Didier, E., Riechmann, M. E. (1986). *Cloning and characterization of a canine oral papillomavirus.* Am J Vet Res. 47 (5), 1142–1144.

Suzuki, M., Kimura, M., Imaoka, K., Yamada, A., (2010). *Prevalence of Capnocytophaga canimorsus and Capnocytophaga cynodegmi in dogs and cats determined by using a newly established species specific PCR.* Vet Microbiol. 144, 172–176.

Talan, D. A., Citron, D. M., Abrahamiam, F. M., Moran, G. J., Goldstein, E. J. C., (1999). Bacteriologic analysis of infected dog and cat bites. New Engl J Med. 340, 85–92.

Taplitz, R. A., (2004). Managing bite wounds. Currently recommended antibiotics for treatment and prophylaxis. Postgrad Med. 116, 49–52.

Thomas, N. and Brook, I. (2011). *Animal bite-associated infections: microbiology and treatment.* Expert Rev Anti Infect Ther. 9, 215–226.

Van den Baar, M. T., Van der Palen, J., Vroon, M. I., Bertelink, P., Hendrix, R. (2010). *Is time to closure a factor in the occurrence of infection in traumatic wounds? A prospective cohort study in a Dutch level I trauma centre.* Emerg Med J. 27, 540–543.

Wacharapluesadee, S., Tepsumethanon, V., Supavonwong, P., Kaewpom, T., Intarut, N., Hemachudha, T. (2012). *Detection of rabies viral RNA by Taqman real-time RT-PCR using non-neural specimens from dogs infected with Rabies virus.* J Virol Methods. 184, 109–112.

Wald, K., Martinez, A., Moll, S. (2008). *Capnocytophaga canimorsus infection with fulminant sepsis in an asplenic patient: diagnosis by review of peripheral blood smear.* Am J Hematol. 83, 879.

Ward, M. A., (2013). *Bite Wound infections.* Clin ped emergency med. 14, (2), 88–94.

Wareham, D. W., Michael, J. S., Warwick, S., Whitlock, P., Wood, A., Das, S. S. (2007). *The dangers of dog bites.* J. Clin. Path. 60, 328–329.

Warrell, M. J. (2012). *Current rabies vaccines and prophylaxis schedules: preventing rabies before and after exposure.* Travel Med Infect Dis. 10, 1–15.

Weese, C., van Duijkeren, E. (2010). *Methicillin resistant Staphylococcus aureus and Staphylococcus pseudintermedius in veterinary medicine.* Vet Microbiol. 140, 418–429.

Wilson, B. A., Ho, M. (2013). *Pasteurella multicida: from zoonosis to cellular microbiology.* Clin Microbiol Rev. 26, (3) 631–655.

Windahl, U., Reimegard, E., Holst, B. S., Egenvall, A., Fernstrom, L., Fredriksson, M., Trowald-Wigh, G., Andersson, U. G. (2012). *Carriage of methicillin resistant Staphylococcus pseudintermedius in dogs – a longitudinal study.* BMC Veter Res. 8, 34.

Xie, G., Chain, P., Lo, C., Liu, K., Gans, J., Merritt, J., Qi, F., (2010). *Community and gene composition of a human dental plaque microbiota obtained by metagenomic sequencing.* Mol Oral Microbiol. 25, 391–405.

5

Zaura, E., Keijser, B. J., Huse, S. M., Crielaard, W., (2009). *Defining the healthy "core microbiome" of oral microbial communities*. BMC Microbiol. 9, 259.

Zehtabchi, S., Tan, A., Yadav, K., Badawy, A., Lucchesi, M. (2012). *The impact of wound age on the infection rate of simple lacerations repaired in the emergency department*. Injury. 43, 1793–1798.

# CHAPTER 21

# Dog Bite Injuries:
# Surgical Management of the Wound

*Christopher Mannion*

**This chapter contains graphic photographs that some readers may find distressing.**

## 21.1 Introduction

Dog bite injuries (DBI) are a common presentation to hospital accident and emergency departments. The type of wounds presenting at hospital ranges from superficial punctures of the skin to significant life- and limb threatening injuries. While death from attacks by dogs are given high prominence in the media, the scale of non-fatal injuries sustained by adults and children is probably only appreciated by those working in general medical practice, emergency medicine and the specialties that go on to treat these patients. There is some debate over the role of surgery in certain types of wound and so this chapter focuses on the decisions to be made regarding this and factors influencing these.

## 21.2 Presentation of dog bite injuries for surgical consideration

The exact number of dog bite injuries sustained each year is poorly documented in the UK, as a significant proportion of wounds may not present to any medical practitioner at all, but in countries where rabies is endemic, data may be more reliable as it may be a statutory requirement to report these incidents (Chapter 22). However, it is perhaps questionable as to whether bites from family dogs are necessarily reported.

Patients sustaining dog bite injuries requiring surgical assessment often present at an accident and emergency department, although some referrals come directly to specialists via their GP. Where direct referral from primary care occurs, it is frequently as a result of multiple wounds, or complex wounds that involve deep tissue layers, resultant tissue loss, or due to complications to a bite wound such as infection or scarring.

Many wounds may be seen and treated while in accident and emergency, only requiring simple medical follow up (Chapters 19 and 20), although psychological follow up may be

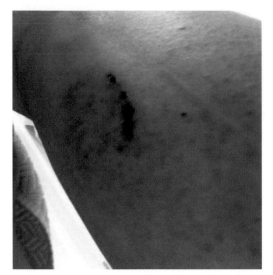

**Figure 21.1** Clinical Case: This patient (MT) was bitten while out walking in a city park in the UK. She sustained a superficial bite wound to her right calf and did not seek a medical opinion.

warranted in some cases (Chapter 23). Other wounds may require a referral for specialist management and admission.

In a recent audit of fifty patients attending our paediatric A&E department, 30% of cases required specialty input, the overwhelming majority therefore being managed within the department and then discharged.

Wounds frequently requiring admission are complicated hand or limb injuries commonly referred to orthopaedic or plastic surgery services, or head, facial and neck injuries requiring specialist input by oral and maxillofacial surgeons, plastic surgeons and occasionally ophthalmology experts if involving the delicate structures of the eye. Only those requiring admission overnight may be included in national statistics, such as those produced for the NHS in the UK, and these actually relate to dog bites or strikes.

These include injuries sustained from dogs in other ways, such as tripping over an animal, although this is not recognised by reports in the popular media of these figures. These are, nonetheless, the injuries more likely to require some form of surgery. Dog bite wounds at the 'minor end' of the scale may range from simple abrasions and may involve penetration of the superficial skin layer. Puncture of the skin and exposure of subcutaneous tissues is of greater concern and usually requires more involved treatment to wash and debride the wound. Damage to muscle, vessels, nerves, bone or joints constitutes a serious injury and requires a thorough inspection. In these cases, general anaesthesia is frequently required to allow a more thorough review of the wound.

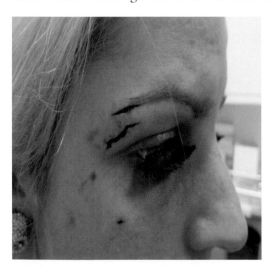

**Figure 21.2** Clinical Case: Patient A injured by her pet dog while arguing with her partner. On closer inspection, two small puncture wounds were present with two superficial skin lacerations. This required careful irrigation and debridement under local anaesthetic and not surgery.

## 21.3 Surgical assessment of the dog bite patient and wounds

### *21.3.1 Assessment of the patient*

A clear and structured approach should be followed when dealing with DBI patients, but in a recent retrospective study of dog bite injuries, the history regarding the incident, together with a detailed wound assessment, was considered inadequate in approximately 70% of cases (Mannion et al. 2015).

Assessing the patient who has been bitten by a dog requires patience and time. A clear and concise history must be obtained, together with a thorough examination. A specific and detailed wound assessment should also be documented. Treatment will then be commenced depending on the clinical findings.

All major injuries resulting from dog bites should be treated in accordance with the US College of Surgeons' Advanced Trauma Life Support guidelines (ATLS 2012). A primary survey should commence with control of the airway and the cervical spine being protected. This is especially important in the case of young children, who may have been shaken and thrown. Following ATLS principles, therefore, assessment should involve the principles as laid out:

- Primary survey:
    A.   Airway with cervical spine protection
    B.   Breathing and ventilation
    C.   Circulation and arrest of haemorrhage
    D.   Disability and neurological status
    E.   Exposure of extremities and environment.

- Investigations and resuscitation.

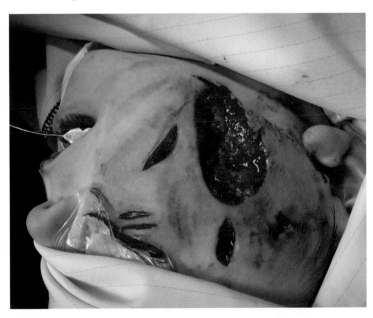

**Figure 21.3** Clinical Case: A young boy bitten by the family dog. Examination under anaesthetic allowed extensive assessment for injury to the facial nerve, parotid duct and estimation of the degree of tissue loss.

Then:

- Secondary survey: This involves a top-to-toe examination to exclude further injuries.

To aid in correct information gathering, a simple proforma can be followed (e.g. Text box 21.1) that identifies key areas for history taking.

## Text box 21.1  Sample proforma for dog bite patient evaluation

Key questions that must be considered are:

- Where and when did the bite occur?
- How? The context of the situation that resulted in the bite and (if a child) was there supervision of the child and animal?
- What is the patient's tetanus status?
- Is rabies a consideration?
- Is there any associated relevant medical history of which you should be aware?

Certain predisposing medical factors should be borne in mind when dealing with the specifics of wound management:

- For example, the diabetic patient is at an increased risk of a wound infection
- A history of alcohol dependence, smoking and/or substance misuse can also affect wound healing and infection risk, and may have been a precipitant to the bite injury
- Chronic liver or lung disease and immunosuppressive states
- Asplenic individuals
- Patients with prosthetic valves or prosthetic joints.

Any of these can reduce the patient's capacity to heal optimally, and lead to a raised risk of infection.

Consideration should also be given to:

- Current medications
- Pregnancy
- Diabetes
- Nutritional state
- Extremes of age.

- The timing of the injury is vital as delay in presentation and treatment has been identified as a significant risk factor for a resulting wound infection (Maimaris and Quinton, 1988). This will therefore affect the overall management of the patient and such wounds are recommended to be washed and debrided as soon as possible.

## 21.3.2 Assessment of the wound

The force delivered by the jaws of a biting dog can be as high as 400lb/sq inch (Barr, no date). Such power delivered by a dog's sharp dentition may result in specific injuries to both the soft (e.g. skin) and hard tissues (e.g. bone) and therefore both of these should be considered in the case of punctures, lacerations and avulsions with or without an actual tissue deficit. A typical dog bite consists of a combination of puncture wounds with adjacent tearing of tissue – 'hole and tear' effect. Some degree of crush injury often results. These 'puncture' wounds are at a higher risk of infection as they harbour micro-organisms deep within the wound (Chapter 20), and have a narrow entry point, making thorough cleaning difficult. Crush injuries can also precipitate infections because of the resulting ischaemic damaged tissue. A significant size of devitalised tissue in severe injuries, such as full thickness wounds, also predisposes to bacterial colonisation and growth, leading to infection.

The Lackmann classification (Table 21.1, Lackmann et al., 1992) of bite wound injury is useful for the description of and communication about a wound, and aids in audit and research.

With an avulsion injury, tissue at the wound site may be displaced from the underlying tissue layers yet still be partially attached (avulsion flap or partial avulsion), or it may be totally detached from the wound site (complete avulsion). Thus, the clinical examination of the wound should highlight:

- Site, size, shape and number of wound(s)
- Depth, tissue involved/tissue avulsion
- State of deep structures (nerves, vessels, tendons, joints and bone)
- Condition of the wound (clean, dirty, infected).

A full and thorough neurovascular examination should be performed, with particular attention to excluding tendon and bony injuries, fractures and joint involvement. In especially young children or babies, bones are soft and these can fracture easily.

Injuries at multiple locations are characteristic of dog bites (Mitchell et al., 2003). Any facial wounds should be examined for penetration into the oral cavity and possible damage to underlying structures and/or avulsion of teeth (Figure 21.3). Bite injuries to the scalp and head should be examined carefully to exclude skull bone fractures, which could precipitate intracranial bleeding with catastrophic consequences (Chapter 11).

Where bite injuries involve the limbs, special consideration should address the various facial compartments. If during examination of the wound pus is evident, a swab must be

**Table 21.1** The Lackmann classification of wounds.

| Lackmann Classification | Definition |
| --- | --- |
| Type I | Superficial lesion without muscle involvement |
| Type II | Deep lesion with muscle involvement |
| Type III | Deep lesion with muscle involvement and tissue defect |
| Type IVa | Class III combined with vascular damage or nerve lesions |
| Type IVb | Class III combined with bone damage or organ involvement |

taken for microbiological culture and sensitivity and appropriate surgical management and antibiotics commenced.

Where there is a clinical concern that a possible underlying bony injury exists, appropriate radiological examinations should be organised.

## 21.4 Initial management

### 21.4.1 Wound cleansing

Following taking a history and performing a clinical examination, the wound must be cleaned. Irrigation and debridement is important in preventing subsequent infection and should be instigated at the earliest opportunity. High-pressure irrigation must be undertaken with care to avoid the risk of driving material deeper into the wound, especially in the case of puncture wounds. Normal saline, a 20ml syringe and a 19-gauge needle is suitable for the purpose. There is no consensus on the volume of irrigant that should be used, however, the quantity of solution should reflect the site, size and nature of the injured tissue. Judicious use of local anaesthetic may be administered through uninvolved adjacent skin and away from the damaged tissue. Elevation of an involved limb can reduce subsequent tissue oedema and swelling. The tetanus immunisation status of the patient should also be addressed at this stage, together with rabies consideration where appropriate.

### 21.4.2 Antibiotic use

Controversy surrounds the use of prophylactic antibiotics in non-infected animal bites (Chapter 20). The risk of infection of a dog bite is reportedly between 2 and 20% (Morgan and Palmer, 2007; Jha et al., 2014). Their use in high-risk wounds (i.e. combinations of wound, location on the hand, deep puncture wounds, or patient factors such as an immunocompromised host – see above) should be considered strongly, together with those cases presenting late (>24 hours since injury).

The antibiotic most commonly recommended for first choice prophylaxis is co-amoxiclav. For patients allergic to penicillin, metronidazole plus doxycycline, or metronidazole plus oxytetracycline (National Institute for Health and Care Excellence (NICE), UK, 2012) is recommended. Oral antibiotics should be prescribed for seven days for those wounds that are infected. If the patient is systemically unwell or has a severe infection, admission and treatment with intravenous antibiotics will be required and a pus sample must be taken.

## 21.5 Surgical management

It may be decided that surgical management is required. The first principle in the surgical management of dog bites should be to fully inspect the wound with a good light, and then to clean and debride this thoroughly, prior to any attempt to close the wound. It is this effective cleaning in combination with the debridement of devitalised tissue that reduces the risk of a wound infection and improves outcome for the patient. The closure and repair of damaged structures can then be considered.

## 21.5.1  Surgical options

There are a number of options for allowing cutaneous healing in surgical defects. These include:

- No repair – healing by secondary intention
- Primary closure
- Skin grafting
- Local tissue transfer with random pattern or axial flaps
- Free tissue transfer.

The choice of which reconstructive option to use is based on:

- The patient's needs and wishes
- The size and location of the wound
- Associated partial or total tissue loss/avulsion
- The type of tissue that has been lost – its form and function
- Patient comorbidities
- The complexity of the options of reconstructive technique.

Consideration to the principles of reconstruction and the reconstructive ladder used by surgeons should achieve the best cosmetic and functional outcome for the patient. In severe injuries, especially those in children, this process is frequently performed in the operating theatre environment and under a general anaesthetic. In considered situations primary repair and closure may be appropriate.

## 21.5.2  Primary closure

Traditional practice regarding dog bite wounds has led to many being left open to heal by secondary intent; the concern being that closure of a potentially infected wound could lead to abscess formation, tissue breakdown and systemic sepsis. This approach still has a place in certain wounds whose location, associated patient and wound factors and propensity for infection spread outweigh any cosmetic concerns. However, low risk wounds (<six hours and no risk factors for infection) for example, lacerations, puncture wounds, and abrasions, can often be managed best with primary repair when appropriate (Kountakis et al., 1998). The literature suggests that there is no statistically significant increase in the wound infection rate when low risk dog bites are closed primarily after adequate washout and debridement (Evgeniou et al., 2013). Special care should be given to high-risk wounds such as those identified below:

- Wounds to the arm and hands
- Delay in seeking treatment >twenty-four hours
- Older patients (>fifty years)
- Deep puncture wounds
- Full-thickness wounds
- Extensive crush injuries/devitalised tissue.

*Primary closure of facial wounds*: Head and neck injuries represent a major cosmetic concern, therefore to achieve an optimal outcome, it is generally accepted that non–infected cases can be closed primarily, after debridement and washout, without any significant increase in the infection rate. The rich vascularity of the face and scalp reduces this risk of infection, but antibiotics are commonly prescribed following primary closure, although there is no universal agreement within this opinion (Herford and Ghali, 2012). Primary closure of facial wounds should be undertaken by specialists to minimise healing times and improve cosmetic outcomes (National Institute for Health and Care Excellence (NICE) 2012).

*Complex wounds of the head and neck:* When there have been serious bite injuries to the head and neck region, exploration under general anaesthetic is required to exclude damage to the major structures such as the vasculature, motor nerves to the facial muscles or the airway. Extensive tissue loss can be especially challenging for the surgeon in this situation. These injuries may require multistage procedures, for example those involving significant soft tissue loss such as avulsion injuries, which should be attempted secondarily after adequate wound care.

The most frequently bitten areas to the face are the upper and lower lips, the cheeks, nose and ears (Mannion et al., 2015). It is worth emphasising that, together with soft tissue damage, penetration into the oral cavity, underlying injuries and fractures to the teeth, facial skeleton and skull should be examined for and managed accordingly. Each particular subunit of the face has its own reconstructive challenge, the detail of which lies outside the scope of this text (Baker, 2014).

*Primary closure of injuries to the limbs and hands:* Dog bite injuries to the hand have a higher incidence of infection, in comparison to those wounds in the head and neck, when closed primarily. In some instances, infection rate of 25% after primary suture has been shown (Aigner et al., 1996) and is therefore seldom recommended. The traditional management following initial irrigation and debridement is to leave these wounds open for twenty-four to forty-eight hours before a second-look procedure.

The possible complications from injuries to the hands are infections, fractures, neurovascular damage, tenosynovitis, septic arthritis, and osteomyelitis. When there is evidence of joint involvement or clinical evidence of septic arthritis, arthrotomy and copious joint washout is required. Postoperative immobilisation of the hand in a plaster splint for up to seventy-two hours is recommended, followed by aggressive physiotherapy in the case of cat bites (Mitnovetski and Kimble, 2004), but is equally advisable in the case of dog bites to the hand.

*Complex wounds of the limbs or hands:* Complex limb and hand injuries frequently involve fractures, tendon and nerve injuries. The repair of these injuries should be managed as any open/contaminated injury. With bony injuries and fractures, permanent fixation should be carried out at a secondary stage after the initial wound washout and after further inspections (Evgeniou et al., 2013). This is a similar approach to that taken for the repair of tendon and nerves injuries. Multiple wound washes and debridement should be required in cases where infection is evident before repair of complex structures is carried out.

## 21.5.3 Delayed presentation

The time elapsed from injury to presentation should be considered. Some advocate managing a wound several hours old differently to one presenting immediately following injury;

the concern being an older wound will have had time to become colonised with pathogenic bacteria and could be deemed at greater risk of subsequent infection. These patients have a significantly increased likelihood of requiring surgical intervention (Bach et al., 2005). A delay of over twenty-four hours before necessary surgical debridement has also been shown to be a risk factor for the development of osteomyelitis (Gonzalez et al., 1993).

## 21.6 Complications

Following initial treatment, the most common complication of a dog bite injury is infection due to micro-organisms (See Chapter 20). Reported infection rates for dog bite wounds lie somewhere between 2% and 30% (Capellan and Hollander, 2003; Morgan and Palmer, 2007). Infection in dog bite wounds tends to result from polymicrobial contamination. Talan et al. (1999) found up to sixteen different bacterial isolates in purulent wounds resulting from dog bites. The most commonly identified bacteria were *Pasteurella, Streptococci, Staphylococci,* and anaerobes. Traditionally it is thought that deep, piercing or puncture wounds are more likely to develop infection, with one study of 769 dog bite wounds finding wound depth, patient gender, and wound debridement were the clinical variables that best predicted the likelihood of developing infection (Dire et al., 1994).

Those wounds that present early (<twelve hours) already with clinical signs of infection are likely to be caused by *Pasteurella* species and this species is present in perhaps more than 50% of dog bites (Talan et al., 1999). This is an aggressive Gram negative pathogen, causing early intense inflammatory response with considerable tissue involvement, and it is likely to cause metastatic infection with severe systemic sequelae (Weber et al., 1984).

The site of injury is important in assessing infection risk, with the hands particularly prone (Rothe et al., 2002). The lowest risk of wound infection is found in facial injury in children (Boenning et al., 1983). It is generally accepted that head and neck wounds carry a relatively low risk of infection due to the improved blood supply to the face (Wu et al., 2011).

When treating an infected animal bite, a pus or deep wound swab should be sent for culture and treated empirically with oral antibiotics for seven days. It is recommended that anyone with a severe infection or who is systemically unwell is admitted for intravenous antibiotics and treatment as required. Inpatient treatment must cover *Pasteurella,* anaerobes, and staphylococci, and be modified according to culture results. Microbiological advice should be sought early because if septicaemia develops, the mortality may be as high as 30%. (HPA, 2006).

## 21.7 Follow-up

Medical follow-up should be arranged for all dog bite injuries. The timing of review will depend on the size, site and infection risk of the wound involved. Wounds left open to heal by secondary intent will require earlier review. Where secondary reconstruction for cosmesis is anticipated, review several months later may be required. Injuries, especially to the face, can leave lasting scars, and act as a permanent physical reminder. Thus it is important to consider that such injuries, especially in children, could also leave psychological scars (Chapter 23). The opportunity to obtain post-traumatic counselling should be available.

## 21.8 Conclusions

The surgical management of dog bite injuries involves careful evaluation of both the patient and the wound, with careful consideration given to the risk of infectious complications. These injuries take many different forms and treatment must be tailored to the individual case. Although surgeons are often focused on repairing the immediate damage caused by the bite, they should be aware of the wider implications of these injuries, including the psychological trauma suffered by the patient and the need to prevent recurrence of injury. A more coherent and collaborative approach between both the veterinary and medical professions should be adopted with a firm emphasis on education and prevention.

## 21.9 References

Aigner, N., Konig, S., Fritz, A. (1996). Bite wounds and their characteristic position in trauma surgery management. *Unfallchirurg* 99 (5):346–50.

ATLS 2012, American College of Surgeons Committee on Trauma (2012). *Advanced trauma life support program for doctors*, 9th edn. American College of Surgeons, Chicago.

Bach, G., Shah, N. A., Mejia, A., Weinzweig, N., Brown, A., Gonzalez, M. H. (2005). Upper extremity dog bite wounds and infections *J. Surg Orthop Adv* 14 (4):181–4.

Baker, S. R. (2014). *Local Flaps in Facial Reconstruction*, 3rd Edition, Elsevier, Saunders.

Barr, D. B. (no date). Dangerous Encounters: Bite Force. www.nationalgeographic.com/siteindex/customer.html

Boenning, D., Fleisher, G., Campos, J. (1983). Dog bite in children: epidemiology, microbiology and penicillin prophylactic therapy. *Am J Emerg Med*1:17–21

Capellan, O., Hollander, J. (2003). Management of lacerations in the emergency department. *Emerg Med Clin N Am.* 205–231.

Dire, D., Hogan, D., Riggs, M. (1994). A prospective evaluation of risk factors for infections from dog-bite wounds. *Acad Emerg Med.* 1:258-66.

Evgeniou E, Markeson D, Iyer S, Armstrong A. (2013). The management of animal bites in the United Kingdom. *Eplasty* 13:e27.

Gonzalez, M. H., Papierski, P., Hall, R. F. (1993). Osteomyelitis of the hand after a human bite *J Hand Surg Am.* 18(3):520–2.

Herford, A., Ghali, G. E. (2012). Soft tissue injuries, in Miloro M. (ed): Peterson's Principles of Oral and Maxillofacial Surgery (ed 3). Oak Park, IL, People's Medical Publishing House, 2012, pp.357–372.

HPA Health Protection Agency (2006). Animal bites and Pasteurella multocida: information for healthcare staff. www.hpa.org.uk

Jha, S., Khan, W. S., Siddiqui, N. A. (2014). Mammalian bite injuries to the hand and their management. *Open Orthop J.* 27(8):194–8.

Kountakis, S. E., Chamblee, S. A., Maillard, A. A., Stiernberg, C. M. (1998). Animal bites to the head and neck. *Ear Nose Throat J.* 77(3):216–20.

Lackmann, G. M., Draf, W., Isselstein, G., Töllner, U. (1992). Surgical treatment of facial dog bite injuries in children. *J Craniomaxillofac Surg.* 20(2): 81–6.

Maimaris, C., Quinton, D. N. (1988). Dog-bite lacerations: a controlled trial of primary wound closure. *Arch Emerg Med.* 5(3):156–61.

Mannion, C. J., Graham, A., Shepherd, K., Greenberg, D. (2015). Dog bites and maxillofacial surgery: what can we do? *Br J Oral Maxillofac Surg.* 53(6):522–5.

Mitchell, R. B., Nanez, G., Wagner, J. D., Kelly, J. (2003). Dog bites of the scalp, face, and neck in children. *Laryngoscope* 113:492e5.

Mitnovetski, S., Kimble, F., (2004). Cat bites of the hand. *ANZ J Surg* 74(10):859–62.

Morgan, M., Palmer, J., (2007). Dog bites *BMJ* 334:413–7.

National Institute for Health and Care Excellence (NICE) (2012) Bites human and animal. Available from: http://cks.nice.org.uk/bites-human-and-animal

Rothe, M., Rudy, T., Stanković, P. (2002). Treatment of bites to the hand and wrist – is the primary antibiotic prophylaxis necessary? *Handchir Mikrochir Plast Chir.* 34(1):22–9.

Talan, D. A., Citron, D. M., Abrahamian, F. M., Moran, G.J., Goldstein, E .J. C. (1999). Bacteriologic analysis of infected cat and dog bites. *N Engl J Med* 340:285–92.

Weber, D., Wolfson, J. S., Swartz, M. N., Hooper, D. C. (1984). Pasteurella multocida infections: report of 34 cases and review of the literature. *Medicine* 63:133–54.

Wu, P. S., Beres, A., Tashjian, D. B., Moriarty, K. P. (2011). Primary repair of facial dog bite injuries in children. *Pediatr Emerg Care.* 27(9):801–3.

# CHAPTER 22

# Dog Bites and Rabies

## Lorraine McElhinney

## 22.1 Introduction

Zoonotic diseases are directly transmissible from vertebrate animals to humans and have been recognised as a public health threat since the beginning of the domestication of animals more than 10,000 years ago. Of the 1,415 infectious organisms recorded as pathogenic for humans in 2001, 61% were deemed zoonotic (Taylor et al., 2001) and approximately 75% of emerging infectious diseases are believed to be due to zoonoses (Woolhouse and Gowtage-Sequeria, 2005). A variety of bacteria in the oral cavity of dogs have been reported to cause zoonotic infections via dog bites (Chapter 20, Zambori et al., 2013, Esposito et al., 2013). While *Echinococcus* species are known zoonotic pathogens in dogs, they are unlikely to be transmitted via dog bites. However, a recent report highlighted the immunosuppressive effect of a primary dog-mediated zoonotic infection (*E.granulosa* – cystic echinococcosis) which subsequently led to sepsis and death when *Capnocytophaga canimorsus* was transmitted to the victim via the bite of her pet dog (Matulionytė et al., 2012).

With the highest case–fatality rate of any infectious disease, rabies remains the most feared dog-borne threat to public health (Fooks et al., 2014). Although human rabies is entirely preventable through highly effective post-exposure prophylaxis (PEP), deaths are still reported in more than 150 countries worldwide (Figure 22.1). While a growing number of regions have controlled the disease through targeted vaccination campaigns, countries maintain their rabies free status at considerable cost and with a continual risk of re-importation. For example, the cost of setting up a *cordon sanitaire* along the entire eastern border of the European Union to prevent incursions into rabies free areas is estimated to exceed US$6.5 million per year (Johnson et al., 2011, Demetriou and Moynagh, 2011).

Many of the 50,000–70,000 humans estimated to die from this disease every year, particularly in Asia and Africa, are children under the age of fifteen years (Abubakar and Bakari, 2012; Anderson and Shwiff, 2013; Liu and Ertl, 2012; Hampson et al., 2015). In addition to the human burden, millions of animals suffer and die, in some cases posing a direct threat to endangered wildlife (Johnson et al., 2010).

Distribution of risk levels for humans contacting rabies, worldwide, 2013

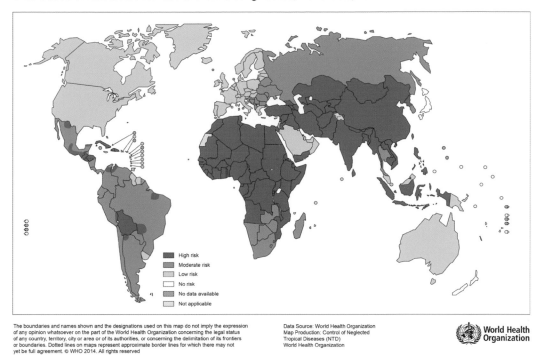

**Figure 22.1** Global distribution of risk to humans of contracting rabies. Reprinted from: www.who.int/rabies/Global_distribution_risk_humans_contracting_rabies_2013.png?ua=1 Accessed: 31 August 2016.

## 22.2 History of rabies

Records dating back to Ancient Mesopotamia support the existence of rabies in humans and dogs for more than four millennia (Rosner, 1974; Neville, 2004). For example, a pre-Mosaic Eshnunna Code, issued in about the twenty-third century BC, specified a fine of two-thirds of a mina of silver (40 Shekels) to an owner who failed to confine his mad dog should it bite and lead to the death of another man (Rosner, 1974).

The domestication of dogs and human colonisation has substantially contributed to the spread of rabies and its present day global distribution (Nel and Rupprecht, 2007). Molecular epidemiological studies of currently circulating rabies virus (RABV) isolates show ancestral roots in Europe in the eighteenth century before its widespread dispersal to Asia, Africa and the Americas as a result of the importation of infected dogs via European exploration and colonisation (Smith et al., 1992; Bourhy et al., 1999; McElhinney et al., 2006; McElhinney et al., 2011; Horton et al., 2015; Talbi et al., 2009, 2010; Vos et al., 2011).

Pet ownership has continued to rise in many countries and international pet travel is increasing with the ease of programmes such as the EU Pet Travel Scheme. Such schemes, intended to bypass quarantine measures for the control of rabies for imported dogs, cats and ferrets, have continued to be extremely popular with pet owners. For example, dogs represented more than 90% of the 1.3 million pets entering the UK under pet movement schemes between 2000 and 2014. However, the rabies-focused schemes do not offer sufficient controls for other diseases such as leishmaniasis, babesiosis, ehrlichiosis and dirofilariasis (of which leishmaniasis and ehrlichiosis are zoonotic).

## 22.3 Rabies virus

Rabies is a fatal encephalitis caused by RNA viruses belonging to the genus lyssavirus within the family *Rhabdoviridae*, order Mononegavirales. Rabies virus (RABV) is the type species and is responsible for the large majority of human and animal cases. Human cases of encephalitis caused by non-RABV lyssavirus species are clinically indistinguishable from RABV-associated cases but extremely rare. The International Committee on Taxonomy of Viruses (ICTV, 2014) classifies the lyssavirus genus into fourteen different virus species based on genetic distance, antigenic properties, geographic distribution and host range (Table 22.1). Antigenic and genetic profiles of the lyssavirus genus allow further delineation into phylogroups (Table 22.1) that predict the likely efficacy of the currently available RABV derived post-exposure prophylaxis (phylogroup I). Protection against the diverse phylogroup II and III viruses is likely to be partial or absent (Hanlon et al., 2005; Horton et al., 2010).

Bats are believed to be the ancestral reservoir species for lyssaviruses. Molecular clock analysis suggests that lyssaviruses may have originated and evolved in the order Chiroptera (i.e. bats) and then later spilled over into the order Carnivora (i.e. terrestrial carnivores) (Badrane and Tordo, 2001). While RABV is detected extensively in various bat species throughout the Americas, it is not detected in bats elsewhere. In contrast, the non-RABV bat lyssaviruses have only been detected in Africa, Europe and Asia (Banyard et al., 2011). Furthermore, RABV is present extensively in terrestrial carnivore species worldwide, whereas the other lyssaviruses are rarely detected in non-flying species. All mammals are susceptible to infection but relatively few are capable of acting as significant reservoirs for disease (Fooks et al., 2014). Only three lyssavirus species have been attributed to rabies disease in dogs (RABV, Lagos bat Virus and Mokola Virus) (Table 22.1).

## 22.4 Pathogenesis

Rabies virus is most commonly transmitted via the bite of an infected animal or by direct contact with mucosal surfaces. Transmission of rabies virus by other means has been reported but is considered rare, e.g. aerosol exposures (Johnson et al., 2006) or via organ transplantation (Maier et al., 2010). The virus cannot penetrate intact skin, so the bite mechanically allows the virus to traverse the dermal barrier and initiate infection.

The virus replicates in the muscle and neuronal cells travelling by fast retrograde transport along motor axons to reach the central nervous system (CNS) and brain (Hemachudha et al., 2013). Until the virus enters the CNS the patient shows no clinical signs and there is no evidence of a localised immune response (Hunter et al., 2010). The associated long and variable incubation period is a key feature of rabies. It can vary from five days to several years (average two to three months), depending on the strain, species, viral dose and the proximity of the site of virus entry to the CNS. A short incubation period would be expected for a deep bite or multiple bites near to the head of the victim. Clinical signs are evident

**Table 22.1** Classification of the Lyssavirus Genus. Fourteen lyssavirus species classified (ICTV, 2014). Three lyssavirus species have been attributed to rabies disease in dogs (RABV, LBV and MOKV).[1] Except in Australia, Antarctica and several islands; bats in the New World only.[2] Most of Europe from Spain to Ukraine. *LBLV and GBLV reported but not yet accepted by ICTV.

| Virus Species | Abbreviation | Phylogroup | Distribution | Species Affected |
|---|---|---|---|---|
| Classical Rabies Virus | RABV | 1 | Worldwide[1] | Wide range of mammals |
| Lagos Bat Virus | LBV | 2 | Sub-Saharan Africa | Fruit bat, dog and cat |
| Mokola Virus | MOKV | 2 | Sub-Saharan Africa | Shrew, cat, dog, rodent and human |
| Duvenhage Virus | DUVV | 1 | Sub-Saharan Africa | Insectivorous bat and human |
| European Bat Lyssavirus Type-1 | EBLV-1 | 1 | Europe[2] | Insectivorous bat, cat, sheep, stone marten and human |
| European Bat Lyssavirus Type-2 | EBLV-2 | 1 | Europe | Insectivorous bat and human |
| Australian Bat Lyssavirus | ABLV | 1 | Australia | Fruit and insectivorous bat, and human |
| Aravan Virus | ARAV | 1 | Central Asia | Insectivorous bat |
| Khujand Virus | KHUV | 1 | Central Asia | Insectivorous bat |
| Irkut Virus | IRKV | 1 | Eastern Asia | Insectivorous bat |
| West Caucasian Bat Virus | WCBV | 3 | South Eastern Europe | Insectivorous bat |
| Shimoni Bat Virus | SHIBV | 2 | Kenya | Insectivorous bat |
| Bokeloh Bat Virus | BBLV | 1 | Germany, France | Insectivorous bat |
| Ikoma Lyssavirus | IKOV | 3? | United Republic of Tanzania | African civet |
| Lleida Bat Lyssavirus | LBLV | * | Spain | Insectivorous bat |
| Gannoruwa Bat Lyssavirus | GBLV | * | Sri Lanka | Insectivorous bat |

5

following substantial infection of the brain and the subsequent centrifugal dissemination of virus through neurons to peripheral organs including muscle spindles, skin, hair follicles and other non-nervous tissues, such as salivary glands, heart muscle, lung and abdominal visceral organs (Hemachudha et al., 2002; Hemachudha et al., 2013). This extensive infection and dissemination also results in the hypersalivation and aggressive behaviour generally responsible for the onward transmission of the virus to new hosts.

Three stages are typically described for rabies; prodromal, encephalitic (excitement or furious rabies) and paralytic (dumb rabies) (Table 22.2). However, not all stages are observed in individual cases. The first clinical symptom reported is usually neuropathic pain, paraesthesia, or pruritus at the site of infection (bite wound) followed by non-specific signs typical

**Table 22.2** Clinical stages of rabies in humans and non-human animals. Disease progression is variable and, although most cases conclude in the paralytic phase, some do not show many of the signs associated with the excitement phase.

| Stage | Clinical Signs |
|---|---|
| Prodromal | • Pyrexia, dyspnoea, tremors<br>• Altered personality (loss of fear, increased nervousness, hyperactivity, disorientation)<br>• Loss of appetite<br>• Hypersensitivity to noise or light, rubbing<br>• Itching, pain or paraesthesia near the site of the healed bite wound (animals may repeatedly bite the wound) |
| Excitement (furious) | • Increased aggression,<br>• Hyper salivation, sweating and lacrimation (poor temperature control)<br>• Abnormal vocalisations (high pitch howl in canines, characteristic bellowing in ruminants)<br>• 'Fly snapping' at imaginary targets<br>• Wandering long distances<br>• Hyper sexuality<br>• Head butting (particularly ruminants)<br>• Staring eyes<br>• 'Bone in throat' syndrome<br>• Acute colic with abdominal straining (horses and ruminants).<br>• Hydrophobia (in man): violent involuntary muscle spasms and hyperextension, combined with terror at sight, sound or mention of water<br>• Aerophobia (in man) : as for hydrophobia but when faced with a blast or draft of air<br>• Brainstem and limbic system defects<br>• Cycling phases of excitation (hallucinations, fear, aggression) and lucidity<br>• Cardiac tachyarrhythmias<br>• Coma<br>• Paralysis<br>• Axonal neuropathy |
| Paralytic (dumb) | • Ascending paralysis, hind limb paralysis, partial paralysis of tongue and lower jaw with excessive drooling of saliva<br>• Dysphagia, inability to drink or swallow<br>• Convulsions<br>• Sphincter dysfunction<br>• Bulbar/respiratory paralysis, respiratory arrest<br>• Coma<br>• Death |

of viral encephalitis. The disease may then progress to either or both the excitement and/or paralytic forms of the disease. Some forms of disease may be observed more commonly in a particular species, with most progressing to the paralytic form in the final stages of infection. In some cases, including humans and dogs, clinical signs are unobserved and rabies virus has only been identified post-mortem as the cause of death. Such atypical rabies is likely to contribute to under-reporting.

In humans, classical signs of rabies infection include involuntary spasms in response to tactile, auditory, visual or olfactory stimuli (e.g. aerophobia and hydrophobia). Such signs occur during the encephalitic stage of infection and are often combined with periods of agitation, lucidity, fear and confusion. However, signs of excitation are less evident in paralytic rabies. Remarkably, cases of fatal encephalitic rabies may not necessarily be accompanied by a substantial inflammatory response in either humans or dogs.

Without intensive care interventions, death usually occurs between one to ten days following the onset of neurological signs. In dogs, the clinical phase can be much shorter at three to four days (Tepsumethanon et al., 2004).

## 22.5 Diagnosis

Although testing for evidence of hydrophobia is sometimes used diagnostically, clinical signs are not generally considered pathognomonic for rabies, particularly in the prodromal phase of disease. A history may raise the index of suspicion, e.g. pet travel especially smuggling, contact with infected wildlife including bats, lack of vaccination. If rabies is suspected in a pet, owners and veterinarians must contact the competent authority in their country.

Clinical diagnosis in animals is based on the observation of clinical signs, the first of which usually appear after the variable incubation period and can vary depending upon species. Differential diagnosis can often be difficult due to commonalities with various diseases, including transmissible spongiform encephalopathies, tetanus, listeriosis, poisoning and other viral non-suppurative encephalitidies. Paralytic rabies in humans can also be mistaken for Guillain-Barré Syndrome (Solomon et al., 2005). In addition, secondary infections, e.g. malaria, can mask the presence of rabies leading to misdiagnosis (Mallewa et al., 2007).

Consequently, diagnosis can only be confirmed by laboratory tests, preferably conducted post-mortem on central nervous system (CNS) tissue removed from the cranium. Post-mortem application of the direct fluorescent antibody technique is the gold standard for rabies diagnosis in animals and humans and is recommended by both WHO and OIE. It is a rapid, sensitive and specific method for detecting the rabies virus antigen in the brain using fluorescently labelled anti-rabies antibodies (Dean and Abelseth, 1973). The WHO and OIE recommend the use of a confirmatory virus isolation test.

Historically, the mouse inoculation test (intracerebral inoculation of mice with a homogenate of brain material) was commonly used as a confirmatory test. However, this in vivo test is time-consuming, expensive and involves the use of animals. Hence, in vitro virus isolation tests such as the Rabies Tissues Culture Inoculation Test (the inoculation of the sample into a neuroblastoma cell line) are now more commonly employed. Molecular techniques, such as polymerase chain reaction (PCR)-based assays, are also becoming more widely accepted and accessible for the diagnosis of rabies with subsequent typing/sequencing used to confirm the origin of the virus isolate (Fooks et al., 2012).

Ante-mortem diagnosis of rabies encephalomyelitis is possible by immunofluorescent staining of skin biopsy sections (nape of neck or wound site) or by PCR on saliva, cerebrospinal fluid, respiratory secretions, tears and skin biopsies. However, due to the transient and intermittent excretion of rabies virus, daily samples must be tested until a diagnosis is confirmed. The presence of specific RABV neutralising antibodies in an unvaccinated host may be indicative of infection, although post-infective rabies antibodies are rarely detectable before death. In general, antibody detection methods such as the rapid fluorescent focus inhibition test or the fluorescent antibody virus neutralisation are employed to determine post-vaccinal immunity in vaccinated animals and humans.

## 22.6 Epidemiology

Rabies virus is largely maintained in two ecologically inter-related disease cycles; sylvatic (wildlife) and urban rabies. Sylvatic rabies remains widespread throughout parts of Eastern Europe, Africa and North America and is maintained in a variety of species including the red fox, raccoon dog, raccoon, skunks, wild dogs and bats.

Dog-mediated rabies is widespread throughout many developing countries, accounting for more than 99% of all human deaths from rabies (Figure 22.1). However, canine rabies has been eliminated from Western Europe, Canada, the USA, Japan, Malaysia and a few Latin American countries. Australia, New Zealand and many Pacific island nations are also free from canine rabies. In Western Europe, North America and Japan, approximately two human deaths per year from rabies are reported and these are mainly restricted to those exposed while visiting rabies endemic areas (Malerczyk et al., 2011). However, it is likely that rabies could be under-reported in developed countries where it has been absent for a considerable length of time and there is thus a low suspicion of disease and clinicians are unfamiliar with the clinical features (Carrara et al., 2013).

More human deaths from rabies occur in Asia than anywhere else in the world. In India, an estimated 20,800 human rabies deaths, accounting for more than 35% of the global rabies burden, and 17.4 million animal bite cases occur annually, representing an incidence rate of 1.7% (Anon, 2003; Hampson et al., 2015). The majority of the human rabies victims are from rural areas and belong to lower socio-economic classes. Two-thirds of the Indian population live in rural areas and are thus at risk of exposure to rabies-infected dogs (Anon, 2003). While there have been improvements with regards to supplies of PEP in India, the incidence of human rabies and access to vaccine across rural areas are uncertain. Similarly, the true incidence of human rabies in rural China is unclear (WHO, 2013).

The 2005 and 2010 estimates of >23,000 annual human rabies cases in Africa are considered highly uncertain due to the paucity of available data (Knobel et al., 2005; WHO, 2013). In areas of Africa and Asia with high general mortality, hospitalisation offers little palliative care. As rabies is inevitably fatal, many victims (>75%), particularly those from poor socio-economic backgrounds, die at home or in the local community and are not represented in official records (Hampson et al., 2015; Tenzin et al 2011; Suraweera et al., 2012).

## 22.7  Disease burden

The annual global burden of canine rabies is estimated to be approximately $124 billion (Anderson and Shwiff, 2013) and while rabies has been identified as a key One Health issue by the World Organisation for Animal Health (OIE), World Health Organisation (WHO) and Food and Agriculture Organisation of the United Nations (FAO), it is still considered a neglected zoonotic disease (Fooks et al., 2005; Pastoret et al., 2014). Rabies is believed to be greatly under-reported, exacerbated by an absence of reliable surveillance data for rabies endemic countries. It is not a notifiable or reportable disease in most developing countries and because many victims belong to lower socio-economic groups, the true number of annual rabies deaths that occur is likely to be much higher than officially documented (Lembo et al., 2011; Sudarshan and Ashwath Narayana, 2010). In addition, paralytic rabies can often be misdiagnosed in cases of co-infection, such as malaria, thus helping to further mask the true global burden (Mallewa et al., 2007). Under-reporting of rabies cases, while sometimes confounded by local cultures and poor education, is in part due to a lack of surveillance and laboratory facilities. Such under-reporting serves to lower the disease as a national health priority, which in turn limits the available resources to determine the true burden of the disease.

To break this cycle and promote rabies awareness, mathematical models are employed to estimate the national and global burden of rabies. Rabies burden is multi-factorial and includes societal, direct and indirect costs. Societal costs are expressed as disability-adjusted life years (DALYs) and include mortality, lost productivity from premature death, morbidity from adverse events of vaccination using nerve tissue vaccines (NTVs) and the psychological effects of exposure to this fatal disease. Direct costs include human losses, livestock losses and post-exposure prophylaxis (PEP). Indirect costs include surveillance, vaccination control programmes, pet movement schemes and multiple journeys to clinics for PEP. The models estimate disease burden using data from literature searches, international databases (e.g. official rabies reports, incidence of dog bites), market data for vaccine use and expert opinion (Anderson and Shwiff, 2013; Shwiff et al., 2013; Hampson et al., 2015). The burden of rabies disproportionately affects countries in Asia, which are estimated to account for more than half of human rabies deaths and approximately 65% of cattle losses, while administering more than 90% of PEP and just under 50% of dog vaccinations (Shwiff et al., 2013).

## 22.8  Post-exposure prophylaxis (PEP)

While no unvaccinated patient showing clinical signs of rabies encephalitis following infection by a dog or other terrestrial mammal is known to have recovered (Warrell and Warrell, 2015), disease progression can be prevented by the prompt administration of PEP to victims of bites by rabid animals. In July 1885, Louis Pasteur recorded the first successful rabies vaccination of a human. Joseph Meister, a nine year old French boy who had been severely bitten by a rabid dog, was successfully treated with the crude vaccine. The subsequent provision of PEP for rabies is believed to have saved more than 20 million lives (Meslin, 2012). As rabies is preventable by PEP, subsequent deaths reflect a health system failure (Dodet et al., 2014). Unfortunately, many dog bite victims do not receive timely or complete post-exposure prophylaxis. A recent study from Bangalore, India, reported the compliance rate for intradermal rabies vaccination was 77.0% while that for intramuscular rabies vaccination was only 60.0% (Shankaraiah et al., 2015). Poor compliance of individuals to complete the PEP course can be due to several factors, including loss of wages, forgotten appointments, the travel costs incurred and the distance from the hospital (Shankaraiah et al., 2015). Such barriers, a poor understanding of the disease and the proportion of dog bites that would not have resulted in an exposure to rabies virus appear to encourage and endorse the use of folk remedies to prevent the disease (Jemberu et al., 2013; Admasu and Mekonnen, 2014). Ultimately, failures in public health intervention are due to poor education and a lack of resources (Dodet et al., 2014). In addition, minor bites to children may remain unnoticed or unreported.

Vaccination offers the principal protection to at-risk human and animal populations. There are several regimens recommended by the WHO for human pre- and post-prophylaxis (Table 22.3). Pre-exposure prophylaxis is recommended for anyone at risk of exposure to the virus via contact with a rabid domestic or wild mammal. Travellers should consider pre-immunisation and avoid contact with dogs, cats and wild mammals in rabies endemic areas (Gautret et al., 2013). In addition, pre-exposure prophylaxis is recommended for those at risk via occupational (e.g. veterinarians, diagnosticians, researchers, clinicians) or leisure activities. As rabies is undoubtedly a significant paediatric disease in endemic areas, incorporation of rabies vaccination into existing childhood immunisation programmes is currently being considered by the WHO (WHO, 2013). This would be particularly applicable in low income, rural areas.

**Table 22.3** Vaccination regimens (pre-exposure and post-exposure) recommended by the World Health Organisation and the Advisory Committee on Immunization Practices. Vaccines must be prequalified by WHO for the administration route employed.

| | Regimen | Vaccine doses | Clinic visits | Administration Route | Schedule of injections |
|---|---|---|---|---|---|
| Pre-exposure | Routine Intra-muscular | 3 | 3 | Intra-muscular | Days 0, 7 & either 21 or 28 (1 dose each) |
| | Routine Intra-dermal | 3 | 3 | Intra-dermal | Days 0, 7 & either 21 or 28 (1 dose each) |
| Post-exposure | Essen | 5 | 5 | Intra-muscular | Days 0, 3, 7, 14 & 28 (1 dose each) |
| | Zagreb | 4 | 3 | Intra-muscular | Days 0 (2 doses), 7 & 21 (1 dose each) |
| | Reduced Four dose | 4 | 4 | Intra-muscular | Days 0, 3, 7 & 14 (1 dose each) |
| | Modified Thai Red Cross | 8 | 4 | Intra-dermal | Days 0, 3, 7 & 28 (2 doses each) |
| Post-exposure for previously vaccinated persons | Two-dose Intra-muscular | 2 | 2 | Intra-muscular | Days 0 & 3 (1 dose each) |
| | Four-dose Intra-dermal | 4 | 1 | Intra-dermal | Day 0 (4 doses) |

Post-exposure prophylaxis (washing the wound with detergent, rabies vaccination and rabies immunoglobulin RIG) is recommended for humans following a potential exposure, e.g. if a rabies susceptible mammal bites, scratches or licks a mucous membrane. It should be started as soon as possible. The RIG offers passive immunisation and neutralises the virus directly in the wound, preventing its spread. This provides rapid protection prior to the vaccine induced immunity (approx. seven to ten days later). Unfortunately, due to the prohibitive costs of producing human-derived products, there is a global shortage of RIG. It is thus not available in several rabies endemic countries and is unlikely to be accessible in many rural areas (Warrell and Warrell, 2015). The shortage of RIG has driven a search for alternatives and a cocktail of selected rabies monoclonal antibodies are currently undergoing clinical trials (Bakker et al., 2008). For pre-immunised patients subsequently exposed to rabies, RIG is unnecessary as the immune system is pre-primed but booster vaccinations are administered.

The increasingly frequent detection of rabid animals imported from enzootic areas into rabies-free areas leads to a precautionary over-prescription of significant numbers of rabies PEP, including the expensive rabies immunoglobulin (RIG), particularly in Western European countries (Bourhy et al., 2009; Gautret et al., 2013). In contrast, a recent survey in the King Edward Memorial Hospital, Mumbai, reported fewer than 2% of severe bite victims in a rabies endemic urban area were prescribed RIG irrespective of its availability (Gogtay et al., 2014). The lack of RIG combined with a likelihood of incomplete vaccine course compliance will significantly reduce the efficacy of PEP, leading to disease (Meslin, 2012).

While pre-immunisation is recommended for animals, particularly cats and dogs, there is little evidence to show the effectiveness of vaccination for post-exposure prophylaxis, and this is not generally recommended in these species.

## 22.9 Management

While the mortality for clinical rabies in general is believed to be 100%, a small number of cases of human rabies survival have been reported over the last forty years, raising hopes that rabies encephalomyelitis might be treatable (Warrell and Warrell, 2015; Willoughby et al., 2005; Jackson, 2014). However, no specific treatment has proved effective and canine rabies remains 100% fatal in unvaccinated people (i.e. in the absence of either pre- or post-exposure immunisation). Patients should be admitted to hospital for palliative care with analgesia and sedation. Although human-to-human transmission of rabies is considered to be unlikely, hospital staff, family or carers may be offered vaccination for reassurance. Intensive care is unlikely to be of benefit in the vast majority of rabies encephalitic cases but may be considered for previously vaccinated patients, especially if presenting early with detectable rabies antibodies (Warrell and Warrell, 2015).

## 22.10 Dog bites and rabies

The severity of the dog bite and likely risk of exposure are categorised by the WHO (Table 22.4). In Africa and Asia, where more than 99% of all human cases occur, the domestic dog is the most important source of transmission and between 45 and 72% of all dog

**Table 22.4** Categories of contact and recommended post-exposure prophylaxis (PEP). Reprinted from: World Health Organisation Rabies Factsheet no. 99 September 2014 Accessed: 31 August 2016.

| Categories of contact with suspect rabid animal | Post-exposure prophylaxis measures |
|---|---|
| Category I – touching or feeding animals, licks on intact skin | None |
| Category II – nibbling of uncovered skin, minor scratches or abrasions without bleeding | Immediate vaccination and local treatment of the wound |
| Category III – single or multiple transdermal bites or scratches, licks on broken skin; contamination of mucous membrane with saliva from licks; contact with bats. | Immediate vaccination and administration of rabies immunoglobulin; local treatment of the wound |

All category II and III exposures assessed as carrying a risk of developing rabies require PEP. This risk is increased if:

- The biting mammal is a known rabies reservoir or vector species;
- The animal looks sick or has an abnormal behaviour;
- A wound or mucous membrane was contaminated by the animal's saliva;
- The bite was unprovoked; and
- The animal has not been vaccinated.

In developing countries, the vaccination status of the suspected animal alone should not be considered when deciding whether or not to initiate prophylaxis.

Recommended first-aid procedures include immediate and thorough flushing and washing of the wound for a minimum of 15 minutes with soap and water, detergent, povidone iodine or other substances that kill the rabies virus.

bites and human rabies cases occur in children less than fifteen years of age (Abubakar and Bakari, 2012; Alabi et al., 2014; Lembo et al., 2010; Liu and Ertl, 2012; WHO, 2013). Unfortunately, children who have been bitten or scratched by suspect rabid dogs may not inform their parents or are unaware of how the disease is transmitted (Cleaveland et al., 2003).

In a survey of 195 recorded dog bite victims between 2006 and 2008 in Jos Plateau State, Nigeria (Alabi et al., 2014), most were less than sixteen years old (n=141, 72.3%) and males accounted for 128 reports (65.6%). Bites were apparently unprovoked in 184 cases (94.4%) and most victims were bitten on the arm (85%). Complete PEP was administered to 54.4% victims. The majority of the biting dogs were owned (housed) but unvaccinated. Similar patterns were observed in Kerman Province, Iran, where animal bites were more common in younger age groups (ten to nineteen years) (Eslamifar et al., 2008). In contrast, in a survey of 245 dog bite victims between 2007 and 2010 in the rabies–free city of Marseille, France, 75.9% of injured patients were over fifteen years of age (Gautret et al., 2013) and in 56.3% of cases the dog was not known or stray. In Marseille, the complete course of rabies PEP was provided as a precautionary measure in 63.7% of dog bite victims as the attacking dogs were not available for observation.

In Lebanon, eight cases of human rabies and 5,280 animal bites to humans were reported to the Lebanese Ministry of Public Health between 2001 and 2012. Although the highest incidence of animal bites was in older children and adults, there was still a marked level of bites in children < fifteen years old, with an average of 134 bites reported per year (Bizri et al., 2014). Dogs were the only vector of rabies infection and were responsible for most reported animal bites to humans. An average of 3 doses of vaccine per bite was administered as post-exposure prophylaxis.

In Pakistan, Zaidi et al. (2013) introduced a mobile phone reporting system for dog bites and rabies surveillance across nine emergency rooms (ER). The system enabled the recording of patient health-seeking behaviours, access to care and the spatial distribution of rabies cases. A total of 6,212 dog bite incidents were reported between 2009 and 2011, with the greatest number of bites reported in Karachi (59.7%), followed by Peshawar (13.1%) and Hyderabad (11.4%). The mobile phone technologies for health (mHealth) allowed for the operation of a national rabies reporting and surveillance system at a relatively low cost. The system identified foci of rabies infections, which could be then targeted for rabies control and highlighted differences in victim behaviours and access to medical care at the local level.

## 22.11 Concluding comments on rabies control

Vaccination is the mainstay of control for both human and animal rabies. As dog rabies accounts for than 99% of all human cases, controlling rabies in dogs is the first priority for prevention of human rabies. Eliminating canine rabies globally would save tens of thousands of lives annually and reduce the economic burden attributed to PEP. Decades of parenteral vaccination campaigns in the industrialised countries of Latin America, Africa and Asia have demonstrated that elimination of rabies in dogs is achievable. A large number of efficacious canine rabies vaccines are produced and batch tested globally. Most provide specific recommendations regarding the age of dogs at primary vaccination and booster intervals. However, when implementing mass dog vaccination programmes in developing countries, all dogs, including puppies less than three months old, should be vaccinated wherever possible to ensure inclusive coverage (Lembo et al., 2012; Morters et al., 2015).

However, resource limited countries often prioritise funds towards the purchase of human rabies biologicals rather than the implementation of a co-ordinated canine vaccination programme (Meslin and Briggs, 2013). Unfortunately, the infrastructures in place to administer PEP are far from optimal and a lack of awareness from the victims in seeking medical intervention hinder the appropriate management of the disease and result in wasted resources (Jemberu et al., 2013; Banyard et al., 2013). For many years the WHO and OIE have recommended a 'One Health' approach, combining the resources of both animal and public health departments to control rabies, fully reflecting the zoonotic nature of the disease (WHO, 2013; Fooks et al., 2011 ). The tools and knowledge exist to eliminate canine rabies and thereby control human rabies incidence. To this end, the WHO, OIE, and FAO have proposed a strategy for the elimination of dog-mediated rabies in rabies endemic countries by 2030.

## 22.12 References

Abubakar, S. A., Bakari, A. G. (2012). Incidence of dog bite injuries and clinical rabies in a tertiary health care institution: a 10-year retrospective study. *Annals of African Medicine*. 11, 108–111.

Admasu, P. and Mekonnen, Y. (2014). Rabies and its Folk Drugs Remedies in Ethiopia: A Review. *International Journal of Basic and Applied Virology* 3(2): 22–27.

Alabi, O., Nguku, P., Chukwukere, S., Gaddo, A., Nsubuga, P., Umoh, J. (2014). Profile of dog bite victims in Jos Plateau State, Nigeria: a review of dog bite records (2006–2008). The Pan African Medical Journal 21;18 Suppl 1:12.

Anderson, A., Shwiff, S. A. (2013). The Cost of Canine Rabies on Four Continents. *Transboundary and Emerging Diseases*. 62; 4, 446–452.

Anon. (2003). Assessing the burden of rabies in India. WHO sponsored national multi-centric rabies survey 2003. Final report. Bangalore: Association for Prevention and Control of Rabies in India; Agu.

Badrane, H., Tordo, N. (2001). Host switching in Lyssavirus history from the Chiroptera to the Carnivora orders. *Journal of Virology*; 75: 8096–104.

Bakker, A. B., Python, C., Kissling, C. J., Pandya, P., Marissen, W. E., Brink, M. F., Lagerwerf, F., Worst, S., van Corven, E., Kostense, S., Hartmann, K., Weverling, G. J., Uytdehaag, F., Herzog, C., Briggs, D. J., Rupprecht, C. E., Grimaldi, R., Goudsmit, J. (2008). First administration to humans of a monoclonal antibody cocktail against rabies virus: safety, tolerability, and neutralizing activity. *Vaccine*; 26: 5922–27.

Banyard, A. C., Hayman, D., Johnson, N., McElhinney, L. M., Fooks, A. R. (2011). Bats and lyssaviruses. *Advances in Virus Research* 79: 239–89.

Banyard, A. C., Horton, D. L., Freuling, C., Müller, T., Fooks, A. R. (2013). Control and prevention of canine rabies: the need for building laboratory-based surveillance capacity. *Antiviral Research*; 98: 357–64.

Bizri, A., Alawieh, A., Ghosn, N., Berry, A., Musharrafieh, U. (2014), Challenges facing human rabies control: the Lebanese experience. *Epidemiology and Infection*. 142(7):1486–94.

Bourhy, H., Goudal, M., Mailles, A., Sadkowska-Todys, M., Dacheux, L., Zeller, H. (2009). Is there a need for anti-rabies vaccine and immunoglobulins rationing in Europe? *Eurosurveillance*. 2;14(13). pii: 19166.

Bourhy, H., Kissi, B., Audry, L., Smreczak, M., Sadkowska-Todys, M., Kulonen, K., Tordo, N., Zmudzinski, J. F., Holmes, E. C. (1999). Ecology and evolution of rabies virus in Europe. *Journal of General Virology* 80, 2545–2557.

Carrara, P., Parola, P., Brouqui, P., Gautret, P. (2013). Imported human rabies cases worldwide, 1990–2012. PLoS Neglected Tropical Diseases. May 2;7(5):e2209.

Cleaveland, S., Kaare, M., Tiringa, P., Mlengeya, T., Barrat, J., (2003). A dog rabies vaccination campaign in rural Africa: impact on the incidence of dog rabies and human dog-bite injuries. *Vaccine* 21, 1965–1973.

Dean, D. J., Abelseth, M. K. (1973). The fluorescent antibody test. In: *Laboratory Techniques in Rabies*. 3rd edn. Eds Kaplan, M. M., Kowprowski, H. Geneva. World Health Organisation. Pp.73–84.

Demetriou, P., Moynagh, J. (2011). The European Union strategy for external co-operation with neighbouring countries on rabies control. *Rabies Bulletin Europe*, 35(1):5–7.

Dodet, B., Durrheim, D. N., Rees, H. (2014). Rabies: underused vaccines, unnecessary deaths. *Vaccine*. 11;32(18):2017–9.

Eslamifar, A., Ramezani, A., Razzaghi-Abyaneh, M., Fallahian, V., Mashayekhi, P., Hazrati, M., Askari, T., Fayaz, A., Aghakhani, A. (2008) Animal bites in Tehran, Iran. *Archive of Iranian Medicine* 11(2):200–2.

Esposito, S., Picciolli, I., Semino, M. and Principi, N. (2013). Dog and cat bite-associated infections in children. *European Journal of Clinical Microbiology and Infectious Diseases* 32:971–976.

Fooks, A. R. Rabies remains a 'neglected disease'. (2005). *Eurosurveillance* ; 10: 211–212.

Fooks, A. R., Hiby, E., Leanes, F., Meslin, F.X., Miranda, M. E., Mueller, T., Nel, L.H., Rupprecht, C. E., Tordo, N., Tumpey, A., Wandeler, A. and Briggs, D. J. (2011). Renewed global partnerships and redesigned roadmaps for rabies prevention and control. *Veterinary Medicine International*, 923149.

Fooks, A. R., Banyard, A. C., Horton, D. L., Johnson, N., McElhinney, L. M., Jackson, A. C. (2014). Current status of rabies and prospects for elimination. *Lancet*. 11;384(9951):1389–99.

Fooks, A. R., McElhinney, L. M., Horton, D., Banyard, A. C., Johnson, N., Marston, D., Freuling, C., Hoffmann, B., Tu C., Fehlner-Gardiner, C., Sabeta, C. T., Cliquet, F., Müller, T., Rupprecht, C.E. (2012). Molecular tools for rabies diagnosis in animals. In: Fooks, A. R., Müller, T., eds. *OIE, Compendium of the OIE Global Conference on Rabies Control* 75–87.

Gautret, P., Le Roux, S., Faucher, B., Gaudart, J., Brouqui, P., Parola, P. (2013). Epidemiology of urban dog-related injuries requiring rabies post-exposure prophylaxis in Marseille, France. *International Journal of Infectious Diseases*. 17(3):e164–7.

Gogtay, N. J., Nagpal, A., Mallad, A., Patel, K., Stimpson, S. J., Belur, A., Thatte, U. M. (2014). Demographics of animal bite victims & management practices in a tertiary care institute in Mumbai, Maharashtra, India. *Indian Journal of Medical Research*. 139(3): 459–462.

Hampson, K., Coudeville, L., Lembo, T., Sambo, M., Kieffer, A., Attlan, M., Barrat, J., Blanton, J. D., Briggs, D. J., Cleaveland, S., Costa, P., Freuling, C. M., Hiby, E., Knopf, L., Leanes, F., Meslin, F. X., Metlin, A., Miranda, M. E., Müller, T., Nel, L. H., Recuenco, S., Rupprecht, C. E., Schumacher, C., Taylor, L., Vigilato, M. A., Zinsstag, J., Dushoff, J. Global Alliance for Rabies Control Partners for Rabies Prevention. (2015). Estimating the global burden of endemic canine rabies. PLoS Neglected Tropical Disease. 16;9(4):e0003709.

Hanlon, C. A., Kuzmin, I. V., Blanton, J. D., Weldon, W. C., Manangan, J. S., Rupprecht, C. E. (2005). Efficacy of rabies biologics against new lyssaviruses from Eurasia. *Virus Research* 111: 44–54.

Hemachudha, T., Laothamatas, J., Rupprecht, C. E. (2002). Human rabies: a disease of complex neuropathogenetic mechanisms and diagnostic challenges. *Lancet Neurology*, 1(2):101–109.

Hemachudha, T., Ugolini, G., Wacharapluesadee, S., Sungkarat, W., Shuangshoti, S., Laothamatas, J. (2013). Human rabies: neuropathogenesis, diagnosis and management. *Lancet Neurology*, 12(5):498–513.

Horton, D. L., McElhinney, L. M., Marston, D. A., Wood, J. L. N., Russell, C. A., Lewis, N., Kuzmin, I. V., Fouchier, R. A. M., Osterhaus, A. D. M. E., Fooks, A. R., Smith, D. J. (2010). Quantifying antigenic relationships among the lyssaviruses. *Journal of Virology* 84: 11841–48.

Horton, D. L., McElhinney, L. M., Freuling, C .M., Marston, D. A., Banyard, A. C., Goharrriz, H., Wise, E., Breed, A. C., Saturday, G., Kolodziejek, J., Zilahi, E., Al-Kobaisi, M. F., Nowotny, N., Mueller, T., Fooks, A.R. (2015). Complex epidemiology of a zoonotic disease in a culturally diverse region: phylogeography of rabies virus in the Middle East. *PLoS Neglected Tropical Diseases*. 26:9 (3):e0003569.

Hunter, M., Johnson, N., Hedderwick, S., McCaughey, C., Lowry, K., McConville, J., Herron, B., McQuaid, S., Marston, D., Goddard, T., Harkess, G., Goharriz, H., Voller, K., Solomon, T., Willoughby, R. E., Fooks, A. R. (2010). Immunovirological correlates in human rabies treated with therapeutic coma. *Journal of Medical Virology*; 82: 1255–65.

International Committee on Taxonomy of Viruses (ICTV, 2014) 2014 Release www.ictvonline. org/virusTaxonomy.asp

Jackson, A. C. (2014). Rabies. *Handbook of Clinical Neurology*.123:601–18.

Jemberu, W. T., Molla, W., Almaw, G., Alemu, S. (2013). Incidence of Rabies in Humans and

5

Domestic Animals and People's Awareness in North Gondar Zone, Ethiopia. *PLoS Neglected Tropical Diseases.* 7(5): E2216–E.

Johnson, N., Phillpotts, R., Fooks, A. R. (2006). Airborne transmission of lyssaviruses. *Journal of Medical Microbiology;* 55: 785–90.

Johnson, N., Mansfield, K. L., Marston, D. A., Wilson, C., Goddard, T., Selden, D., Hemson, G., Edea, L., van Kesteren, F., Shiferaw, F., Stewart, A. E., Sillero-Zubiri, C., Fooks, A. R. (2010). A new outbreak of rabies in rare Ethiopian wolves (Canis simensis). *Archives of Virology* 155(7):1175–7.

Johnson, N., Freuling, C., Horton, D., Müller, T., Fooks, A. R. (2011). Imported Rabies, European Union and Switzerland, 2001–2010. *Emerging Infectious Diseases.* 17(4): 751–753.

Knobel, D. L., Cleaveland, S., Coleman, P. G., Fevre, E. M., Meltzer, M. I., Miranda, M. E., Shaw, A., Zinsstag, J., Meslin, F.X. (2005). Re-evaluating the burden of rabies in Africa and Asia. *Bulletin of the World Health Organisation.* 83, 360–368.

Lembo, T., Hampson, K., Kaare, M. T., Ernest, E., Knobel, D., Kazwala, R. R., Haydon, D. T., Cleaveland, S. (2010). The feasibility of canine rabies elimination in Africa: dispelling doubts with data. *PLoS Neglected Tropical Diseases* 4: e626.

Lembo, T. (2012). The blueprint for rabies prevention and control: a novel operational toolkit for rabies elimination. *PLoS Negleted Tropical Diseases.* 6, e1388.

Lembo, T., Attlan, M., Bourhy, H., Cleaveland, S., Costa, P., de Balogh, K., Dodet, B., Fooks, A. R., Hiby, E., Leanes, F., Meslin, F. X., Miranda, M. E., Mueller, T., Nel, L. H., Rupprecht, C. E., Tordo, N., Tumpey, A., Wandeler, A., Briggs, D.J. (2011). Renewed global partnerships and redesigned roadmaps for rabies prevention and control. *Veterinary Medicine International,* 923149.

Liu, Q., Ertl, H.C. (2012). Preventative childhood vaccination to rabies. *Expert Opinion on Biological Therapy.* 12, 1067–1075.

McElhinney, L. M., Marston, D. A., Stankov, S., Tu, C., Black, C., Johnson, N., Jiang, Y., Tordo, N., Müller, T., Fooks, A. R. (2006). Molecular epidemiology of lyssaviruses in Eurasia. *Developments in biologicals* (Basel). 2008; 131:125–31.

McElhinney, L. M., Marston, D. A., Freuling, C. M., Cragg, W., Stankov, S., Lalosevic, D., Lalosevic, V., Müller, T., Fooks, A. R. (2011). Molecular diversity and evolutionary history of rabies virus strains circulating in the Balkans. *Journal of General Viroogyl.* 92(Pt 9):2171–80.

Maier, T., Schwarting, A., Mauer, D., Ross, R. S., Martens, A., Kliem, V., Wahl, J., Panning, M., Baumgarte, S., Müller, T., Pfefferle, S., Ebel, H., Schmidt, J., Tenner-Racz, K., Racz, P., Schmid, M., Strüber, M., Wolters, B., Gotthardt, D., Bitz, F., Frisch, L., Pfeiffer, N., Fickenscher, H., Sauer, P., Rupprecht, C. E., Roggendorf, M., Haverich, A., Galle, P., Hoyer, J., Drosten, C. (2010). Management and outcomes after multiple corneal and solid organ transplantations from a donor infected with rabies virus. *Clinical Infectious Diseases.*15;50(8):1112–9.

Malerczyk, C., DeTora, L., Gniel, D. (2011). Imported human rabies cases in Europe, the United States, and Japan, 1990 to 2010. *Journal of Travel Medicine* 18:402–407.

Mallewa, M., Fooks, A. R., Banda, D., Chikungwa, P., Mankhambo, L., Molyneux, E., Molyneux, M. E., Solomon, T. (2007). Rabies encephalitis in malaria-endemic area, Malawi. *African. Emerging Infectious Diseases* 13, 136–139.

Matulionytė, R., Lisauskienė, I., Kėkštas, G., Ambrozaitis, A. (2012). Two dog-related infections leading to death: overwhelming Capnocytophaga canimorsus sepsis in a patient with cystic echinococcosis. *Medicina (Kaunas).* 48(2):112–5. Epub 23 March 2012.

Meslin, F. M. (2012). The Louis Pasteur Oration. Paper presented at the Association for the Prevention of Rabies in India Conference, Kolkata, India. July 6–8, 2012.

Meslin, F.X., Briggs, D.J. (2013). Eliminating canine rabies, the principal source of human infection: what will it take? *Antiviral Research*; 98: 291–96.

Morters, M. K., McNabb, S., Horton, D. L., Fooks, A. R., Schoeman, J. P., Whay, H. R., Wood, J. L., Cleaveland, S. (2015). Effective vaccination against rabies in puppies in rabies endemic regions. *Veterinary Record.* Jun 24. pii: vetrec-2014-102975.

Nel, L. H., Rupprecht, C. E. (2007). Emergence of lyssaviruses in the Old World: the case of Africa. *Current Topics in Microbiology and Immunology.* 315:161–93.

Neville, J. (2004). Rabies in the ancient world. In: *Historical perspectives of rabies in Europe and the Mediterranean Basin*, Eds., King, A. A., Fooks, A. R., Aubert, M., Wandeler, A. I. OIE, Geneva, Switzerland, pp: 1–13.

Pastoret, P.-P., Van Gucht S., Brochier B. (2014) Eradicating rabies at source. *Revue scientifique et technique (International Office of Epizootics).* 33 (2), 509–519.

Rosner, F. (1974). Rabies in the Talmud. *Medical History* 18: 198–200.

Shankaraiah, R. H., Rajashekar, R. A., Veena, V., Hanumanthaiah, A. N. (2015). Compliance to anti-rabies vaccination in post-exposure prophylaxis. *Indian journal of public health* 59: (1) P 58–60.

Shwiff, S., Hampson, K., Anderson, A. (2013). Potential economic benefits of eliminating canine rabies. *Antiviral Research*; 98: 352–56.

Smith, J. S., Orciari, L. A., Yager, P. A., Seidel, H. D., Warner, C. K. (1992). Epidemiologic and historical relationships among 87 rabies virus isolates as determined by limited sequence analysis. *Journal of Infectious Diseases* 166, 296–307.

Solomon, T., Marston, D., Mallewa, M., Felton, T., Shaw, S., McElhinney, L. M., Das, K., Mansfield, K., Wainwright, J., Kwong, G. N., Fooks, A. R. (2005). Paralytic rabies after a two week holiday in India. *British Medical Journal.* 3, 331, 501–3.

Sudarshan, M. K., Ashwath Narayana, D. H. (2010). A survey of hospitals managing human rabies cases in India. *Indian Journal of Public Health.* 54(1):40–1.

Suraweera, W., Morris, S. K., Kumar, R., Warrell, D. A., Warrell, M. J., Jha, P. (2012). Deaths from Symptomatically Identifiable Furious Rabies in India: A Nationally Representative Mortality Survey. *PLoS Neglected Tropical Diseases.* 6(10):e1847.

Talbi, C., Holmes, E. C., de Benedictis, P., Faye, O., Nakouné, E., Gamatié, D., Diarra, A., Elmamy, B. O., Sow, A., Adjogoua, E. V., Sangare, O., Dundon, W. G., Capua, I., Sall, A. A., Bourhy, H. (2009). Evolutionary history and dynamics of dog rabies virus in western and central Africa. *Journal of General Virology* 90: 783–791.

Talbi, C., Lemey, P., Suchard, M. A., Abdelatif, E., Elharrak, M., Nourlil, J., Faouzi, A., Echevarría, J. E., Vazquez Morón, S., Rambaut, A., Campiz, N., Tatem, A. J., Holmes, E. C., Bourhy, H. (2010). Phylodynamics and human-mediated dispersal of a zoonotic virus. *PLoS Pathogens.* 28:6(10):e1001166.

Taylor, L. H., Latham, S. M., Woolhouse, M. E. (2001). Risk factors for human disease emergence. *Philosophical Transactions of the Royal Society of London. Series B: Biological Sciences* 356, 983–989.

Tenzin, Dhand N. K., Gyeltshen, T., Firestone, S., Zangmo, C., Dema, C., Gyeltshen, R., Ward, M. P. (2011). Dog Bites in Humans and Estimating Human Rabies Mortality in Rabies Endemic Areas of Bhutan. *PLoS Neglected Tropical Diseases.* 5(11):e1391.

Tepsumethanon, V., Lumlertdacha, B., Mitmoonpitak, C., Sitprija, V., Meslin, F. X., Wilde, H. (2004). Survival of naturally infected rabid dogs and cats. *Clinical Infectious Diseases* 39 (2):278–80.

Vos, A., Nunan, C., Bolles, D., Müller, T., Fooks, A. R., Tordo, N., Baer, G. M. (2011). The occurrence of rabies in pre-Columbian Central America: an historical search. *Epidemiology and Infection* 139(10):1445–52.

Warrell, M. J., Warrell, D. A. (2015). Rabies: the clinical features, management and prevention of the classic zoonosis. *Clinical Medicine.* 15(1):78–81.

Willoughby, R. E. Jr, Tieves, K. S., Hoffman, G. M., Ghanayem, N. S., Amlie-Lefond, C. M., Schwabe, M. J., Chusid, M. J., Rupprecht, C. E. (2005). Survival after treatment of rabies with induction of coma. *New England Journal of Medicine* 352: 2508–14.

Woolhouse, M. E., Gowtage-Sequeria, S. (2005). Host range and emerging and re-emerging pathogens. *Emerging Infectious Diseases* 11, 1842–1847.

World Health Organisation (2013). WHO Expert Consultation on Rabies: Second Report (*WHO Technical Report Series; No. 982*). World Health Organisation, Geneva.

Zaidi, S. M. A., Labrique, A. B., Khowaja, S., Lotia-Farrukh, I., Irani, J., Salahuddin, N., Khan A.J. (2013). Geographic Variation in Access to Dog-Bite Care in Pakistan and Risk of Dog-Bite Exposure in Karachi: Prospective Surveillance Using a Low-Cost Mobile Phone System. *PLoS Neglected Tropical Diseases* 7(12): e2574.

Zambori, C., Cumpanasoiu, C., Bianca, M., Tirziu, E. (2013). Biofilms in Oral Cavity of Dogs and Implication in Zoonotic Infections. *Scientific Papers: Animal Science and Biotechnologies*, 46 (1) 155.

# CHAPTER 23

# Impact of Dog Aggression on Victims

## Carri Westgarth and Francine Watkins

## 23.1 Introduction

The impact of dog bites on victims is difficult to grasp for two main reasons:

1.  Firstly, we do not really know how often they occur or how to collect data on it. For example, in 2009–10 being 'bitten or struck by a dog' was responsible for 5,914 episodes of admitted patient care in England, accounting for 11,503 occupied bed days (HES, 2012). However, the number of unreported dog bites, especially if not severe enough to cause a hospital visit, is significantly more (Beck and Jones, 1985); for example, it has been estimated that each year 1.8% of the US population are victims of dog bites, however only 0.3% of the population seek medical care for a dog bite (Sacks et al., 1996). That means at least six times more do not seek medical attention than do, and, in the UK at least, we only routinely collect records on those who are actually admitted into hospital, and not those who attend emergency departments, walk-in centres or GP surgeries. A random telephone survey in Belgium suggested that of twenty-six children bitten the preceding year, only one was hospitalised; ten presented to a GP and five to a hospital emergency department (Kahn et al., 2004). Therefore, if we are interested in the impact of dog bites on victims across the severity scale, there is likely a very large sample of the population missing from most records.
2.  The second issue concerns where the research has been concentrated so far. While the issue of dog bites is in some respects a highly researched topic, there are also large gaps in the literature. When a dog bites a person, there will be varying degrees of both physical and psychological injury. While there is a plethora of useful information available concerning prevalence of physical injury and best treatment, including surgical and infection (see Chapters 20 and 21), there is little published evidence regarding the wider impact on victims, such as psychological trauma. Further, evidence concerning bites not severe enough to require medical treatment is practically non-existent.

Considering that dog ownership is high (approximately 24% of households in the UK (Murray et al., 2010,  Westgarth et al., 2007); possibly 47% in the USA (HumaneSociety, 2014) the potential for future contact between victims and dogs is high; it is not a situation that can be easily avoided. Further, as it is often cited that people are most often bitten by dogs familiar to them (Voith, 2009), victims are likely to be exposed to that dog again, and they may even still own it. Finally, young children are known to comprise a significant proportion of victims of dog bites receiving medical treatment and are often bitten in the face (Hon et al., 2007; Kahn et al., 2003). Thus, the implications of being bitten by a dog for them are even more far reaching: they have a lifetime ahead to have to deal with the consequences of the experience; they may have received a significant facial injury; and they may come across pet dogs belonging to friends and family while visiting houses to play. Thus there is potential for considerable psychological as well as physical consequences to being bitten by a dog and victims will continue to experience dog contact as it is not easily avoided.

It is also important to fully consider the impact of dog bites on victims because of the balance between positive and negative impacts of dog ownership on individuals and wider society. Owning pets has been reported to confer both physiological and psychological benefits and has implications for economical savings for health services (see Headey, 2003; McNicholas et al., 2005; O'Haire, 2010). Hypotheses as to why dog ownership may positively impact health are that they provide emotional protection from the stresses and strains of life (the 'buffer' effect) (McNicholas et al., 2005), facilitate social interaction (Messent, 1983) and encourage a more active lifestyle (Christian et al., 2013). However, dog owners, and the wider community, may also find ownership detrimental to health, due to behavioural issues, zoonoses and noise pollution (Voith, 2009; Jackson, 2005). Thus, policy concerning dog ownership needs to consider the complexity of dogs in our communities in terms of both benefit and risk. The impact of dog bites on victims is a central part of this that has received little evidence-based assessment.

This chapter aims to summarise the currently available evidence concerning the impact of dog bites on victims (excluding fatalities – see Chapter 11), from a review of the published literature.

In the absence of previous detailed study into this area, we also present the unpublished findings from a pilot investigation into the experiences of eight female dog bite victims. Some of the findings relating to this study have been previously published, along with the methodology (Westgarth and Watkins, 2015), but here we will specifically address extra unpublished findings about the impact on the victims of being bitten. As it was essential to understand in more detail how victims perceived the events immediately before, during and after the bite, a qualitative approach was chosen. Detailed one-to-one interviews allowed scope for the participant to tell their story in depth and for the researcher to ask questions to understand the circumstances (Green and Thorogood, 2009). Further detail of the study methodology can be found in the published paper (Westgarth and Watkins, 2015). It must be noted that the participants were all females, as these were who came forward. Further research is required to target the viewpoints of male bite victims.

## 23.2 Physical trauma related to dog bites (see also Chapter 21)

### 23.2.1 Physical trauma in adults

In adults, UK hospital admission data describes open wounds of wrist or hand as the most common 'dog bite or strike, injury (HSCIS, 2014); plastic surgery is the most common reason for hospital admission. However, many other dog bite victims may not seek medical attention, let alone be admitted to hospital after attending an emergency department; a survey estimated that of ninety-four adult dog bites only twelve (13%) sought any medical treatment (Sacks et al., 1996). Secondary infections requiring antibiotic treatment are a cause of some emergency room admissions some time after the event, especially when bites occur on the hands (Pfortmueller et al., 2013). Our qualitative study of eight dog bite victims (Westgarth and Watkins, 2015) also described physical consequences of being bitten by a dog; these bites were generally considered by the participants to be non-serious and did not require any or significant medical treatment (Box 23.1).

### 23.2.2 Physical trauma in children

UK hospital admission data describes open wound of head as the most common 'dog bite or strike' injury to children causing admission, and accordingly plastic surgery as the most frequent and oral or maxillo facial surgery as next frequent treatments (HSCIS, 2014). Physical trauma documented in children often focuses on the issue of facial bites and average healing time can be more than ten months (Hersant et al., 2012). However, studies of emergency room entrance in children and adolescents also document many bites to limbs and torso, usually single site. Most bites treated, 82%, do not require hospitalisation; 20% are only minor scratches and bruises (Hon et al., 2007; Kahn et al., 2003). This concurs with other evidence that, of twenty-six children bitten, only one was hospitalised; five presented to a hospital emergency department, ten to a GP and ten did not seek medical attention (Kahn et al., 2004). Thus, although it is frequently stated that children are most/more likely to be bitten on the face, this effect may partially reflect the majority of data on the subject coming from serious hospital admission records rather than simply a case of dogs directing bites towards this area. However, there is also data to support younger children being at higher risk of facial injuries than older children where, similar to adults, arms and hands become more common (Hon et al., 2007; Kahn et al., 2003).

### 23.2.3 Indirect physical effects

The psychological repercussions of being bitten by a dog may also have further physical effects. Fear leading to a reduction in physical activity has also been reported in children due to bites from free-roaming dogs (Vargo et al., 2012) and avoidance of areas such as parks was also reported in children suffering post-traumatic stress disorder (PTSD) from dog bites (De Keuster et al., 2006). Reduced physical activity was also reported in our qualitative study (Box 23.1).

> **Box 23.1  Physical effects of dog bites and medical treatment required in a qualitative study of eight dog bite victims (Westgarth and Watkins, 2015)**
>
> The bites discussed usually resulted in pain, puncture and bruising, taking at most a few weeks to heal but leaving scars. Yet surprisingly, the physical effects of the bites were portrayed as minor by the participants and quickly dismissed, with downplaying of the seriousness of the injury:
>
> > *Not very deep at all. It did draw blood but it just sort of looked like scratch marks. Yeah so it wasn't, wasn't serious at all [...] I put some Savlon on it. But I have lots of friends who are doctors and I contacted one of them and they said 'no, you'll be fine'. And I had a tetanus within the time limit, so I didn't think there was a problem. (Ellie – bitten while running)*
>
> Four participants received medical attention, which involved cleaning and dressing the wound, a tetanus vaccination or a course of antibiotics. However, none of the participants reported that during their interactions with health practitioners were their psychological responses or fears addressed, even when the mental health effects of being bitten were significant, and in some cases resulted in behaviour changes and lifestyle changes. The consequence of the psychological impact could also impinge on physical health as they reported changes to their physical behaviour. For example, reduced activity due to fear of going out on walks was reported:
>
> > *Well I used to take the dog to the park each day. My husband now takes it once, and now, only now am I starting to take him again. (Annie – bitten by neighbour's dog)*

## 23.3  Psychological trauma related to dog bites

It has been recognised that adverse psychological impacts of dog bites are typically not documented in hospital cases (Hon et al., 2007). If they are not documented, it is also unlikely that they are being addressed in the hospital setting. Our qualitative study of eight dog bite victims also demonstrated psychological consequences of being bitten by a dog. In contrast to their downplaying of the physical consequences of the bite, there was an emphasis by the participants on the mental health consequences of being bitten (Box 23.2). These bites were generally considered by the participants to be non-serious and did not require any or significant medical treatment, but even if they did seek this out, psychological health impacts were not addressed.

### 23.3.1  Fear and PTSD in adults

Even in what might be considered a minor bite, fear and wariness of dogs can be a consequence but this is often directed at specific dogs or situations (Box 23.2).

It seems reasonable to assume that the psychological consequences of being bitten by a dog may scale up with the seriousness of the bites, thus we may expect to find these effects in

**Box 23.2 Fear and wariness effects of dog bites in a qualitative study of eight dog bite victims (Westgarth and Watkins, 2015)**

Almost all participants spent a great deal of time directing the discussion towards the non-physical health consequences of the bite. This invariably ranged from increased 'wariness' or 'cautiousness' around dogs to a more significant fear, especially when coming into contact with dogs and relating it to their bite situation, to the specific dog itself, or dogs that looked like they may behave similarly:

> *Just specifically to that dog really, I just didn't want to go near him and I was very wary of him [...] Maybe if I came across a dog with similar problems to him, maybe I would see (Name) in that dog and I would be a bit more careful. (Claire – bitten by family member's dog)*

However, it was unusual for fears to be generalised to all dogs. Several participants expressed that they 'still loved dogs' after being bitten, and that it was important to them that the bite did not affect their general view of dogs as this would be upsetting to them.

hospital-treated bites. There are a few published studies concerning bites from free roaming dogs that mention fear of dogs as a consequence (Shen et al., 2014; Vargo et al., 2012). However, fear of free-roaming dogs is a different context to that of owned pet dogs in a typical developed society. There are also a few reports in the form of case studies of PTSD resulting from a dog bite, for example causing selective mutism in a child (Anyfantakis et al., 2009) and PTSD activation in an elderly woman who was not actually bitten but 'knocked over aggressively' by unleashed dogs (Jovanović et al., 2011). This latter example highlights that the psychological effects of a dog bite may not strictly relate to the physical aspect of being bitten by a dog but be related to the frightening nature of the experience, and concurs with evidence that having been actually attacked by a dog is less strongly related to fear of dogs than having been threatened by a dog (Boyd et al., 2004). This was also found in our qualitative interviews, when discussing the experience of dog–dog attacks (Box 23.3).

## 23.3.2 Fear and PTSD in children

Where psychological consequences are documented the studies have focused mainly on the effects on children. One longitudinal study followed fifty-seven children who had received mutilating traumatic facial injuries, including from dog bites (but did not discuss these specifically); almost all children were symptomatic for PTSD after five days of the event and 44% continued to report symptoms at one year follow-up (Rusch et al., 2000). Another study of seventy-seven child victims of facial dog bites requiring plastic surgery suggested that at least 35% had psychological problems afterwards (Hersant et al., 2012). Thus, there is certainly evidence of psychological consequences for children from serious dog bites.

An in-depth Belgian study followed twenty-two children who were treated in emergency departments but not admitted to the hospital and again found that approximately seven months later twelve had reported PTSD symptoms for more than one month (De Keuster et al., 2006). Six of the children with PTSD but none of the children with no PTSD symptoms

> ## Box 23.3  The effect of threatening situations with dogs in a qualitative study of eight dog bite victims (Westgarth and Watkins, 2015)
>
> Another source of fear was experiences of dog–dog attacks, even if the person had not been bitten themselves:
>
> *It's a horrible feeling inside. Her biting me was nothing in comparison with that other dog coming to get her, to attack her. That, even now, when I see people with those similar types of dogs [...] I'm absolutely scared right the way through, the whole of my body. It's just hard to describe it. (Debra – speaking about when her dog was attacked)*

had suffered multiple and deep wounds, whereas children with minor bites had only one or no PTSD criteria (De Keuster et al., 2006). It is not known if children from these studies who scored positive for PTSD symptoms were also offered treatment and support. PTSD symptoms included:

- Vivid recollection and reliving – constant questioning and extreme fear reactions in presence of dog
- Avoidance behaviours – refusal to go out unaccompanied to a park, street or at school
- Numbing – lack of interest in games and school activities
- Increased arousal – Shy and aggressive with siblings and peers
- Hypervigilance – fear of potential accidents, the dark, and anxiety when left alone, difficulty going to bed, nightmares, and night-time arousals.

In summary, there is good evidence of psychological trauma suffered, at least in children. However, there appears to be less evidence available concerning the effects of bites on adults, in particular males. There is also little published evidence concerning the psychological consequences of less serious bites – those that do not require medical attention – but our interviews of dog bite victims suggest this is still an issue.

## 23.4  Understanding further psychological consequences of dog bites

Our qualitative investigations of dog bite victims highlighted further psychological consequences of dog bites beyond the expected fear, caution and wariness. These emotional issues were often complex and centred around perceived breaks in the human–animal relationship and societal issues of blame and stigmatisation. Themes described included:

- Guilt, shame and embarrassment (Box 23.4)
- Blame (Box 23.5)
- Anger (Box 23.5)
- Betrayal and broken trust (Box 23.6)

## Box 23.4 Guilt, shame and embarrassment in a qualitative study of eight bite victims (Westgarth and Watkins, 2015)

For two victims there was a longer term emotional response brought on by their immediate reaction to the bite, which had resulted in them striking out in pain or anger and hitting the dog. This conflict often resulted in feelings of shame and guilt, which clearly played heavily on the participants' minds:

*I was disappointed in myself [...] but the minute it hit me I reacted completely emotionally and I think that really shook me to some extent, because I think, you know, yes it was painful, but you haven't solved the problem by shouting and screaming at them, and shaking them and putting them on the ground, that doesn't solve the problem. (Barbara − rescues and rehabilitates dogs)*

*... and it just went for me, and I don't like hitting the dog at all, but in the end [...] I just had to knock him with the (newspaper), and I told him to go, and then some. One of the boys came, one of the boyfriends came out, and he was swearing at the dog and, 'I'm going to hit him,' and I said, 'Oh please don't hit him, I think he's been through enough.' (Annie − bitten by neighbour's dog)*

When participants were bitten by their own dogs, they also reported feelings of embarrassment and concern about how others would react to their dog bite. One immediate response was to cover for the dog to avoid getting the dog in trouble or to avoid it being perceived as a 'dangerous dog':

*I made up a story, that Dave's mum's cat, who is fifteen and is really old, had chomped on me when I was stroking her [...] because I think people think, dangerous dogs, you know, dog bites are all, the media's all over it [...] And I just wouldn't want anybody to think, 'Oh, Helen's got a savage dog, she's got a dangerous dog, she needs to get rid of that dog.' (Helen − bitten on face by own dog)*

Apart from obvious medical implications of receiving a dog bite, living with an aggressive dog is stressful (Voith, 2009) and owners may invest considerable time and costs into treating the problem or deciding on an alternative course of action. Aggression towards humans is the most common reason for referral to an animal behaviourist (Appleby and Magnus, 2005; Westgarth et al., 2012). Aggressive behaviour also has welfare implications for the dog. It will no doubt weaken the owner–animal bond and may cause considerable stress to the animal, for example through restricted activities and specialised management and training (Voith, 2009). It may lead to rehoming, relinquishment to an animal shelter or ultimately euthanasia. When a dog that you love and cherish bites you, there is, not surprisingly, considerable emotional turmoil (Box 23.6).

## Box 23.5  Issues of blame and anger in a qualitative study of eight bite victims (Westgarth and Watkins, 2015)

None of the participants blamed the dog, and many felt the need to state this clearly. Any discussion of blame towards the dog was indirect in that the perception was that it was acting on natural instinct and just being an animal. More often than not the participants in this study blamed themselves in some way and viewed it as their fault. This was especially the case for participants who perceived themselves as 'experienced' with dogs, through ownership, employment or voluntary work. In these situations participants felt they were responsible and they should have behaved differently in order to prevent the bite:

> *Yes, I'm to blame. I still hold that my reactions to his [dog] aggression are what caused the bite. In almost every circumstance that I have been bitten, I have been to blame. And I don't just say that because I love dogs (laughter) and I don't blame dogs for anything. [...] But I can't think of any occasion that I've been bitten where I couldn't have handled it better. (Barbara – bitten by dog that she knew well)*

> *At the time, me and my sister [were to blame] because we should have been a bit more careful and a bit more sensible about it. I mean it could be one of those things that you could never know, I suppose any dog could bite you. But I don't really believe that. I think, because we were both experienced with dogs ... that we should have known better. I did at the time think that maybe she should have been a bit more careful about who she was letting alone with the dog that she probably didn't know particularly well, but I don't really blame, I certainly don't blame the dog, at all.' (Claire – bitten by family member's dog)*

However, if the dog was not the participant's own dog, he or she tended to blame the owner. There was a perception that the owner's (in)actions led to the bite and therefore it should have been his or her responsibility to take action to prevent it by using knowledge and experience of the dog to intervene:

> *Well ... they shouldn't have let the dog out. And they should have had gates up. So yes I do blame them all really. (Annie – bitten by neighbour's dog)*

Issues of blame can cause mental stress through feelings of guilt that the victim somehow 'caused' the bite and the dog may suffer as a consequence. In contrast, there may be anger towards whoever else they felt was responsible for the incident. Participants felt 'anger' in particular if the owners were not apologetic about the incident:

> *Humiliated, devastated, I thought. 'Why would I lie about such a thing?' Why would I lie about this dog biting me, what would be in it for me to do that? I was really humiliated about the whole episode of me having to stand there in my underwear in front of this lady who I didn't know to prove what*

*I was saying. That was what I think upset me more than anything else. More than the bite, more than anything else. It was the fact that she didn't believe me. (Gina – bitten by neighbour's dog)*

During the rare situation when the incident was reported to authorities, participants were also angered if the consequence of this was that the victim did not feel that it was taken seriously enough:

*I thought [the police] would just come and say, 'It's okay, we'll sort it out,' or, 'They're going to have to get it trained,' or that sort of thing, but they didn't even come to see us, though they said they would [...] I was cross about that. (Annie – bitten by neighbour's dog)*

This had particular significance because making the decision to report was a difficult process for the participants in the first place and most did not want to; it was even described as a reason for not wanting to seek medical attention for the wound. Further negative consequences reported were neighbourly disputes or tension resulting in increased stress, not just to the victim but within the whole community.

**Box 23.6  Issues of betrayal and broken trust in a qualitative study of 8 bite victims (Westgarth and Watkins, 2015)**

There were several emotional responses expressed by dog bite victims in the study when describing being bitten by their own dog, including feelings of 'failure and betrayal', particularly due to perceiving a breakdown of relationship with the dog:

*I should have known better, and I knew he'd go for me but you kind of expect that when you've got that trust bond with your dogs that they maybe wouldn't, even if you do something to upset them, so that's probably why it upset me because I was maybe expecting him not to be like that even though I knew that he would kind of thing, so. It's silly really. (Claire – when bitten by her own dog).*

## 23.5  Special consideration – dog bite victims that work with dogs

Many professions may involve contact with dogs, whether occupations directly involved (groomers, kennel workers, rescue organisations, veterinarians, dog trainers) or indirectly (postal workers, police, social services, midwives, health visitors). Many other people also 'work' extensively with dogs as a hobby such as through dog training classes, dog sports or agility. However, these people are at particular risk of dog bites through their increased interactions with them.

At particular risk are postal workers: 3,311 postmen and women were attacked across the UK by dogs from April 2013 to April 2014 (Nicholas Burns of Royal Mail Group, personal communication 2015) and incidence is now estimated at nine per day (Turnbull, 2014).

Again, short- and long-term physical consequences of these bites to postal workers and other 'communication workers' have been documented (Anon, 2014) but discussion of the emotional and psychological consequences is lacking. However, it is likely that there were psychological consequences, in line with the two victims in the qualitative study reported here who were bitten while delivering to neighbour's houses. Personal communication with these organisations also evidences that consequences can range from fear of delivering to that house to forced changes of shift to a new area due to intimidation by local residents (Dave Joyce of Communication Workers Union, personal communication 2013).

People who work closely with dogs may come to accept the risk of dog bites as just 'one of those things' that must be presented as part of the job (Westgarth and Watkins, 2015). However, whether the development and implementation of coping strategies to negotiate the daily risk of dog bites are deemed acceptable in that profession does not negate the fact that this requires considerable mental effort and is likely to be an added stress to the working lives of many. One published study did examine the perceptions and beliefs of veterinary surgeons about the risk of dog bites in practice and described a number of stressful situations where the veterinarian has to repeatedly negotiate risk of being bitten by 'problematic' patients and dealt with the challenge with varied emotional stability (Sanders, 1994). However, this study does not specifically explore the consequences of being bitten in this population.

## 23.6 Conclusion

In conclusion, the psychological repercussions may be significant even in minor bites and also wider ranging than may be thought on first glance, incorporating issues of shame, guilt, embarrassment, anger and community tensions. Even if the physical injury is not severe, the stressful experience of a potential 'dog attack' can affect victims deeply. Research into this area is extremely limited, and consideration of the treatment and support for the psychological consequences of dog bites (as opposed to physical injury) is largely missing. This is likely related to the generalised stigma in society of talking about mental as opposed to physical health issues. Not only is this insufficient in terms of meeting the needs of an individual who has been bitten and may require help, but it is also a completely missed opportunity for intervention to prevent future bites through discussion of the bite incident. Considering that it has been reported that often hospitalised cases are due to repeat biters (Hersant et al., 2012), this needs addressing.

## 23.7 References

Anon. (2014). *Dangerous Dogs – Bite Back: Case Studies* [Online]. Communication Workers Union. Available: www.cwu.org/52211/case-studies.html [Accessed 11 February 2015].

Anyfantakis, D., Botzakis, E., Mplevrakis, E., Symvoulakis, E. K., Arbiros, I. (2009). Selective mutism due to a dog bite trauma in a 4-year-old girl: A case report. *Journal of Medical Case Reports*, 3.

Appleby, D., Magnus, E. (2005). APBC Annual Review of Cases 2005. Association of Pet Behaviour Counsellors.

Beck, A. M., Jones, B. A. (1985). Unreported dog bites in children. *Public Health Reports*, 100, 315–321.

Boyd, C. M., Fotheringham, B., Litchfield, C., Mcbryde, I., Metzer, J. C., Scanlon, P., Somers, R., Winefield, A. H. (2004). Fear of dogs in a community sample: effects of age, gender and prior experience of canine aggression. *Anthrozoös*, 17, 146–166.

Christian, H., Westgarth, C., Bauman, A., Richards, E. A., Rhodes, R., Evenson, K., Mayer, J. A., Thorpe, R. J. (2013). Dog ownership and physical activity: A review of the evidence. *Journal of Physical Activity and Health*, 10, 750–759.

De Keuster, T., Lamoureux, J., Kahn, A. (2006). Epidemiology of dog bites: A Belgian experience of canine behaviour and public health concerns. *Veterinary Journal*, 172, 482–487.

Green, J., Thorogood, N. (2009). Chapter 4 – In-Depth Interviews. Qualitative Methods for Health Research. London: Sage.

Headey, B. (2003). Pet ownership: good for health? *Medical Journal of Australia*, 179, 460–461.

Hersant, B., Cassier, S., Constantinescu, G., Gavelle, P., Vazquez, M. P., Picard, A., Kadlub, N. (2012). Facial dog bite injuries in children: Retrospective study of 77 cases. *Annales De Chirurgie Plastique Esthetique*, 57, 230–239.

HES. (2012). HES on ... dog bites and strikes. [Online]. Available: https://catalogue.ic.nhs.uk/publications/hospital/monthly-hes/hes-on-dog-bite/hes-on-dog-bite.pdf [Accessed 24 April 2013].

Hon, K. L. E., Fu, C. C. A., Chor, C. M., Tang, P. S. H., Leung, T. F., Man, C. Y., Ng, P. C. (2007). Issues associated with dog bite injuries in children and adolescents assessed at the emergency department. *Pediatric Emergency Care*, 23, 445–449.

HSCIS. (2014). Provisional monthly topic of interest: admissions caused by dogs and other mammals. [Online]. Health and Social Care Information Centre, available: www.hscic.gov.uk/catalogue/PUB14030/prov-mont-hes-admi-outp-ae-April%202013%20to%20January%202014-toi-rep.pdf

Humane Society. (2014). *Pets By the Numbers* [Online]. The Humane Society of the United States., available: www.humanesociety.org/issues/pet_overpopulation/facts/pet_ownership_statistics.html [Accessed 25 November 2014].

Jackson, T. (2005). Is it time to ban dogs as household pets? *British Medical Journal*, 331, 1278.

Jovanović, A. A., Ivković, M., Gašić, M. J. (2011). Post-traumatic stress disorder in a World War II concentration camp survivor caused by the attack of two German shepherd dogs: Case report and review of the literature. *Forensic Science International*, 208, e15–e19.

Kahn, A., Bauche, P., Lamoureux, J., Dog Bites Research Team (2003). Child victims of dog bites treated in emergency departments: a prospective survey. *European Journal of Pediatrics*, 162, 254–258.

Kahn, A., Robert, E., Piette, D., De Keuster, T., Lamoureux, J., Leveque, A. (2004). Prevalence of dog bites in children: a telephone survey. *European Journal of Pediatrics*, 163, 424–424.

McNicholas, J., Gilbey, A., Rennie, A., Ahmedzai, S., Dono, J.-A., Ormerod, E. (2005). Pet ownership and human health: a brief review of evidence and issues. *BMJ*, 331, 1252–1254.

Messent, P. R. (1983). Social facilitation of contact with other people by pet dogs. In: Katcher, A. H., Beck A. M. (ed.) *New perspectives on our lives with companion animals*. Philadelphia: University of Pennsylvania Press.

Murray, J. K., Browne, W. J., Roberts, M. A., Whitmarsh, A., Gruffydd-Jones, T. J. (2010). Number and ownership profiles of cats and dogs in the UK. *Veterinary Record*, 166, 163–168.

O'Haire, M. (2010). Companion animals and human health: Benefits, challenges, and the road ahead. *Journal of Veterinary Behaviour*, 5, 226–234.

Pfortmueller, C. A., Efeoglou, A., Furrer, H., Exadaktylos, A. K. (2013). Dog Bite Injuries: Primary and Secondary Emergency Department Presentations 2014; A Retrospective Cohort Study. *The Scientific World Journal*, 2013, 6.

Rusch, M. D., Grunert, B. K., Sanger, J. R., Dzwierzynski, W. W., Matloub, H. S. (2000). Psychological adjustment in children after traumatic disfiguring injuries: A 12-month follow-up. *Plastic and Reconstructive Surgery*, 106, 1451–1458.

Sacks, J. J., Kresnow, M., Houston, B. (1996). Dog bites: how big a problem? Inj Prev, 2, 52–4.

Sanders, C. R. (1994). Biting the Hand that Heals You: Encounters with problematic patients in a General Veterinary Practice. *Society and Animals*, 2, 47–66.

Shen, J., Li, S., Xiang, H., Lu, S., Schwebel, D. C. (2014). Antecedents and consequences of pediatric dog-bite injuries and their developmental trends: 101 cases in rural China. *Accident Analysis and Prevention*, 63, 22–29.

Turnbull, M. (2014). Biting back against dog attacks: MPs support Royal Mail's Dog Awareness Week [Online]. Royal Mail Group. Available: www.royalmailgroup.com/biting-back-against-dog-attacks-mps-support-royal-mail%E2%80%99s-dog-awareness-week [Accessed 11 February 2015].

Vargo, D., Depasquale, J. M., Vargo, A. M. (2012). Incidence of dog bite injuries in American Samoa and their impact on society. *Hawai'i journal of medicine & public health: a journal of Asia Pacific Medicine & Public Health*, 71, 6–12.

Voith, V. L. (2009). The Impact of Companion Animal Problems on Society and the Role of Veterinarians. *Veterinary Clinics of North America-Small Animal Practice*, 39, 327–345.

Westgarth, C., Pinchbeck, G. L., Bradshaw, J. W. S., Dawson, S., Gaskell, R. M., Christley, R. M. (2007). Factors associated with dog ownership and contact with dogs in a UK community. *BMC Veterinary Research*, 3.

Westgarth, C., Reevell, K., Barclay, R. (2012). Association between prospective owner viewing of the parents of a puppy and later referral for behavioural problems. *Veterinary Record*, 170.

Westgarth, C., Watkins, F. (2015). A qualitative investigation of the perceptions of female dog-bite victims and implications for the prevention of dog bites. *Journal of Veterinary Behavior: Clinical Applications and Research*, epub ahead of print.

# Section 6
# Handling the Aggressive Dog

In Section 6 we consider issues relating to the handling of potentially aggressive dogs. Many professionals are handling such dogs on a daily basis; not only is this a risk to the person, but also it impacts on the welfare of the dog. In Chapter 24, Kevin McPeake guides us through protocols for situations where we need to handle an aggressive dog, for example in the veterinary clinic, outlining physical and chemical restraint methods. With an emphasis on using the minimum restraint needed, he highlights the importance of avoiding the risk of making matters worse, increasing the risk of either the probability or severity of a bite in either the short or longer term. To this end, early chemical restraint should be considered. Strong physical handling and punishment are not recommended.

Many dog owners will also encounter a situation where their own dog becomes aggressive and a bite risk. In Chapter 25, Esther Schalke provides thoughtful counselling advice directed towards owners of dogs who have bitten as to the available options and short-term management. Her empathetic but realistic approach allows the stressful impact of owning an aggressive dog to be recognised and useful practical solutions employed. This chapter will be a useful first-line resource to manage the situation before specific professional behavioural help can be received. Knowledge of how to prevent and manage aggressive behaviour is useful to the pet owner and also to those working in shelters. In Chapter 26, Lynn Hewison and Graham Turton provide practical 'first aid' behavioural guidance as to the types of approaches that can be taken in order to prevent overtly aggressive behaviour, retrain a dog that is starting to show signs of an overt physical threat, and handle aggressive behaviour by dogs in everyday situations in the home or in kennels. Useful tips are also given as to what to do in the event of a dog fight. Again, the central theme is to avoid confrontation where possible and show or teach the dog that alternative behaviour is preferable.

In summary, this sixth section contains many practical resources that should be of use to anyone owning or working with dogs, who wish to be informed of current thinking and best practice behind how to both prevent aggressive behaviour from developing, or how to minimise the risk to both human and animals when it is already present.

6

# CHAPTER 24

# Physical and Chemical Restraint of the Aggressive Dog

*Kevin McPeake*

## 24.1 Introduction

Restraint can be defined as 'a measure or condition that keeps something under control' (Oxford Dictionaries, 2015) and can be used to limit some or all of an animal's movement (Pines, 2010). Restraint is often used purportedly to prevent dog bites. Many people who routinely handle dogs want to know 'how to handle an aggressive dog', and feel that the answer lies in some form of physical restraint. The answer is actually much simpler: stop, work out why the dog is being aggressive, and change it. In an ideal scenario this would occur, however sometimes the dog must be handled there and then, for its own good, if the procedure cannot be postponed.

It is important to appreciate that restraint does not resolve the underlying problem that is leading to the risk of a dog bite, but rather that it restricts the problem and so is a temporary measure. In the longer term an individualised treatment programme should be developed by a relevant professional to resolve the underlying issue. Aggressive behaviour is part of the normal canine behavioural repertoire (See Chapter 1). Restraint will limit a dog's movement, including its ability to move away from a situation it perceives as a threat, and thus can exacerbate the problem. Furthermore, the act of restraining may be taken as a threat in a dog that was not until that point a risk of biting. As such, restraint should only be carried out if absolutely necessary. Although those dogs already displaying aggressive behaviour may require careful restraint in emergency situations, many principles described within this chapter can be applied to all dogs to minimise the chance of those animals that have not yet shown aggressive behaviour from feeling the need to do so.

Restraint is used in a variety of professions from those working in grooming parlours, rehoming centres and boarding kennels to the police force and dog wardens. In the veterinary context, a dog may be restrained for a physical examination, blood sampling or a minor procedure such as an ear clean. In the veterinary clinic, there is free access to a full range of handling adjuncts, medications for chemical restraint and additional staff as required.

6

Handling and restraint of dogs can be more challenging when in other locations, such as in the home of an owner.

In the UK, chemical restraint (sedation) is a medical treatment that amounts to an act of veterinary surgery, even if it is to be administered by a person acting under veterinary direction, such as an owner or suitably qualified nurse (RCVS, 2015). This chapter therefore focuses on the chemical and physical restraint of the aggressive dog in the veterinary context, but some of the information can be extrapolated and applied to those handling dogs in other contexts.

## 24.2  Prevention is better than cure

Efforts should be made to try to minimise the risk of a dog displaying aggressive behaviour when being handled. It is important that owners work with dogs from a young age to establish positive associations with handling, including being groomed and handled all over (for a video guide, see Pupblog 11), holding of feet for nail clipping, lifting ears as if to administer topical medication, etc, to prepare a dog for that which may be encountered in the veterinary context (protocols for which have been developed, see Zulch and Mills, 2012). This should be continued in the veterinary and other potentially threatening environments where the focus should be on a dog having positive experiences, which can be facilitated by the use of food treats (or potentially play with access to a favourite toy if this is more motivating for the dog) (Moffat, 2008). The use of high value food (value depends on the individual dog, but typically, highly palatable food such as cheese or soft dog treats, etc.) can help form a positive association with visits and handling to reduce risk of problems, as well as counter-condition a dog requiring a change in emotional state during a visit.

In those dogs where difficulty in handling has already been established, assistance should be provided to owners in working to improve this. Such advice may include handling exercises at home, guidance on use of handling tools (including muzzles) (see Chapter 25, visits to the vets for desensitisation and counter-conditioning, Shaw, 2015) and may even include addressing any issues associated with travel to the clinic, if this is an additional stressor (Mills et al., 2013). This will typically culminate in reintroduction to staff and handling in the veterinary clinic (Herron and Shreyer, 2014). For a detailed client handout on desensitisation and counter-conditioning to the veterinary clinic, see Palestrini (2009), but where possible, advice should be tailored to the individual patient and client's needs, and the clinician should consider referral to a suitably qualified behaviourist to formulate a behaviour modification programme to facilitate this process if such advice cannot be offered in-house.

## 24.3  Set up of the veterinary clinic

Various studies suggest that a trip to the veterinary clinic can be particularly distressing for dogs (Döring et al., 2009; Stanford, 1982). There are a multitude of characteristics of stimuli (triggers) and environmental cues that can be perceived as more threatening for dogs in the veterinary context, such as increased speed of movement and invasion of personal space (Mills and Zulch, 2010). The accumulation of different stressors has been referred to as 'trigger stacking' (Donaldson, 1996) and may contribute to the use of aggressive behaviour in various contexts including the veterinary clinic, where, if the dog had presented with individual triggers with time to recover in between, aggressive behaviour may have been avoided (Hedges, 2014).

As an example, take a dog that is fearful meeting other dogs and has been taken to the veterinary clinic for a routine booster vaccination. The veterinarian is running late and the dog spends ten minutes sitting in a waiting room in close proximity to an unfamiliar dog, which barks regularly. When eventually called into the consulting room there are strong chemical smells, and the veterinarian proceeds hurriedly to approach and examine the dog, triggering a biting incident.

Now look at this scenario with a few changes: the dog is permitted to wait outside in a quiet area until the veterinarian is ready and is taken into the consulting room via an alternative entry (which avoids encountering the unfamiliar dog); the consulting room had been cleaned with a neutrally scented disinfectant and time has been allowed for it to dissipate (which minimises the strong smells); the dog is given time to approach the veterinarian, and provided with some food rewards for doing so (which gives the dog time to relax and form a positive association with the vet and situation). The dog allows handling, and receives the vaccination without a biting incident.

Veterinary clinics should therefore strive to create an environment minimising potential stressors for visiting patients. Attention should be paid to every area from waiting room and consultation room to kennel and hospitalisation areas and the prep room. Some measures relate to the design and layout of the building and may be more challenging to change, but many are straightforward measures that can be implemented easily. Table 24.1 summarises some hints and tips to minimise stressors within the veterinary clinic.

In addition, there are tools that can be used on a dog to minimise visual (Calming cap) and auditory (cotton balls in ears, Mutt Muffs) stimuli that may be used consciously in dogs where they have been successfully introduced to them, or after chemical restraint (if it is safe to do so), to help maintain the level of sedation.

## 24.4 Body language

### 24.4.1 Human

A dog can feel threatened by sudden movements, a person looming over, giving direct eye contact, or approaching them from the front. It is important that all staff involved in handling dogs are aware of how their body language may impact on the dog's perception of the interaction. Appropriate measures to adjust body language to be less threatening for dogs and which may in turn encourage an approach in a fearful dog include:

- Avoiding prolonged eye contact
- Allowing the dog to approach (where safe to do so)
- Crouched posture, bending at the knees not waist to prevent a perception of looming over the dog
- Turn side on to the dog
- Ensure any movements are slow and deliberate rather than fast and erratic.

**Table 24.1** Hints and tips to minimise stressors within the veterinary clinic.

| Feature | Hints and tips |
|---|---|
| Arrival at clinic | Consider leaving a dog in the car or outdoors in a safe area with the owner until the clinician is ready (Shepherd, 2009), or even a spare consulting room |
| | Use an alternative door for entry and exit to avoid dogs passing through a busy waiting room (Martin et al., 2015) |
| | Appointment times at quiet times of the day for more challenging dogs allowing sufficient extra time for dealing with them |
| Visual stimuli | Use of softer lighting, avoiding bright lights (Herron and Shreyer, 2014) or fluorescent lights with a flicker frequency dogs can detect. |
| | Partitions in waiting rooms to block visual stimuli of other dogs/owners (could simply be clever placement of food stands) |
| | Waiting rooms large enough to increase distance between different owners/dogs |
| | Separate entry/exit from waiting rooms (Overall, 2013) |
| | Kennels designed to avoid animals facing each other directly (Shepherd, 2009) |
| | Block visual access in kennels e.g. towel over kennel door, clothes drying maiden in middle of room with sheet over it |
| Auditory stimuli | Separate kennel room for dogs more sensitive to noise OR to prevent those dogs making noise from impacting on others |
| | Half-glass fronted kennels with lower half opaque to minimise noise (Beesley and Mills 2010) |
| | Speak softly/quietly, avoid making loud noises (Herron and Shreyer, 2014) |
| | Use sound-absorbing surfaces in practice design |
| | If music permitted in clinic, avoid loud music, consider quiet music to mask background noise (Herron and Shreyer, 2014) |
| Olfactory stimuli | Clean areas thoroughly between seeing patients to reduce the impact of any deposited alarm pheromones, allowing time for the chemical smell to dissipate (Herron and Shreyer, 2014) |
| | Use of air ventilation units between consultations to remove stress pheromones (Hedges, 2015) |
| | Limit the use of strong smelling substances such as air fresheners, and use surgical spirit sparingly (Herron and Shreyer, 2014) |
| | The use of dog appeasing pheromone diffusers throughout the practice including waiting room, consultation room, kennel and prep-room areas to create a greater chemical sense of security (Mills et al., 2013) |
| Tactile stimuli | Ensure all surfaces a dog will walk on are non-slip for the dog, solid floor being preferred Overall (2013) |
| | Rubber non slip mats on examination tables and weighing scales – the addition of a towel or blanket may provide a more comfortable surface (Herron and Shreyer, 2014) and preferably one owned by the animal |
| | Rubber backed mats or fleeces for kennels and resting areas |

For a useful video demonstrating these points please see APBC video: Approaching a dog in practice to reduce fear and defensive aggression.

### 24.4.2 Dog

It is important for all those dealing with dogs to have an understanding of body language and what it may mean, including veterinary staff and owners (see Chapter 2).

Treats can be tossed to dogs while being given lots of space, which may be enough to start to create a positive association with the clinician and may encourage approach. In those dogs reluctant to take treats, if the owner is able to cue a behaviour with a history of being rewarded, such as a 'sit', then this may provide a window of opportunity for the dog to relax where they have an expectation of a reward, and may take a food treat. However, avoid luring the very fearful dog close with food in the hand, as a sudden bite may occur. Use food to reward relaxed and approachable behaviour instead.

Where possible, examining dogs on the floor may be easier, reducing the need to lift the dog on to the table. Hydraulic tables if available may be easier for larger dogs IF examination on a table is essential (Shepherd, 2009).

## 24.5 Physical restraint

### 24.5.1 Important considerations

The ability to safely handle and restrain animal patients while maintaining safety of others is listed as a day one competency under the RCVS guidelines (RCVS, 2014).

During handling and restraint, it is paramount that whichever methods are chosen prioritise the welfare of the dog to maintain their physical safety as well as their emotional well-being, as aggressive behaviour is usually a sign of a negative emotional state. Guidelines recognise the equal importance of ensuring animals are kept free from emotional and physical harm (Rooney et al., 2009; Act, A. W. 2006; Farm Animal Welfare Council, 1992).

Maintaining the safety of those involved in any part of the restraint process is also vital, including the owner, as the impact of any injury, particularly from dog bites, can be great both to those injured (see Chapter 23) and from the associated costs to employers of these injuries, including any liability.

### 24.5.2 What level of restraint is necessary?

The minimum level of restraint required for that individual in that circumstance should always be used. If careful attention is paid to the factors described in this chapter, very little restraint should be required in typical situations.

If further restraint is required, handling tools such as muzzles, and then chemical restraint should be considered. It should be remembered that veterinary visits, handling and restraint can all become predictive of a negative experience for dogs. Consideration should be given for the management of that dog in the future in the veterinary context and any other context in which that dog may be handled. As such, choosing to use chemical restraint to facilitate handling is often preferable to heavy physical restraint to minimise the degree to which learning can occur from that situation (Moffat, 2008). Previous experiences with that patient should be noted on the clinical records so a suitable handling plan can be created for each visit. This should detail the handling tools, chemical restraint and other medication to be administered (Overall, 2013). If a dog is to be sedated or anesthetised as part of this plan, it is advisable to maximise the number of procedures that the dog requires to be performed at that visit where safe to do so listed to be performed in order of priority from most to least important in case time does not permit everything to be completed. This may include other diagnostics (e.g. radiographs if there is a suspected focus of pain that may be influencing behaviour), and collection of blood and urine samples to screen for disease and/or to obtain normal baseline values if consideration is being given to using behaviour modifying medications in the future (Fatjó and Bowen, 2009).

## 24.5.3 Low stress handling and restraint

Handling and restraint techniques aimed at minimising stress for the patient and maximising safety for those dealing with them should always be used (for a detailed illustrated text and DVD on this subject for dogs (and cats), please see Yin, 2009). Although the handling of each dog should be tailored to the individual, some important general factors to consider include:

- **Do not over-restrain** as this may cause unnecessary stress to the animal that leads to aggression. Use the lightest touch required, knowing that pressure can be increased if required if the animal starts to struggle.
- **Do not lean over** the dog as this may be interpreted as threatening.
- **Control a dog's movement** by reducing the length of the lead and/or requesting an appropriate behaviour such as a sit or lie down. This may help prevent those excited dogs from being more highly aroused and those fearful dogs from becoming increasingly anxious.
- **Support the dog so it feels secure and balanced** using your hands and body. This helps to limit it struggling and injuring itself, particularly when moving it into different positions such as lying on its side.
- **If a dog does struggle** for more than two to three seconds, stop what you are doing and wait for the animal to relax while reassessing how the handling can be improved and try again.
- **Wait for the dog to relax** while being restrained before performing any procedures.
- **Avoid unnecessary discomfort** where possible, e.g. if it may be painful for an elderly arthritic dog to have its neck extended for jugular venipuncture for a blood sample, then consider using another site such as the lateral saphenous while the dog is standing if this is more comfortable. If discomfort is unavoidable, ensure appropriate analgesia is provided BEFORE the procedure.
- **Use food and praise** where possible, at times as a distraction to facilitate the procedure being performed, as well as to reinforce compliant and relaxed behaviour.

## 24.5.4 Handling tools

Handling tools are available to assist in the restraint and handling of dogs to maximise safety and welfare of staff and patient. It is important that all staff members involved in the restraint of dogs are trained and well-rehearsed in the approach being taken for each individual case, including the use of specific handling tools.

### 24.5.4.1 Muzzles

Every dog should be trained to accept and enjoy wearing a muzzle so in the event that it is required to use one, it is less distressing for the dog to have one fitted (for a video guide, see University of Lincoln Life Skills for Puppies: Muzzle training video). The main aim of a muzzle during handling is to reduce the risk of a bite (to veterinary staff and/or the dog's owner). Various types of muzzle are available with pros and cons for each type.

- **Fabric- and mesh sleeve-type muzzles** (see Figure 24.1) work by closing a dog's mouth so do not allow vomiting, drinking, or panting, which may cause distress if used for long periods. They are only suitable for short-term use while supervised, and not in conjunction with chemical restraint with agents, which may cause vomiting. These muzzles can make it more difficult to administer food if being used as part of a behaviour modification programme, and those muzzles open at the front do not stop a dog from 'nipping' with incisors.

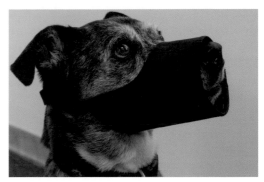

**Figure 24.1** Fabric muzzle.

- **Basket type muzzles** (see Figure 24.2) do not have the limitations that occur with the fabric muzzles and are the author's preferred muzzle of choice, allowing a dog to eat, drink and pant while wearing it (Horwitz and Pike, 2014). However, in situations where presented with a dog requiring muzzling for the first time and muzzle training will be recommended for future visits, then the use of a fabric muzzle in the short term may be best to minimise the impact on any subsequent training to accept a basket-type muzzle. If a dog is known to use aggressive behaviour during handling and has been taught to wear a basket-type muzzle, it should be fitted before the visit to veterinary clinic, to prevent the need to attempt to fit it when the dog may have already become distressed by the visit. It is important though that the muzzle is used at other times at home, for example before enjoyable activities, so it is not predictive of a veterinary visit.

- Other types of muzzle such as the Air Muzzle (see Figure 24.3) are available and offer an option for brachycephalic dog breeds where conventional muzzles do not fit appropriately.

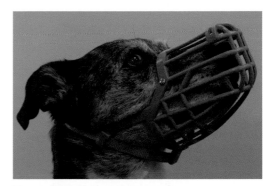

**Figure 24.2** Basket-type muzzle.

When placing a muzzle in an emergency it is advisable to position yourself side on to the dog, scooping the muzzle from under the chin and securing to the side/behind the dog's head (Herron and Shreyer, 2014). As many dogs will try to reverse, use a person or wall (ideally a corner) as a 'bum stop' to prevent this. It is important the person fitting the muzzle is confident and efficient at doing so, as any hesitation will complicate the procedure.

If it is safe to do so, time permitting

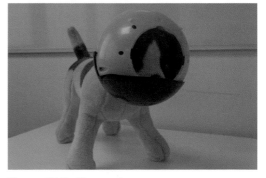

**Figure 24.3** Air muzzle.

6

and the patient is allowed to eat, it is advisable to spend some time offering some food to the dog for seeing the muzzle, then investigating the muzzle, before fitting it in the above manner. This will likely be insufficient to form a positive association with the use of the muzzle but may minimise the impact of the procedure, which may in turn make introduction or fitting of a muzzle at future visits an easier task.

### 24.5.4.2 Alternative methods of head restraint

The use of an Elizabethan collar, head collars tightened to close the mouth, a lead wrapped around the muzzle of a dog (see Figure 24.4) or a towel wrapped around its neck (see Figure 24.5) may offer some protection (Herron and Shreyer, 2014) but are not as effective as muzzles. In some situations the fitting of a tape muzzle (Atkinson et al., 2011) or the sliding of a fabric muzzle over the lead attached to a head collar (Yin, 2009) may reduce the risk of a bite by ensuring more distance between the operator's hands and the dog's teeth.

### 24.5.4.3 A note on owner involvement

Whether the owner should be allowed to fit a muzzle in this situation and his or her involvement in physical restraint of the dog requires a risk assessment in itself, as there is the possibility of litigation should an owner be injured. This risk assessment should be based on

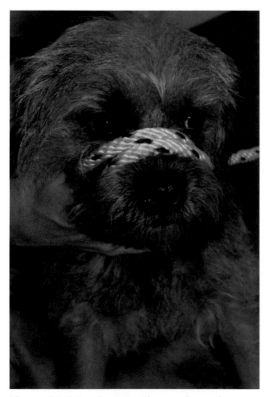 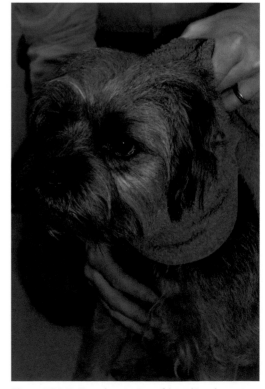

**Figure 24.4** Lead wrapped around muzzle.    **Figure 24.5** Towel restraint of head/neck.

the dog's behaviour at that time and historically to the owner, his or her confidence and capability to fit the muzzle, and on the ability to follow directions. The clinician should be present to supervise this and should halt the procedure if it appears there is risk that the dog may direct aggressive behaviour to the owner, or the owner is not capable of fitting the muzzle (Herron and Shreyer, 2014).

For general handling, where safe to do so, if the dog seems to be more tolerant with the owner present, then it is preferable to allow this. Some animals that may be easier to manage away from their owners while others may actually be more distressed without the support of their owner (Herron and Shreyer, 2014).

It should be explained to owners why reprimands (physical or verbal) should be avoided if their dog does display any unwanted behaviour, including aggression. All clinic staff dealing with or giving advice on patients should be briefed to the same effect so a consistent message is delivered by the practice, led by the example of those people the owners see dealing with their dogs.

### 24.5.4.4 Maximising safety with inpatients

Moving dogs that have shown aggressive behaviour around the clinic, particularly from their kennel, can be a particularly high-risk situation. To reduce the need to clip a lead on to a dog's collar to remove it from a kennel, a long trailing lead can be left on with the handle end accessible outside the kennel. These dogs need to be supervised to ensure they do not chew the lead or get caught up in it (this should be less of a problem if also wearing a muzzle). Double leashing a dog (Beaver, 2009), and considering two people to be involved (one lead per person) may increase control of the dog.

### 24.5.4.5 Severe cases

In severe cases, where a muzzle cannot be fitted safely, and often to facilitate intramuscular injection with a sedative, other techniques may be required. One handler can walk the dog on a lead up to a doorway (see Figure 24.6) so the dog is on one side of the closed door and the lead kept taut at the level of the dog's head on the other side of the door to ensure safe control of the dog (see Figure 24.7). The handler in the room with the dog can then safely inject the dog from behind (see Figure 24.8) (Yin, 2009). In smaller dogs where a muzzle cannot be fitted, the use of a 'crush' or squeeze cage to facilitate safe intramuscular injection may be required. When handling at such times the use of padded gauntlets may minimise the risk of a bite damaging the hands and forearms. Dog catcher poles (Beaver, 2009) should be available for use if required, and if using them, the dog's head should be kept at a level where it can still bear weight on its front feet, which minimises any potential injury or discomfort around its neck.

In the author's experience it is extremely rare to encounter severe cases requiring the above methods and they should be reserved as a last resort as they can be traumatic for the dog. Often they are only used briefly to facilitate injection with a suitable chemical restraint combination. In these rare situations where they are required, the aim is to be efficient, and minimise any distress to the dog while maintaining the safety of those involved in the handling process.

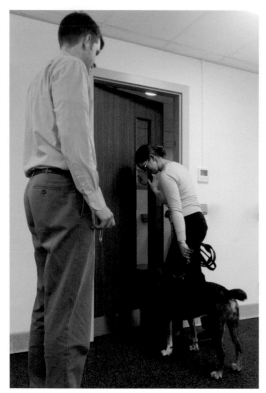 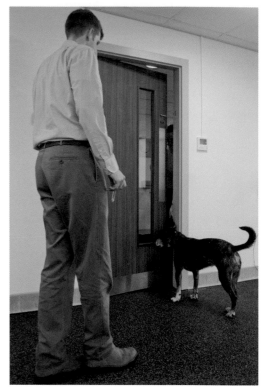

**Figure 24.6** Handler leads dog to doorway.

**Figure 24.7** Dog restrained with lead through door, kept at level of dog's head.

## 24.6 Chemical restraint

### 24.6.1 *When to use chemical restraint*

The use of chemical restraint should complement and not replace the above advice on setting up the veterinary clinic environment and appropriate physical restraint. Where chemical restraint is to be used, it is best to make the decision to use it sooner in the restraint process. This ensures that the physical restraint required to administer the chemical restraint can be minimal. Using chemical restraint as a last resort when the patient is already highly distressed can also reduce the efficacy of certain medications used due to endogenous catecholamine release (Sinclair, 2003) and potentially increase the risk of adverse events (Pinson, 1997). If such a situation does occur in elective or non-emergency procedures, then it is always worth considering delaying the procedure to another day. This will give the chance to create a revised protocol for handling to address the problems encountered and consider the earlier use of chemical restraint next time round.

### 24.6.2 *Considerations in using chemical restraint*

When considering the dose of chemical restraint to be used, the clinician must take into account the individual's age, health status, current or previous medical problems, as well as the behaviour of the patient in previous visits and on the day of presentation (Moffat,

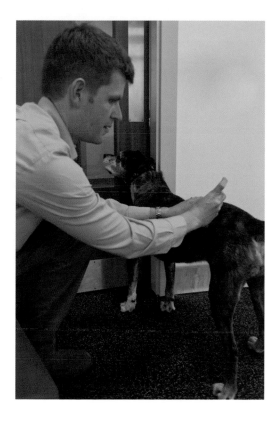

**Figure 24.8** Handler safely administers an intramuscular injection.

2009). Consideration should be made as to whether it is desirable to use a reversible medication and, if so, ensuring the reversal agent is available. The aim is to dose appropriately to achieve the required plane of sedation – avoiding low doses that may require 'topping up', which can prolong patient distress with repeated handling and injections and may reduce the efficacy of the agents used.

It is important to always assess for potential contraindications and drug interactions before combining medications (refer to the compendium of datasheets: NOAH, 2015 and current drug formulary: Ramsey, 2014). This is especially important if the dog displaying aggressive behaviour is already being treated with any other medications (including psychoactive medications), as there can be potential drug interactions with some of the agents used for chemical restraint. If the initial chemical restraint protocol is to be used as a premedication to a general anaesthetic (e.g. those patients that may present for surgical procedures or more invasive diagnostics where sedation is insufficient) the clinician should be familiar with the sparing effects of the premedication agents chosen on both induction and anaesthetic drugs being used thereafter. It is sensible to ensure that the chosen protocol for chemical restraint incorporates and does not interfere with any specific analgesic agent likely to be required.

It should be remembered that patients that appear sedated may become suddenly aroused (particularly as a result of external auditory stimuli such as a cage door being opened, being moved, or the handling of a painful area) and as a result may show 'sudden' aggressive behaviour such as lunging or snapping (Yin, 2013). Appropriate physical restraint to ensure the safety of those handling the patient is key and continued use of a muzzle in these patients during handling and moving can reduce the risk of injuries from biting. If it is deemed appropriate that a muzzle is to be left on while chemical restraint takes effect, then given the potential side effects of nausea with some of the agents used, it is recommended that a basket-type muzzle is used, which allows the dog to vomit. If a dog vomits wearing a fabric muzzle that restricts the opening of the mouth, there is a significant risk of aspiration and other associated complications.

Many sedative agents are licensed to be given by various routes and the dose can vary depending on the route given (often reduced doses for intravenous administration). When dealing with dogs displaying aggressive behaviour, often the intramuscular route is the easiest and safest to use, and when using a combination of injectable agents, it is easiest if they can be administered mixed in the same syringe (Quandt, 2013).

If the dog is more relaxed with the owner (and it is deemed safe for them to be present) then permitting the owner to be present while the dog is injected and until it is sedated can be useful, before the dog is admitted. For those dogs where the presence of the clinician increases their distress, it is the author's preference to leave the room while still monitoring the patient via a window if available – one-way mirror tinting on such a window reduces the impact of the viewing clinician on the patient. In this scenario it is important that the owner is briefed on what agents have been used in the chemical restraint protocol, how and when they are likely to take effect and if there are any potential side effects such as vomiting. If they are prepared for what to expect, the process should be predictable and less distressing for the owner.

## 24.6.3 Oral medications

For certain patients it may be sufficient to use oral medications, generally in tablet form, prescribed by the veterinary surgeon to be administered before elective visits. In the author's experience, these are best reserved for those patients at the milder end of the spectrum of difficulty in handling.

Although unlicensed by this route, certain agents such as medetomidine and dexmedetomidone can be absorbed across mucus membranes, and administering the injectable formulation via the orotransmucosal route has been described (see table for dosing). A detomidine gel formulation licensed for the transmucosal route for sedation in horses has been available for some time, and a recent study looked at its application to facilitate handling in a group of six dogs (Hopfensperger et al., 2013). At the time of writing, a dexmedetomidine oromucosal gel (Sileo) has been licensed and has been recently released in the UK and Europe (European Commission, 2015).

The use of oral medications can also be considered following a particularly negative experience through physical restraint. Benzodiazepines such as alprazolam may be useful to block long-term memory formation from the event (Overall, 2013) thus potentially reducing the impact on learning for future visits, therefore consider administering it before the patient leaves or by the owner soon after leaving. If it is thought that such medication may be required, it is preferable to administer it in advance of the situation.

## 24.6.4 Recovery period

The period from recovery from a procedure to the patient being collected by the owner is also very important. Consideration should be given to sending patients home as soon after recovery as is safe to do so, balancing the close monitoring of their recovery with the time in which they may be potentially distressed while waiting to go home. In some situations if it is safe to do so, having the dog's owner remove the dog from the kennel can be useful, particularly in those dogs who show aggressive behaviour towards staff whilst being kennelled. In some situations the use of a basket type muzzle from admittance to recovery and the patient going home may be required to manage the risk of a biting incident sufficiently.

## 24.6.5 Severe cases

When considering chemical restraint in any patient the potential side effects of the agents used and risks to the dog must be balanced with the aforementioned benefits to the patient and those dealing with it. In rare situations, there may be situations where a clinician is faced with a highly aggressive dog that cannot be handled at all that is to be euthanised, and facilities are not as available as at the clinic (e.g. during a home visit). The welfare of the dog is vital to minimise distress although potential side effects of the sedation (such as giving too large a dose) are less important. It is still preferable to provide chemical restraint that will maintain blood pressure and venous access to administer the solution for euthanasia. In such situations there is an option of hiding tablets in food that can be offered to the dog in a secured area, and a combination of medications in tablet form such as phenobarbital, acepromazine and a benzodiazepine can potentially be used (Yin, 2013).

## 24.7 Specific classes of medications

The following section summarises the particulars of specific classes of medications. A good review of the current classes of drugs used in behavioural therapy can be found in Landsberg et al., 2013, Chapter 8: Pharmacologic intervention in behavioural therapy.

### 24.7.1 Benzodiazepines

Benzodiazepines exhibit their effects by binding to a specific benzodiazepine binding site on the inhibitory neurotransmitter GABA ($\gamma$-aminobutyric acid) receptor. They act as anxiolytics, anticonvulsants and muscle relaxants, and the range of different benzodiazepines allow choices in administering them orally or by injection (Landsberg et al., 2013).

Increased appetite can be seen with administration of benzodiazepines, which may be a positive when using food for counter-conditioning procedures, but as they can impair learning there may also be disadvantages if trying to use this class of drugs as an adjunct to behaviour modification. Benzodiazepines can have an amnesic effect (Dodman and Shuster, 1998) – this may be of benefit in cases where blocking the formation of short- to long-term memory from a negative experience is required so can be used as an interventional drug (Overall, 2013).

In patients that are fearful and inhibiting their aggressive behaviour, there is a potential risk of disinhibition, which may result in increased aggressive behaviour, so benzodiazepines should be used with care (Crowell-Davis and Murray, 2006). In patients where the underlying emotion is not fear, and where they are clearly not inhibiting their behaviour, this may be less of a concern.

Paradoxical excitement can be seen in some dogs administered benzodiazepines, which is not desirable when the aim is to facilitate handling. This is more of a concern when it is administered as a sole agent and so has implications for those dogs being administered oral benzodiazepines at home prior to the situation requiring handling. It is therefore recommended that a test dose is performed at home at a time when the owner is able to supervise the dog for the duration of the effect of the benzodiazepine chosen. If paradoxical excitement is seen, it is not recommended that the specific benzodiazepine compound is used, but an alternative can be tried at a test dose, as excitement seen with one type does not mean excitement will be seen with others.

Reversal of benzodiazepines

Lumazenil is available to antagonise the actions of the benzodiazepines effectively if required (Herron and Shreyer, 2014).

## 24.7.2 Phenothiazines

Phenothiazines are neuroleptic tranquilisers that act by blocking dopamine receptors in the brain, resulting in central nervous system depression and reduced motor function (Landsberg et al., 2013). Acepromazine is the most commonly used phenothiazine in veterinary medicine, but it is not advisable to use this as a sole agent, as in the author's experience it is not reliable in facilitating handling when given orally before presentation to the veterinary clinic. Also, although it reduces motor function, it does not change sensory perception of events and so may further sensitise those individuals to whom it is administered (Bowen and Heath, 2005), although there appear to be no case reports documenting this effect in the literature, so the concern may be entirely theoretical.

## 24.7.3 Opioids

Opioids have analgesic effects and may also produce mild sedation and loss of proprioception. A variety of opioids are available for use in veterinary medicine ranging from partial agonists such as butorphanol and buprenorphine, to full agonists such as morphine and methadone. Full agonists have the benefit of providing superior analgesia for moderate to severely painful procedures, however butorphanol can provide superior sedation (Lukasik, 1999).

Reversal of opioids

Naloxone is available to effectively antagonise the actions of all the opioids, in case of overdose, but will also reverse analgesic effects, therefore it is important to ensure that sufficient analgesia is provided by other means. In addition, the partial agonists butorphanol and buprenorphine can be used to partially reverse full opioid agonists (Lukasik, 1999).

## 24.7.4 Alpha-2-adrenergic agonists

Alpha-2-adrenoreceptors are inhibitory receptors widespread throughout the body. Alpha-2-adrenergic agonists primarily work to decrease norepinephrine (noradrenaline), producing sedation, and analgesia. Care should be used in geriatric dogs or those with cardiorespiratory disease; vomiting is a potential side effect (Lukasik, 1999). This class of drug is most commonly administered via injection in combination with other medications, but due to transmucosal absorption can also be administered via this route (European Commission, 2015; Hopfensperger et al., 2013; Yin, 2013), and a transmucosal formulation for dogs is now available commercially (Sileo, Orion Pharmaceuticals).

Clonidine is a selective alpha–2-adrenoreceptor agonist that was originally developed as an anti-hypertensive due to its effects on reducing noradrenaline, but can block autonomic responses and may be useful dosed orally prior to a situation requiring handling and restraint in dog's with fear, anxiety or frustration associated with aggression.

### Reversal of alpha-2-adrenergic agonists

Atipamezole is available to effectively antagonise the actions of the alpha–2-adrenergic agonists. Due to the analgesic properties that are also reversed, it is important to ensure that sufficient analgesia is provided by other means (Lukasik, 1999).

## 24.7.5 NMDA receptor antagonist

NMDA (N-methyl-D-aspartate) receptor antagonists are dissociative anaesthetic agents, and the most commonly used in veterinary medicine is ketamine (Quandt, 2013). Ketamine can be added to the other combination protocols to provide additional sedation and analgesia (Yin, 2013) but should not be used alone as it can cause skeletal muscle hypertonicity (offset by the use of alpha–2-adrenergic agonists). When combined with an alpha–2-agonist, reversal of the latter should be delayed until forty-five minutes after ketamine administration (Ramsey, 2014).

## 24.7.6 Serotonin-2A antagonist/reuptake inhibitor

The atypical antidepressant trazodone has mixed serotonergic agonist and antagonist properties, and has been used as an anxiolytic in veterinary medicine, usually as an adjunct to other behavioural medications (Landsberg et al., 2013). It has been suggested as an option to be given orally prior to veterinary visits to facilitate handling (Herron and Shreyer, 2014).

## 24.7.8 Drug dosage tables

Tables 24.2 to 24.5 display agents, doses and combinations that can be used to chemically restrain dogs. For further details of specific licensed preparations and dosages it is recommended to refer to an up to date compendium of data sheets (NOAH, 2015). For other suggestions on oral and injectable medications (including off-licence products) see the drug formulary (Ramsey, 2014) and www.vasg.org (Veterinary Anesthesia and Analgesia Support Group).

### Key to abbreviations used:

ml = millilitres; mg = milligram; kg = kilogram; $m^2$ = metres squared (body surface area of patient); q = every; h = hour; min = minutes; po = orally; im = intramuscularly; iv = intravenously; sc = subcutaneously; prn = as needed; q24h = SID, every twenty-four hours, once a day; q12h = BID, every twelve hours, twice a day; q8h = TID, every eight hours, three times a day; q6h = TID, every six hours. q4h = every four hours, six times a day; Not licensed = medications which have not been licensed for use in dogs in the UK.

**Table 24.2** Injectable medications – combination protocols.

| Drug | Dose for dogs | Use/comments | References |
|---|---|---|---|
| Benzodiazepine + Opioid | | | |
| Midazolam<br>PLUS opioid of choice | 0.2–0.3mg/kg im | Both relatively safe option in critically ill patients | Ramsey (2014) |
| OR | | | |
| Diazepam<br>PLUS opioid of choice | 0.2–0.3mg/kg im | | |
| Phenothiazine + Opioid ('neuroleptanalgesia') | | | |
| Acepromazine<br>PLUS opioid of choice | 0.01–0.05mg/kg im | Lower dose suggested in Boxers of 0.005–0.01mg/kg im | Ramsey (2014) |
| Alpha-2-adrenergic agonist + Opioid | | | |
| Medetomidine<br>PLUS opioid of choice | 0.005–0.02mg/kg im | Recommended for healthy animals | Ramsey (2014) |
| OR | | | |
| Dexmedetomidine<br>PLUS opioid of choice | 0.0025–0.01mg/kg im | | |
| Other combinations for more challenging patients | | | |
| Alpha-2-adrenergic agonist + Opioid | At above combination doses | | |
| PLUS | | | |
| Acepromazine | 0.01mg/kg im | Deep sedation | Ramsey (2014) |
| | 0.05mg/kg im | Profound sedation, (reserve for large and/or extremely aggressive dogs) | |
| Alpha-2-adrenergic agonist + Opioid | At above combination doses | | |
| PLUS | | | |
| Midazolam | 0.05–0.2mg/kg | Triple combination provides balanced sedation. Not licensed | Yin (2013) |
| PLUS (optional) | | | |
| Ketamine | 3mg/kg | Quadruple combination with addition of ketamine for more fractious patients | |

**Table 24.3** Opioid options to be added to combinations.

| Drug | Dose for dogs | Use/comments | References |
|---|---|---|---|
| Opioids | | | |
| Butorphanol | 0.1–0.4mg/kg im, sc | Most sedating partial agonist | Yin (2013) |
| Buprenorphine | 0.02–0.03mg/kg im, sc | Superior analgesia partial agonist | Ramsey (2014) |
| Methadone | 0.1–0.4mg/kg im, sc | Full agonist | Ramsey (2014) |
| Morphine | 0.2–1.0mg/kg im | Full agonist<br>Not licensed | Yin (2013) |

**Table 24.4** Reversal agents.

| Drug | Dose for dogs | Use/comments | References |
|---|---|---|---|
| Reversal of benzodiazepines | | | |
| Flumazenil | 0.001mg/kg, then work up to 0.01mg/kg) iv | Not licensed | Herron and Shreyer (2014) |
| Reversal of opioids | | | |
| Naloxone | 0.01–0.02mg/kg iv, 0.04mg/kg im, sc | Not licensed | Ramsey (2014) |
| Reversal of alpha-2-adrenergic agonists | | | |
| Atipamezole | Use equal volume of atipamezole to medetomidine or dexmedetomidine administered, im | For full reversal | Ramsey (2014) |
| | Use half volume of atipamezole to medetomidine or dexmedetomidine administered, im | For partial reversal or when medetomidine or dexmedetomidine has been administered at least an hour before | |

## 24.8 Conclusion

Both chemical and physical restraint can be required in dogs using aggressive behaviour. Appropriate handling from a young age may help reduce the need for physical and chemical restraint in dogs, and for those with established problems, appropriate behaviour modification techniques should help improve tolerance of handling. In the veterinary context, a multitude of simple changes to the environment, equipping owners and staff with the knowledge to read their dog's body language and modify their own interactions, including implementation of specific handling techniques, can help minimise stressors and reduce the likelihood of aggressive behaviour being used. A range of handling tools can be used to increase safety when handling. At times, chemical restraint may be required to facilitate handling, and a range of options are available. Overall, the techniques described in this chapter should allow safe management of dogs and minimise the need for them to use aggressive behaviour, which is important for the safety of veterinary staff and owners and also the welfare of the dog.

## 24.9 Further resources

APBC video: Approaching a dog in practice to reduce fear and defensive aggression. APBC. https://www.youtube.com/watch?v=lpecvb9Q7QY

Pupblog 11: Handling and grooming training. Carri Westgarth. https://www.youtube.com/watch?v=mGam8afeBQw

University of Lincoln Life Skills for Puppies: Muzzle training video: www.lifeskillsforpuppies.co.uk/muzzlevideo

Veterinary Anesthesia and Analgesia Support Group: www.vasg.org

Yin, S. (2009). *Low Stress Handling, Restraint and Behaviour Modification of Dogs and Cats*. Cattledog Publishing, Davis, California. (book and DVD)

**Table 24.5** Oral medication for chemical restraint.

| Drug | Dose for dogs | Use/comments | References |
|---|---|---|---|
| Benzodiazepines | | | |
| Diazepam | 0.5–2.0mg/kg po prn, up to q4h, administer 30-60 minutes before required | Test dose recommended<br><br>Not licensed | Ramsey (2014) |
| Alprazolam | 0.01–0.1mg/kg po prn, up to every 6 hours, give 30–60 minutes before required | Test dose recommended<br><br>Not licensed | Ramsey (2014) |
| Phenothiazines | | | |
| Acepromazine | 0.5–2.2mg/kg p.o. up to every 6 hours | Do not use as a sole agent as does not provide anxiolysis – consider combining with trazodone or a benzodiazepine | Herron and Shreyer (2014) |
| Serotonin-2A antagonist/reuptake inhibitor | | | |
| Trazodone | 2–3mg/kg po prn up to every 8 hours, maximum 300mg/dose | Not licensed | Landsberg et al. (2013) |
| Alpha-2-adrenergic agonists | | | |
| Clonidine | 0.01–0.05mg/kg po up to every 12 hours, give 1.5–2 hours prior to event | Not licensed | Landsberg et al. (2013) |
| Dexmedetomidine OR Medetomidine injectable version | 20–40mg/kg transmucosally | Can mix with honey or maple syrup<br><br>Not licensed via this route | Yin (2013) |
| Detomidine oral gel | 0.35–1mg/ m² | Not licensed | Hopfensperger et al. (2013) European Commission (2015) |
| Dexmedetomidine oromucosal gel<br><br>(0.1mg/ml oromucosal gel, Sileo™) | Please refer to manufacturers data sheet for dosing instructions using syringe notches | Administer into the oral mucosa between cheek and gum, for doses >1.5ml, administer half dose inside each cheek | |
| | Can be given every 2 hours up to 5 times within consecutively | Maximum concentration 0.6 hours after administration, so administer approximately 30–40 minutes prior to event | |

# 24.10 References

Atkinson, T., Devaney, J., Girling, S. (2011). Animal Handling, Restraint and Transport. In: Cooper, B., Mullineaux, E., Turner, L. (ed.) *BSAVA Textbook of Veterinary Nursing,* 5th edn. British Small Animal Veterinary Association, Cheltenham, England, pp.228–255.

Beaver, B. (2009). *Canine Behavior – Insight and Answers,* 2nd edn, Saunders Elsevier, St Louis, Missouri.

Beesley, C.H. and Mills, D.S., (2010) Effect of kennel door design on vocalization in dogs. *Journal of Veterinary Behavior: Clinical Applications and Research*, 5, 60-61.

Bowen, J., Heath, S. (2005). *Behaviour Problems in Small Animals – Practical Advice for the Veterinary Team,* Elsevier Saunders, Philadelphia, Pennsylvania.

Crowell-Davis, S. L., Murray, T. (2006). *Veterinary Psychopharmacology*, Blackwell Publishing, Ames, Iowa.

Dodman, H., Shuster, L. (1998). *Psychopharmacology of Animal Behavior Disorders,* Blackwell Science, Malden, Massachusetts.

Donaldson, J. (1996). *The Culture Clash.* James and Kenneth Publishing, Berkeley, California.

Döring, D., Roscher, A., Scheipl, F., Kütchenhoff, J., Erhard, M. H. (2009). Fear-related behaviour of dogs in veterinary practice. *The Veterinary Journal.* 182, 38–43.

European Commission (2015). Summary of product characteristics, Sileo 0/1mg/ml oromucosal gel for dogs. Available at: http://ec.europa.eu/health/documents/community-register/2015/20150610131892/anx_131892_en.pdf (accessed 18 August 2015).

Farm Animal Welfare Council. (1992). Five freedoms. *Vet. Rec,* 131, 357.

Fatjó, J., Bowen, J. (2009). Medical and metabolic influences on behavioural disorders. In: Horwitz, D.F. and Mills, D.S. (eds.) *BSAVA Manual of Canine and Feline Behavioural Medicine,* 2nd edn. British Small Animal Veterinary Association, Cheltenham, England, pp.1–9.

Hedges, S. (2015). Advanced approaches to handling dogs in practice. *The Veterinary Nurse.* 6, 6.

Hedges, S. (2014). *Practical Canine Behaviour: For Veterinary Nurses and technicians.* CABI, Oxfordshire, England.

Herron, M. E., Shreyer, T. (2014). The pet-friendly veterinary practice: a guide for practitioners. *Veterinary Clinics of North America.* 44, 451–481.

Hopfensperger, M. J., Messenger, K. M., Papich, M. G., Sherman, B. L. (2013). The use of oral transmucosal detomidine hydrochloride gel to facilitate handling in dogs. *Journal of Veterinary Behaviour Clinical Applications and Research.* 8(3), 114–123.

Horwitz, D. F., Pike, A. L. (2014). Common sense behaviour modification: a guide for practitioners. *Veterinary Clinics of North America.* 44, 401–426.

Landsberg, G., Hunthausen, W., Ackerman, L. (2013). *Behaviour Problems of the Dog and Cat,* 3rd edn. Saunders Elsevier, Philadelphia, Pennsylvania.

Lukasik, V. M. (1999). Premedication and Sedation. In: Seymour, C. and Gleed, R. (eds.) *BSAVA Manual of Small Animal Anaesthesia and Analgesia.* British Small Animal Veterinary Association, Cheltenham, England, pp.71–85.

Martin, D., Campbell, L. M., Ritchie, M. R. (2015). Problem prevention. In: Shaw, J. K., Martin, D. (eds.) *Canine and Feline Behaviour for Veterinary Technicians and Nurses,* Wiley Blackwell, Ames, Iowa, pp.145–203.

Mills, D., Braem Dube, M., Zulch, H. (2013). *Stress and Pheromonatherapy in Small Animal Clinical Behaviour,* Wiley-Blackwell, Chichester, England.

Mills, D., Zulch, H. (2010). Appreciating the role of fear and anxiety in aggressive behaviour by dogs. *Royal Canin – Veterinary Focus.* 20 (1) 44–49.

Moffat, K. (2008). Addressing canine and feline aggression in the veterinary clinic. *Veterinary Clinics of North America.* 38, 983–1003.

NOAH (2015). National Office of Animal Health Compendium Datasheets A-Z. Available at: www.noahcompendium.co.uk/Compendium-datasheets_A-Z/Datasheets/-23637.html (accessed 18 August 2015).

Overall, K. (2013). *Manual of Clinical Behavioural Medicine for Dogs,* Elsevier, St Louis, Missouri.

6

Oxford Dictionaries (2015). Definition of 'restraint'. Available at: www.oxforddictionaries.com/definition/english/restraint (accessed 19 September 2015).

Palestrini, C. (2009). Treating a fear of the veterinary clinic using desensitization and counter-conditioning. In: Horwitz, D.F., Mills, D. S. (eds.) *BSAVA Manual of Canine and Feline Behavioural Medicine,* 2nd edn. British Small Animal Veterinary Association, Cheltenham, England, p.312.

Pines, M.K. (2010). Restraint. In: Mills, D., Marchant-Forde, J. N., McGreevy, P. D., Morton, D. B., Nicol, C. J., Phillips, C. J. C., Sandoe, P., Swaisgood, R.R. (eds.) *The Encyclopedia of Applied Animal Behaviour and Welfare,* CAB International, Oxfordshire, England, pp.526–527.

Pinson, D. (1997). Myocardial necrosis and sudden death after an episode of aggressive behaviour in a dog. *Journal of the American Veterinary Medical Association.* 211(11), 1371–1372.

Quandt, J. (2013). Analgesia, anesthesia, and chemical restraint in the emergent small animal patient. *Veterinary Clinics of North America.* 43, 941–953.

Ramsey, I. (2014). *BSAVA Small Animal Formulary,* 8th edn. British Small Animal Veterinary Association, Gloucester, England.

RCVS (2014). *RCVS Day One Competences.* Available at: https://www.rcvs.org.uk/document-library/day-one-competences/ (accessed 20 August 2015).

RCVS (2015). *The RCVS Code of Professional Conduct for Veterinary Surgeons.* Available at: www.rcvs.org.uk/advice-and-guidance/code-of-professional-conduct-for-veterinary-surgeons/pdf/ (accessed 19 August 2015).

Rooney, N., Gaines, S., Hiby, E. (2009). A practitioner's guide to working dog welfare. *Journal of Veterinary Behavior: Clinical Applications and Research,* 4(3), 127–134.

Shepherd, K. (2009). Behavioural medicine as an integral part of veterinary practice. In: Horwitz, D. F., Mills, D. S. (eds.) *BSAVA Manual of Canine and Feline Behavioural Medicine,* 2nd edn. British Small Animal Veterinary Association, Cheltenham, England, pp.10–23.

Sinclair, M. (2003). A review of the physiological effects of $\alpha_2$-agonists related to the clinical use of medetomidine in small animal practice. *The Canadian Veterinary Journal,* 44(11), 885–897.

Stanford, T. L. (1982). Behavior of dogs entering a veterinary clinic. *Applied Animal Ethology.* 7, 271–279.

Yin, S. (2009). *Low Stress Handling, Restraint and Behaviour Modification of Dogs and Cats.* Cattledog Publishing, Davis, California.

Yin, S. (2013). Reducing stress and managing fear aggression in veterinary clinics. In: Landsberg, G., Hunthausen, W., Ackerman, L. (eds.) *Behaviour Problems of the Dog and Cat,* 3rd edn. Saunders Elsevier, Philadelphia, Pennsylvania, pp.367–375.

Zulch, H., Mills, D. (2012). *Life Skills for Puppies: Laying the Foundations for a Loving, Lasting Relationship.* Veloce Publishing Ltd, Dorchester, England.

# CHAPTER 25

# Best Advice to a Dog Owner Whose Dog has Bitten Someone

## *Esther Schalke*

## 25.1 Introduction

In the case of a biting incident, the stress for the dog owner is at first great. In addition to the fear that one's dog might bite someone again, there is the personal disappointment that your dog bit someone at all. The most important consideration in this situation is: safety first. The dog owner must do everything possible to avoid or prevent a situation in which his or her dog could hurt someone again. The dog should not be able to learn through repeated incidents that aggressive behaviour is an effective or desirable strategy in a conflict situation. Each time a dog is allowed to show aggressive behaviour there is the risk that the dog will more readily show aggression again, even in less tense situations. A further stress for the dog owner is to encounter other dog owners in the street who often give well-meaning pieces of advice. It is generally best to ignore this advice, and not try to put others' tips into practice. If an owner is given advice that is unsuitable for his or her dog, they are responsible for the consequences and it can also put them in personal danger.

## 25.2 How can conflict situations be avoided?

The correct immediate approach depends on a number of factors: who the dog directs the aggression at; how badly those involved have been injured; and to what extent the dog owner can avoid the situation.

However, the following advice applies to all situations: <u>do not try to physically dominate your dog</u>. In the past, dog owners were advised to physically assert their authority over their dog – but this advice is in all cases inadvisable.

- If an owner tries to hit the dog he or she will put themselves in serious danger of being bitten.
- The dog may also learn that aggression is an acceptable way of resolving a conflict, which might encourage it to choose this response in future.

- Any conflict can lead to the owner sustaining serious injuries. Remember: dog bites can be very painful! If an owner does not know how his or her body reacts under pain, they can be frighteningly helpless in such a situation. It is therefore negligent for an owner to put their dog and themself in this situation. If you have ever confronted a dog that weighs about 30kg that really wants to bite you, then you will know how foolish it would be to physically provoke it, but the same applies even to smaller dogs.
- From the dog's point of view, there is also a good reason to refrain from physical confrontation. If fear is the emotion underlying the aggressive behaviour, this gives the dog a good reason to be afraid of its owner. This is not a good basis for a harmonious relationship or successful behaviour therapy.

Measures for avoiding critical situations can be divided roughly into those that require training and those that do not.

## 25.3  Measures without training

For these measures it is important to differentiate between whether the dog is threatening a stranger or a family member. If a family member is involved, an important question to ask is: how much stress is the dog owner exposed to? If the owner fears his or her own dog and the trust in their relationship has broken down, then other steps must be introduced. When the owner feels confident in his or her ability to implement change, then the problem is much more easily solved. In principle there are always at least three possible choices:

- The first is euthanasia, which should be considered in very serious cases.
- The second is a change of owner, which is a decision that is often also not easy to make. Sometimes it is simply the combination of dog and owner that does not fit. For many dog owners this decision will feel like a personal failure, but it is one that offers both the dog and the dog owner a second chance.
- The third is to seek professional guidance to solve the problem.
- There may also be a fourth, temporary choice. Most dog owners become closely attached to their dog but it can nevertheless cause great stress if the dog bites and seriously hurts a family member. In such a situation it can help for the dog to spend a period of time in a dedicated dog shelter so that everyone is given time to reflect and think calmly about the situation. Some behaviour therapists, for example, offer to look after the dog for a period of time and during this period also give the dog necessary training.

It is much easier to avoid critical situations that risk an aggressive episode if it is an unfamiliar individual that is the focus of the behaviour. Places and times can be chosen for walks where it is possible to avoid problem situations. It may be possible to drive to places where other people and dogs can be avoided. For a period of time it is also possible to let the dog run only in the garden at home or to take it for very short walks. These are not permanent solutions, since a lack of physical and mental activity can also make the problem worse or even be the cause of the problem. But, as initial measures, these can make life much easier.

If the dog is already being taken to a training school or a sports ground, then interrupting this training routine for the time being until specialist advice is received is often a good idea. Some aggression issues can be due to training techniques. Incorrect training does not always mean that too much hardness or antipathy was used to teach the dogs; we have worked with some dogs that had been trained with incorrectly executed impulse control methods that resulted in them biting their owners.

One of the most common triggers for aggressive dog behaviour in the domestic setting is a confrontation over resources. Dogs that are very possessive force one to keep the house tidy. All things that a dog finds interesting and would like to have must be hidden away, to avoid the risk of conflict. Situations in which the dog possesses a resource that needs to be repossessed can become confrontational. In our training with dogs, we introduce this measure before anything else. The dog's environment must be an area in which access to resources can be controlled. With highly dangerous dogs this place could be restricted to a kennel in the garden. With dogs that are clearly less of a problem it is enough to keep them temporarily in an area separated from the rest of the house, using baby gates or latchable doors. In a smaller residence, if it is not possible to devote a whole area to the dog, a fenced corner space is sufficient, perhaps using a child's playpen or similar. If the dog is only to be kept away from certain areas that are used frequently, for example a sofa or a spatial bottleneck where people walk, a trailing leash (houseline) may be sufficient. The leash allows the owner to get the dog out of the way without needing to touch it or getting too close to it. The leash for indoors must be thin and have no loops or knots that the dog can get tangled up in. It should also always be fastened to a harness or a broad collar; otherwise there is a risk of strangulation.

The assigned area must also be practical for dogs to confront strangers who enter the domestic space. If the dog shows aggressive behaviour towards visitors in the house, then it should never be taken to the door. The dog should be shut away securely in a kennel or a room before visitors arrive. If a visitor arrives unexpectedly, the leash can be used to pull the dog away from the door and take it to its assigned place. Sometimes it is difficult to change the old habits of a dog owner, but this is an important immediate measure. If the dog shows aggressive behaviour towards a family member, not only physical contact but also close interaction with that family member, and possibly others, should be avoided in order to prevent any potential conflict situations occurring; stroking, brushing, or cleaning the dog with a towel are habits that must be left for another time.

## 25.4 Measures that require training

Some measures need a small amount of training before one can use them in daily handling. These include containing the dog in a crate, and wearing a muzzle or head halter.

### 25.4.1 Crate training

- The crate serves the same purpose as a kennel or a demarcated area for the dog in the house. It means a safe space for the dog to be contained when required.
- However, the spatial limitation must not frustrate the dog. Rather, it must be a space in which the dog can relax. If dogs showing aggressive behaviour to strangers or children do so because of a feeling of insecurity, they need a place to retreat. It is a place that

they can withdraw to as soon as they do not feel like being elsewhere. The dogs must be taught that in this assigned place nothing will disturb them and everyone in the home as well as visitors must respect this. For this, training with food is particularly effective.

- Consuming food encourages relaxation. Therefore, food the dog can chew on for a while is particularly useful, such as commercially available chews, or special chewing toys that can also be used without problems in a limited space. There are also many ideas on the internet for homemade, food-filled toys.
- It is useful to ask the dog to wait a bit longer for the food each time it is in its space.

- In order for the dog to understand that this place offers security, it is very important for visitors and children not to stroke the dog in this place or sit with it, etc. For small children I strongly recommend setting up a child fence around this place. This will prevent children from sticking their fingers through the fence around the dog's crate.

### 25.4.2 Muzzle training

Good muzzle training is important for every dog. This is not just for safety reasons, since for many dogs it is better for them to wear a pretrained muzzle rather than an Elizabethan collar if they need to be prevented from gnawing at a bandage, wound or sutures. In some countries the law requires a dog to wear a muzzle on public modes of transport, in others dogs of a certain type must be muzzled in a public place. There are a number of different muzzles on the market (see Chapter 24). For exclusive use in a veterinary practice one can use a fabric muzzle. They are simple to store and easy to clean. There is, however, the major disadvantage that such a muzzle prevents a dog from panting easily. They are therefore unsuitable for everyday life. A good muzzle has the following qualities: it sits well on the snout, it allows the dog to pant and to drink, and it reliably prevents the dog from biting. In principle, basket muzzles, whatever they are made of, have the above characteristics, but different types do have different properties:

*Plastic muzzles*
**Advantages:** the dog can drink and pant, and the muzzle is easy to clean.
**Disadvantages:** they are very hard at the contact points beneath the eye and the chin, where they should be stitched with soft material. Many plastic items are not stable and potentially break easily. They are thus a potential safety risk.

*Metal muzzles*
**Advantages:** the dog can drink and pant, and the muzzle is easy to clean, very stable and secure.
**Disadvantages:** also hard at the contact points, therefore stitching is likewise necessary. If the dog pushes someone with the muzzle they can be bruised because of the hardness of the material.

*Leather muzzles*
**Advantages:** the dog can drink and pant, and they are often pleasantly soft.
**Disadvantages:** they remain damp for a long time, which can cause skin infections if the muzzle is always on, and the material is harder to clean.

Whichever muzzle is used, it must sit well on the dog's snout:

- It should be sufficiently wide so that the dog can pant properly and drink
- It should also sit well on the nose, without slipping into the eyes
- Some muzzles are marketed as being made for particular breeds of dog. Our experience is that these muzzles are often made too small for the indicated breed
- A forehead strap, stops the dog from pulling off the muzzle using its paws, and so is essential.

The dog must be trained to wear a muzzle – a process that can be made easier with the help of tasty food. See text box 25.1, also University of Lincoln Life Skills for Puppies: Muzzle training video: www.lifeskillsforpuppies.co.uk/muzzlevideo

The first few steps are nearly always the most difficult regardless of how well the dog has been trained beforehand. Later on, your dog may find the muzzle irritating when it first tries to sniff at something and its nose cannot reach the desired spot. Then it will try to pull it off. It is important to prevent this from happening and continue walking briskly

**Text box 25.1 Muzzle training your dog**

1. As a first step, place a tidbit such as liver sausage directly into the lower part of the muzzle. Hold the muzzle in such a way that the dog places its head into it to lick the treat that is placed there.
2. While it eats the food, stroke your dog on its forehead and neck behind the ears.
3. Repeat every time you put the muzzle on.
4. Remove the muzzle before the dog pulls his/her head back.
5. Once this exercise has been repeated many times and the dog is completely relaxed with the procedure, then you can start to work on doing up the muzzle. Fasten the straps loosely enough that they can easily be pulled free over the ears and later fasten the strap of the muzzle over the head. If the dog is not comfortable being touched, then this may need to be worked on separately but it might be that you can use a helper to calm it by holding and stroking it gently during the process. That way, your hands are out of the way and not in danger of being bitten.
6. If the dog now looks at the muzzle with an expectant expression and finds contact with it pleasant, then you may continue with the following step. Fasten the straps loosely enough that they can easily be pulled free over the ears. Put some more food into the muzzle, wait for the dog to put its nose in there to get the food and then with a stroking movement pull the strap over its head. If the dog accepts the muzzle without any problem, then you have overcome the biggest hurdle.
7. You can now stretch out the time the dog is wearing the muzzle. Distract the dog with some small exercises during this time. If all goes well and the dog has an expectant expression when you get out the muzzle, then you can move on to the last step.
8. Put the muzzle on the dog and take it for a short walk.

and distract the dog. After a while the dog will get accustomed to the muzzle and wear it without any problems.

### 25.4.3 Head halter

The head halter is a very useful article that makes walking with a dog liable to show aggressive behaviour much easier. With the aid of a head halter, the dog can be safely kept in line with a leash and away from troublesome situations. It also enables the owner to control the dog's line of sight. For these reasons it makes life much easier for the owner of an aggressive dog. When a dog wants to threaten or attack something it will first stare at the target and then tense. After that it will move towards the target and may charge at it. With a head halter, the owner can gently but firmly guide the dog's head in the direction wanted, e.g. away from a troublesome stimulus and towards the owner. It also prevents the dog from sighting and staring down a target, and possibly showing aggression. There is only a small chance of the dog threatening a person or another dog if it does not have eye contact with that person or dog. As with the muzzle, the dog must be gradually accustomed to wearing a head halter.

The process follows a similar process to the one used for fitting and acclimatising a muzzle. The final step in the process, however, is for the dog to learn to turn away as soon as the leash tightens even slightly. For this, it is important to reward the dog in training each time it turns its head towards the owner. Even if the owner causes the dog to mechanically turn away, it is important to give it a reward. If the dog is walked with a head halter, the other end of the leash should be fixed to the collar. If the dog should try to pull away from the head harness, this can be prevented with the help of the leash, which is fastened to the collar. A short leash should always be used so the dog is always close by. With a head harness, the leash should never be jerked because of the risk of injuring the dog, and in the case of a dog with a neck problem a muzzle is preferable to a head halter.

## 25.5 Summary

All the measures mentioned here should be understood as initial safety precautions. They are not final solutions. If a dog shows aggressive behaviour, specialist advice should be sought from a suitably qualified professional who uses appropriate methods not designed to intimidate the dog. Owners should be discouraged from trying to diagnose the problem themselves. It is difficult not to do this with your own dog: but owners should not underestimate the problem. Even if the dog has not yet bitten anyone but is only threatening to do so, advice for this threatening behaviour is warranted. The sooner the problem is dealt with, the sooner it will be that the owner does not have to worry about the dog endangering itself and others, which is good for everyone's well-being.

## 25.6 Useful resources

Association of Pet Behaviour Counsellors Advice Sheet – Preparing your dog for a muzzle or head collar
American College of Veterinary Behaviorists, www.dacvb.org
www.apbc.org.uk/system/files/private/advice_sheet_8_preparing_your_dog_for_a_muzzle_or_
  headcollar.pdf

APBC video. Teaching a dog to be happy wearing a head collar, https://www.youtube.com/watch?v=fcCTvEkSS_4

Association of Pet Behaviour Counsellors, www.apbc.org.uk

Certified Clinical Animal Behaviourist Accreditation Scheme, www.asab.org/ccab

European College of Animal Welfare and Behavioural Medicine, www.ecawbm.com

University of Lincoln Life Skills for Puppies: Muzzle training video: www.lifeskillsforpuppies.co.uk/muzzlevideo

# CHAPTER 26

# Behavioural First Aid – Aggressive Behaviours

## *Lynn Hewison and Graham Turton*

## 26.1 Introduction

The first thing to remember is that aggressive behaviours form part of a dog's normal behavioural repertoire and therefore need to be seen as a form of communication (see Chapter 2). The way aggressive behaviours are used and to what degree may vary with the context and individual:

- Dogs usually use aggressive behaviours when they are not comfortable in a situation. Often it is to increase distance between the dog and the other individual/s.
- The dog's motivation in using aggressive behaviours could be to get the person approaching to move further away from it, or it could be to stop the person coming any closer.

Some dogs will not choose to move themselves away from a situation (even if they appear to have the option to do so). There are many different reasons for why this may be, e.g. because they have some form of occult pain (Barcelos et al., 2015):

- If a dog is using aggressive behaviour in a situation, it is vital to pay attention to them and act in a way to avoid or defuse the situation to minimise the risk of injury. Backing down is not a sign of weakness; it could potentially defuse a situation and reduce the risk of a bite.

## 26.2 Common areas of conflict

The scenarios described below are examples of situations where we as humans may want one outcome from a situation and the dog may want another. The reasons behind why the dog may be expressing these behaviours are not discussed here but it must be understood that long-term management of the situation is essential to help reduce the risk of injury. It is also important that the dog learns to communicate with others effectively. If an individual can recognise the more subtle signs of his or her dog being uncomfortable in a situation (such as turning body or head away, staring), it reduces the need for it to use more overt signs (growling, barking, snapping).

1. If you are growled at:

   • Do not move any closer or in any direction that the dog may perceive as towards it.
   • Stop where you are, do not stare at the dog and very slowly move away and out of the room if necessary.
   • Do not go into the room if the dog is there and has growled at you. Go out of the room and after a short period of time, call it to another area.
   • Stop petting and move your hands away slowly. At this time, avoid eye contact and any quick movements.

2. Conflict over getting the dog to move, e.g. off furniture:

   • If you do not have a reliable hand signal to move your dog, avoid conflict by calling it away and then reward it.
   • Do not physically move it in any way.
   • If the dog will not come when called, then use some treats or a toy and toss them away from where the dog is to encourage it move. This luring technique can be used in the short term until hand and verbal cues have been trained effectively.

To prevent this sort of problem the dog needs to learn that being in an alternative location, such as on a bed on the floor, is the best place to be. This place needs to be rewarding, so while the dog is there, a chew or stuffed toy can be provided (as long as the dog is not possessively aggressive over items). It may be necessary to block access to areas by closing doors, using baby gates, etc. to prevent access, in the interim.

It is possible for dogs to learn sequences of behaviour, referred to as behaviour chains. If an owner always calls his or her dog off the furniture and then rewards it, there is a risk of it learning an undesired behaviour chain; going on to the furniture in order to be called off to get a reward. This is why it is important to provide comfortable alternative places to the furniture and to not allow the dog the opportunity to get into a situation that will lead to conflict.

3. Stolen items:

If your dog has hold of something he should not have and you do not have a reliable drop cue for him to release it, the following can be used to manage the situation until he is taught a reliable drop cue:

• Do not be tempted to go and get the item from the dog's mouth as this will not encourage him to willingly give things up in future.
• Entice to swap the item for a piece of food or a toy.

- Do not chase your dog around after the item as this is unlikely to encourage him to drop it.
- Maximise safety at all times by closing doors or stair gates between your dog and the item.

If the dog is likely to keep hold of the item and use aggressive behaviours:

- Let the dog make the decision to leave the item.
- Before any aggressive behaviour, pretend you are not interested in the item and, without making a big fuss, go and find another activity to do that the dog will be interested in. This can be in a different room or the same room if large enough for you to be a good distance away from the item. Most dogs are too nosy to resist coming to see what is happening in another room.
- Ringing the doorbell is another good distraction technique (as long as it is not overused).

If the dog has dropped the item when it comes to you:

- Ask it to do something it already knows how to do, such as sit and reward it.
- Ask it to do a few more tricks and then drop a few treats on the floor to keep it occupied. Close the door to keep it in and to make it safe to go and retrieve the item.

If the dog has NOT dropped the item when it comes to you:

- Ask it to do something, such as sit but drop the reward on the floor.
- Slowly encourage it to move further and further away from the item by dropping the treats further away.
- Continue to do this and ask for occasional responses to cues until it is out of the room. Only then should you or someone else safely retrieve the item.
- Do not bend down to pick the item up until it is out of the room and it is safe to do so or it may learn to rush back to get the item.

4. Reducing the risk around children:

Children often behave less predictably than adults; moving and sounding differently. This can be difficult for dogs. Even dogs that have never shown any aggressive behaviour towards children may not be comfortable with all interactions or even being in the same room. If a dog has been unwell recently or perhaps is a bit sore, it might be less tolerant of interactions with others.

- The best strategy is to keep children and dogs separated from one another whether in the same or different rooms.
- Use physical barriers such as closed doors or stair gates between them if necessary.
- Always actively supervise interactions between any child and a dog. Do not be a few steps away.

- Provide your dog with somewhere comfortable where it will feel safe and secure, such as its bed.
- When in its place, there should always be a rule that nobody should disturb it or go and fuss it there. This way, it will have a place it feels safe and that it has access to at all times. This gives it control over the situation and the choice of where to be, which is important for its welfare.
- If a child cannot understand the rules for interaction then he or she must not be left without direct supervision around dogs.

## 26.3 There are usually warning signs before a bite! – see Chapter 2

If you can see your dog is not comfortable, try to establish what it is uncomfortable with and work to change the situation. In the shorter term this may mean removing your dog from the situation or at least moving it further away. In the longer term, it is important to teach the dog how to behave appropriately and get it used to situations it may need to encounter in the future. For example, if a dog does not like to be patted on its head and you can see it is turning its head away as someone leans over it with their hands outstretched, you can give the dog the space to be able to move away, you can call it away or you can ask the person to interact with it in a different way.

## 26.4 The use of house lines

House lines are long lightweight leads, often without handles, which are designed to be clipped to your dog's flat collar while in the house. At all times while wearing a house line, your dog should be supervised to ensure it does not become injured by the house line becoming trapped under or around anything. Similarly, care needs to be taken if you have multiple dogs or there are children in the house due to risk of injury from entanglement or the house line being used inappropriately to tug the dog.

House lines can be useful in preventing your dog from practising unwanted behaviours. They give you more control to prevent situations from occurring by giving you the opportunity to gently stop it from progressing further, encourage it away and reward it for a more appropriate behaviour. If your dog often steals items, the house line can be used to prevent it from accessing something that is not safe for it to have or could cause conflict between you and the animal. House lines can also be useful when you need to manage your dog in situations where getting closer to it may increase the risk of it using aggressive behaviour as the house line allows you to guide it from a distance away.

## 26.5 Basic principles for managing and handling aggressive dogs in kennels/shelters

Many dogs that enter a shelter/kennels can show aggressive behaviour. For more general information on handling and restraint of aggressive dogs in the short term, see Chapter 24. However looking after an aggressive dog in kennels for a long period adds further challenges as the dog cannot be left to its own devices until it settles; it must be fed, provided with fresh water and cleaned at least.

Effort should be made to avoid any confrontation with the dog unless necessary, for the safety of the worker and also to protect the welfare of the dog and avoid making the situation worse. As far as possible, only one person (or realistically two) should be assigned to work that dog section for the foreseeable future; constant new people will undermine the trust of the dog. These handlers must be calm and confident with dogs, able to move slowly and in a non-threatening manner, and read subtle dog body language (see Chapter 2). To counter-condition the dog to the presence of people near the kennel, food rewards should be tossed in at intervals from a safe and non-threatening distance.

If the dog must be physically handled extensively, use sedation (see Chapter 24), and the quickest and least stressful physical handling method in order to administer the sedation. This may require the use of a catch pole/long arm/grasper by an expert.

One of the highest risk areas for bites is working with a new arrival. Imagine you have a dog that has just come into the kennels and is looking nervous or even trying to bite you. You need to somehow move it safely from one kennel to another or to an outside run.

- One option may be to use a long arm/grasper/catch pole to move the dog but this can be both stressful for both the dog and the kennel staff. Also, some dogs react badly to it and making friends with the dog afterwards becomes a lot harder, especially if the dog is already nervous.
- If a hatch system to let the dog through into a separate run is not available, the dog should be located in an area where the immediate surroundings can be sectioned off, but some sort of windows allow the dog to be observed from a distance or from behind a barrier. Then it is possible to leave the dog to move itself from one dirty kennel to another clean one, via the intermediate area, by leaving a fresh tasty bowl of food in the back of the new kennel as a lure. Once the dog has been observed to enter the kennel fully, the section can be entered and the new kennel door shut behind it.
- When the dog begins to offer approaches confidently, the kennel door can be opened slightly and a loose slip leash slowly threaded over the head of the dog. If the handler is not feeling confident enough to move with the dog at this point, a second handler can thread a second slip lead over the head and provide a second control point in case the dog lunges to bite.
- Dogs often become aggressive at the point that you try to take their leash off to put them in the kennel. It is often possible to get the dog on a lead but you cannot remove the lead safely without provoking an attempted bite. One option is to use a slip lead with a clip lead attached to the large ring on the slip lead. By holding both leads it is possible to slip it over the dog's head, pulling tight on the slip lead to pull the lead tight (see Figure 26.1a) then it is possible to gently walk the dog to an outdoor run or kennel. Once at the destination, let go of the slip lead and gently pull on the clip lead and this will loosen the slip lead, allowing it to be pulled over the dog's head safely (see Figure 26.1b). This method reduces danger to the handler trying to remove the lead or putting the dog at a strangle risk by leaving a lead around a dog's neck while it is unsupervised. In most cases after a few days of doing this the dog becomes more happy

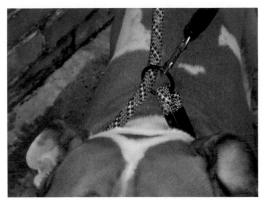 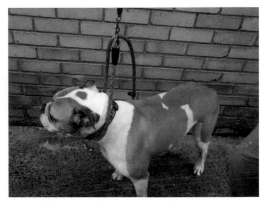

**Figure 26.1a–b The two-lead method (slip and clip lead) for moving highly aggressive dogs**.
Although the pictures demonstrate on a friendly dog so that the method can be seen more clearly,
please in practice remove the leads from behind an almost closed door/gate.

to have a lead put on it and trust can be built up where you no longer have to do this
and can revert back to a normal collar and lead.

Given sufficient space, time and encouragement using rewards, most dogs show significant signs of improvement within a few days, or at most a couple of weeks. If this does
not occur, or a previously friendly dog starts showing aggressive behaviour, the situation
is more serious and requires strategic handling and a decision about the likely future of the
dog and whether rehabilitation is realistic given the resources available (see Chapter 28).

## 26.6 Breaking up a dog fight

Many people get bitten when trying to break up a fight between two dogs. There is no
'best' way to break up a dog fight but the following are suggestions that have been known
to work, although are not without risk of injury. They work best if there are two people
available, to quickly move each dog away from the other once the fight has been interrupted,
otherwise one of the dogs will often restart the fight:

- A loud yell of 'Hey!' in a thundering voice can often startle the dogs enough from what
  they were doing to quickly move them apart. Other loud devices such as rape alarms
  or pet correctors can be carried and used in emergencies but should be directed away
  from the dog as to not cause injury.
- A blast from a hosepipe or emptying of a water bucket over the individuals can have
  the same startling effect.
- Manoeuvring the fight towards a doorway, and slowly closing a door, such as a kennel
  door, between the dogs' heads.
- Inserting an object such as a broom handle between the dogs to prise them apart.
- If nothing else is available, a protected leg inside a Wellington boot could also be used,
  but beware that a bite can still occur through these but will likely be less serious than

356 Handling the Aggressive Dog

if hands were used – never do this, as a savaged hand is no use to you or your dog and the fight will continue.

- Do not pick the dog up as this exposes the vulnerable undercarriage (and yourself) to further and more serious injury. It is more sensible to attempt to gain control of the primary aggressor and let the other dog run away to safety.

If you have successfully separated two dogs after a fight, keep them separate (away from dogs and people) for at least thirty minutes or until they are both calm and relaxed. Any intervention earlier could result in further injury due to still elevated arousal levels. If the fight is between dogs from the same household, professional advice is recommended before considering reintroductions.

## 26.7 Reference

Barcelos, A. M., Mills, D. S., Zulch, H. (2015). *Clinical indicators of occult musculoskeletal pain in aggressive dogs.* Veterinary Record, 176 (18). p.465.

# Section 7
# Managing Future Risk

Section 7 provides practical examples of how we can reduce the risk of dog bites. Although we must acknowledge the many gaps in our scientific understanding of this issue, that does not mean we can, or should, do nothing to reduce the risks associated with dogs. Dog ownership, like many other pastimes, carries with it an inevitable element of risk. We must make best use of the available information and combine this with best professional practice to manage the problem as far as is reasonably practical. This does not mean we eliminate risk, rather we wish to minimise the risk to a socially and societally acceptable level.

In the first of these chapters, Barbara Schöning shows how the careful evaluation of dogs, combined with high standards of professional practice, can produce meaningful assessment with good prognostic value in real-life situations. While it is important to have a degree of standardisation, this is neither a simple nor prescriptive process. Each test, like each dog, is individual, and procedures need to be adapted to the circumstances according to the goal. This theme is very much repeated in the next chapter by Katharina Woytalewicz and Susanne David, who work in the rehabilitation of dogs that have bitten. In their chapter they draw on their experience to show how a solid understanding of scientific principles can be used to behaviourally rehabilitate many of these cases so they pose no greater risk than any other dog. With three case studies they illustrate the practical application of the principles and process they outline in the first half of their chapter. The effective application of science allows this process to be implemented in a compassionate, humane and reasonable way, which respects the needs of all involved. Clearly, as our knowledge and understanding of dog bites grow, so will the ability to more efficiently manage the risk associated with cases brought to our attention.

7

# CHAPTER 27

# Risk Assessment Principles and Procedures in Use

## *Barbara Schöning*

## 27.1 Introduction

Risk assessment means describing the form and level of danger to an individual's well-being that might be related to a given situation. 'Danger' is defined as the probability of suffering, liability to suffer, injury or loss of life, and 'dangerous' means 'with any likelihood of causing danger to somebody or something'. The term 'danger' thus consists of the probability that someone or something (a subject of protection) might come into contact with something hazardous and includes in parallel the probability of the severity of significant consequences.

One could say that risk assessment is occurring throughout life. Every day any ordinary person will compare costs and benefits related to simple actions in simple situations: when to cross a street; when to put the foot on the brake; when/if at all to eat sweets or drink alcohol; or what freedom to allow children when roaming the internet.

Risk assessment procedures are implemented in many fields of everyday human life. For example, in technical areas such as engineering, e.g. measuring how many cars at one time can safely cross a bridge without causing it to collapse. In public health management, risk assessment also comprises the attempts to reduce the probability that an endemic situation involving an infectious disease might become an epidemic one (WHO, 2012, Chapter 22).

In this chapter, the reasons why dogs are risk-assessed is considered, before the processes involved in making this assessment in practice. The reader is referred to Chapter 9 for a more detailed scientific critique of the tests available; in addition, Chapter 18 describes the specific assessment of dogs for the courts, while the current chapter focuses on the practical execution of the processes involved in risk assessment for whatever purpose. In the absence of an agreed and demonstrably valid approach, the following paragraphs are necessarily an opinion on how risk assessment can be performed effectively; to answer the questions 'who, where, when, why and how' it should be done in the most reliable and valid manner, while acknowledging relevant limitations.

## 27.2 Why dogs are risk-assessed

This chapter deals with risk assessment related to dogs. Dogs can inflict injury and pain by biting third parties, be it humans, other dogs or other animals. One solution to these problems would be to get rid of all dogs; problem solved! But this is not the solution we are aiming at, as dogs play an important role in human society, psychologically and as physical aids to our work, e.g. as working or assistance dogs. Dogs can bring great pleasure to their owners, and dog ownership is associated with a wide range of physical and psycho-social benefits (e.g. Bradshaw, 2011; Friedmann, 1995). Furthermore, it is argued that enshrined in the laws of many societies is the idea that dogs should have the right to a 'good life'; the right to well-being and fulfilment of needs, in accordance with current knowledge and practice relating to welfare science.

A dog showing problem behaviour, e.g. biting people, not only has to be considered from a risk assessment perspective, but also as a welfare problem. Welfare compromising breeding and/or living conditions are thought to lead to the development of many behaviour problems – i.e. behaviour considered problematic. This may lead to further welfare compromising conditions (restriction, punishment). Therefore a vicious circle can be quickly established, leading to physically and/or mentally injured, or dead, subjects.

Therefore the risk assessment of a dog must not only try to identify the actual risk a dog poses for others but also (indirectly) to itself and in parallel look at how risk can be decreased, i.e. which measures (management and training procedures) will be necessary to secure a 'good' life for the individual dog and any possible victim.

However, it is a sad truth that sometimes, even after thorough professional scientific investigation, the only rational solution for an individual dog is euthanasia. Of the 1,200 or so dogs assessed by the author in the last fifteen years, about half of them had bitten another dog or a human being, and half belonged to a designated breed listed in a German state's Dangerous Dogs Legislation (DDA), without a history of a previous biting incident. Roughly 1% of these dogs were put to sleep due to a poor prognosis after the assessment, and from the 'surviving' dogs, in only seven cases was a later report received of a significant incident.[1] In these cases, the investigation following the second incident made clear that the owner/keeper had played a major role as a risk factor (Schöning, in preparation).

The European Society of Veterinary Clinical Ethology (ESVCE) states in its position statement on risk assessment (De Meester et al., 2011) that it is unreasonable to expect all risk to be eliminated, but that measures should be taken to protect potential victims as far as 'reasonably practicable'. This concept is often only half-heartily enshrined in the dangerous dog laws of many countries, when they focus on how to deal with dogs that have bitten or otherwise caused injury to third parties. Sadly, in almost all cases where I have had to assess a dog after it had bitten, there was a clear antecedent leading to the final bite bringing the dog to assessment (Schöning, in preparation). Thus I believe that if the dog and its living

---

1  As registers are kept in most German communities on dogs that have been assessed following an incident or because they belong to a DDA-listed breed, any incident that police or regulatory authorities become aware of will be fed back to the particular assessor.

conditions were assessed earlier, or if the owners of the dog had greater awareness of any problems arising, many of these incidents could have been avoided.

Scientifically sound and effective prevention of biting incidents (see Section Three and eight of this book) does not appear to be high on the agenda of authorities, or at least in Germany. Many German states focus on expertise in new dog owners and in owners of a 'dangerous' dog. Apart from the state of Lower Saxony, all German states have certain breeds listed in their DDA, whom they label 'irrefutably dangerous'; meaning these states depend on phenotype of the dog for risk assessment, despite a lack of strong evidence to this effect (Chapter 10). Dogs from these breeds are subjected to measures ranging from being neutered, permanently running muzzled and leashed, or even being euthanised on the spot without having bitten anybody and without been assessed. A similar problem exists in the UK (Chapter 18).

Despite the legislative measures imposed on dogs and owners before and after a biting incident, the number of incidents in Germany over the last ten years does not appear to have reduced (summarised by Schöning, 2014). Risk assessment procedures are currently implemented in all German statutes, however, different German states have not only implemented different procedures but also have different criteria as to who is allowed to undertake risk assessment, and what scientific and/or practical expertise this person requires. Other countries are likely to have similar issues, as internationally so far no 'standard procedure of risk assessment' exists.

## 27.3 General principles of risk assessment

At the heart of any risk evaluation is the assumption that the future can be influenced; making risk assessment is not only important for preventing disaster but also for how best to deal with the disaster when it presents (Renn and Klimke, 1998; WHO, 2012).

Effective risk assessment comprises the following points:

1. Categorisation of possible hazard/danger.
2. Probability of occurrence including any specific scientific background and, in the case of public health, regarding existing control measures.
3. Identification of any additional relevant factors.
4. Implementation of exact criteria, how risk assessment shall be conducted.
5. Any measures for further risk reduction including continuous monitoring of the situation at risk and communication with subjects at risk.

In the case of, 'How many cars at one time can safely cross a bridge without causing it to collapse?':

1. Would mean a list of hazards that might happen, ranging from potholes to a complete collapse that can result in anything from damaged cars to dead drivers.
2. Would comprise data on things like the materials used in construction, ageing processes etc. that affect the likelihood of the hazard.
. Would deal with additional factors, e.g. 'How well did the engineers of the bridge do their maths,' i.e. the track record of the company.

4.  Would detail the exact and possibly most standardised processes to be used for measuring, and inspection that will be conducted.
5.  Would potentially include any necessary repair and maintenance activities.

According to Rodricks (1994), the practice of risk assessment is characterised by the use of specific default assumptions to allow the completion of assessment even when data and knowledge are incomplete.

## 27.4 General principles of risk assessment and how they apply to dogs

When we look at dogs, working through these stages is somewhat more difficult, with probably more incomplete data, as we have to deal with living beings at both ends of the leash. In addition the first four stages will have fluid borders and will not be distinguished so clearly from each other as they would during the evaluation of inanimate objects or problems regarding physics or chemistry (Text box 27.1).

The categorisation of possible hazard/danger may still be relatively easy. Dogs have teeth and they can use them to inflict wounds on another subject or even kill it. Dogs can jump up at individuals, causing damage due to subjects falling over, falling from a bicycle, etc. Dogs can startle, shock or frighten subjects due to 'normal dog behaviour' such as reactive barking, jumping up at visitors, or running after individuals, and the frightened subject might fall over and injure him or herself.

Here all potential risk factors for dog bites, have to be regarded. However, risk assessment always has to deal with an individual dog in individual situations; there are no known 'major or general factors' that make any dog bearing these factors (e.g. being of a certain breed or height) definitely more dangerous than other dogs, when it comes to the likelihood of a bite. Although we know that there are certain elements or factors that require deeper consideration in one individual dog but not the other, we have to evaluate the impact of all possible factors for each individual dog to answer the questions, 'How serious is this situation? How high is the risk that someone might get bitten or might get bitten again?' The possible factors influencing the *probability of occurrence* have been discussed in Chapter 10. They serve to assist in answering the questions of 'where, when, how and why harm might arise' together with a standardised practical evaluation of the dog in question.

### Box 27.1 How to define dangerousness of a dog, a personal example

If 'dangerousness' of a dog was measured by the financial strain on the public health system, my parents in the 1970s had a very dangerous Labrador: he quietly sneaked into the kitchen once and lay down behind granny. She did not notice, stumbled over the dog and needed an artificial hip as a result. Any dog of any size, sex or age can theoretically cause danger for a third party – which leads to the questions on probability of occurrence and identification of any additional relevant factors that will help in addressing 'who is in danger, where, when, why and how might harm arise'.

To answer the question, 'How serious is the situation? How high is the risk that someone might get bitten or might get bitten again?' a standardised protocol should be followed, and acknowledged. Standardised procedures have the advantage that they potentially allow comparison between assessors, dogs and outcomes as much as possible when dealing with living systems. Table 27.1 gives an overview of a logical pathway for conducting a dog risk assessment.

**Table 27.1** Logical procedure and points for consideration in a risk assessment.

| Timeline | What to do / ask for / look for |
|---|---|
| Before seeing the dog | a) Why has the dog to be assessed?<br>  – Is it because it belongs to a certain breed?<br>  – Or because it is going to work as assistance dog or visiting dog in a home for the elderly?<br>  – Is it because there has been an incident? (see also Chapter 18)<br>This information is necessary for the assessor to decide from the beginning, how the risk assessment shall be conducted. Quite a lot of 'service-dog-organisations' for example have their own testing procedures. Knowing about these procedures and putting them in a scientific context will help to decide on further steps.<br>b) Information about any biting incident:<br>  – Where, when, what were the exact circumstances.<br>  – Especially: what did victim, dog, and owner do before, during and after the incident.<br>  – Information about wounds and medical intervention on the victim's side.<br>c) Information about the dog:<br>  – Age, sex, breed, weight, height.<br>  – Past history (where did it come from, how was it socialised and trained, etc.). Try to get as much information as possible to get an overview what you might expect in regard to social competence, fear, frustration and stress tolerance levels, communication skills, bite inhibition, obedience, and former experience with analogous situations to the current biting incident.<br>  – Living conditions at the time around the incident.<br>  – Living conditions after the incident.<br>  – Health status and history.<br>d) Information about the owner, caretaker and/or person who was looking after the dog when the incident occurred. Especially important is any information to assist evaluation of the theoretical and practical expertise in dog behaviour and training of these persons.<br>e) Information about the victim(s): age, sex, health status (when allowed). Anything that might help to evaluate the victim's theoretical and practical expertise with dogs and his/her attitude towards dogs. |
| On seeing the dog | There is no such thing as a 'valid risk assessment' without seeing the dog. 'Seeing the dog' has to be thoroughly planned in advance, utilising the information gained prior to the inspection of the animal. It should happen in as standardised a way as possible and it should include testing for bite inhibition and learning capability. Also a health check as far as reasonably possible should be conducted on the day or a few days before assessing the dog (in the case of dogs that have bitten, a health check as close to this time as possible is also essential). The following aspects should be regarded:<br>a) The ideal location:<br>  – Fenced, plain and non-slippery ground.<br>  – Big enough to allow dog and people some space from others if necessary; big enough to allow the dog to be walked a few metres.<br>  – Have a catch-pole to attach to the dog if necessary; have easy to reach and open doors; access to a water supply. |

On seeing the dog
- Quiet (without too much noise and onlookers around).
- Some space to where the dog can retreat, if it wishes.

b) People
- At least three people are needed: the assessor, the cameraperson, and one person to hold/look after the dog.
- Everything that is done to/with the dog in assessment should be video-taped. The cameraperson needs to move freely to get the best view on the dog and the test-situation. A useful quality for a cameraperson is therefore some experience with dogs, allowing them to find the best distance and angle. The cameraperson should not be too near as this might irritate the dog and confound the assessment.
- At least one helper is necessary to lead the dog on leash. The assessor cannot do this as it would be inconsistent with his/her special role. Sometimes two persons holding the dog might be necessary. Tying the dog to a pole throughout the test should only be a last resort.

c) Dogs
- Many aggression tests involve dog–dog situations and at least when there has been a dog–dog incident, one has to see the dog in a dog–dog encounter.
- Encounters have to be done as thoroughly as possible so that no one gets injured (see below).
- It is important to find 'the right dog' as a stooge dog, in the case of inter-dog incidents. A fearful dog with reduced social competence will not make a good stooge; its welfare will be compromised and there is a risk that the dog will later develop a dog–dog problem itself.

d) Security
- The dog to be assessed has to wear a broad, flat, well-fitting collar or harness (no prong or choke collars). Head halters should only be used when the dog is trained to wear one and there is no other way of control.
- A muzzle can be an important security device but reduces the information to be gained. When not well trained it will be a largely uncontrollable stressor; it obscures the full view on the face; it still leaves the question 'would the dog really have bitten in this special test situation and if yes, how intensely?'.
- A leash should be strong and not too long, allowing the dog a radius of about 1.20m.
- Having the dog on two leashes, held by two people is preferable to tying the dog to a pole. In this case one leash should be attached to a collar and the other to a harness.
- Thick clothes and/or special protective clothes designed for dog sports prevent injury during close contact with the dog. Kevlar sleeves especially help in answering questions on bite-inhibition and 'whether the dog really would have bitten'.

e) Welfare of people and dogs must be taken seriously. Pauses in assessment shall be done when stress levels become or look like becoming unacceptably high, and they shall be as long as individually necessary. In encounter situations start from a longer distance and decrease distance in small increments. Nobody involved in the test should be overstrained and the dog to be assessed should not have a bigger problem with people or other dogs after the test than before as a result of its assessment. Plan some time after the assessment to modify any negative experiences, e.g. via desensitisation, if necessary.

After seeing the dog
Plan enough time to evaluate the video and write the statement. A thorough assessment requires that, first, all observations are taken (which behaviours did the dog show in which situations) and, after this, any interpretation and judgement takes place. Give a clear assessment, following your observation and interpretation, about what risk the dog poses for others and what should be done with the dog. Give advice for handling, training and placement of the dog when applicable, and mention possible no-gos in these fields. Also give advice for any monitoring or retesting.
In summary: try to give the most reliable and valid possible prognosis for the future.

## 27.5 Behavioural testing of the dog

Aggression tests have already been discussed in Chapter 9 and it is clear that there is no such thing as 'the perfect test' for risk assessment. Nevertheless, those tests in use, which have undergone some validation, are a useful tool. They tend to be similar in regard to test situations and stressors inflicted upon the dog. In principle these tests follow the same process: observing the dog in individual and standardised test situations, with a prognosis for the future offered.

- Usually dogs are confronted in as standardised a manner as possible with a certain number of 'everyday situations' (e.g. a running person, a dog passing by, a person kicking a ball or shouting at the dog, etc.).
- In addition test situations involve the dog being deliberately threatened.

A good example for a standardised test is the test in use in the Lower Saxony Statutes,[2] which has been widely assessed and shown to be of sufficient validity and reliability for answering the essential questions concerning risk discussed in this chapter – but only when the assessment is done by a knowledgeable and theoretically and practically qualified person (Mittmann, 2002; Böttjer, 2003; Bruns, 2003; Schöning, 2006; Paroz et al., 2008; Schöning, in preparation).

- When a dog has to be assessed after an incident, such a standardised test should be complemented with situations mimicking the incident. This will not be possible in every case, for safety reasons and/or because of lack of knowledge about the incident. Mimicking the incident as such should never be done purposefully to the extent that the dog really bites; this is not necessary for gaining a complete picture of the dog (see below). When mimicking the incident, this has to be done very carefully so as to not overstrain any individual involved and to not launch 'unwanted' learning processes in the dog.

The goal of testing in risk assessment is not to deliberately trigger the dog to the extent that it bites. Any dog will bite if individually strained to a certain extent. In the test, the individual test situations do not need to permanently and regularly undercut individual distances and/or tolerance levels for biting. This could be necessary for an individual dog with an individual biting history in a special test situation, but should not be done as a general rule throughout the test. In particular in dog–dog test situations all necessary information can be gained even when the dogs have no close contact (Schöning, 2006).

As stated in Table 27.1, at least three persons are necessary for testing a dog – but more than three is advantageous.

- It can be helpful for the assessor to stay back and just watch certain scenes with another person approaching the dog.

---

2 http://www.ml.niedersachsen.de/portal/live.php?navigation_id=1613&article_id=4745&_psmand=7

• Dogs can learn to focus on one individual person and just show aggressive behaviour towards this person whereas another person can freely manipulate the dog in a test situation. Such observations help in completing the overall picture of the dog.

Caution has to be advised with regard to children. Even when children were involved in the incident, they should not be recruited for help in a risk assessment test. Adults have to try to mimic 'childish behaviour'; where necessary, large puppets can be used, and relevant sound can be provided easily via smartphone. Some dogs will discriminate these 'fake children' from the real situation, and again it needs the experienced assessor to compensate for this: it is important to look at the overall picture the dog gives in the test and how its behaviour in a test situation with fake children fits into this.

## 27.6 Generating a prognosis

Opponents of 'aggression tests' used as part of risk assessment often criticise that the number of 'everyday situations' is infinite, and therefore tests consisting of thirty or thirty-five test situations never can give a reliable picture of a dog's temperament and aggressiveness, never mind a prognosis for the future. However, such critics misunderstand what is really examined in such tests.

Standardised tests comprise certain standardised situations, as mentioned above. These situations have in common that the dog is purposefully confronted with specific stressors (*triggers of conflict*). The assessor looks for when the individual tolerance levels for fear, frustration and stress of the dog are reached in each test situation, and which behaviour strategies are then displayed (*conflict solving strategies*). This then is the information, combined with the information on the dog's past and the incident as such, that allows a risk prognosis for the future. Low tolerance levels for stress, fear and frustration, a moderate bite inhibition and a quick escalation into biting in test situations pose a bigger risk for the future, than for example, low tolerance levels combined with fairly good bite inhibition and a tendency to back away when under stress or fear. In both cases the reason why the dog had to be assessed could have been the same: for example the dog, while being walked by the owner, bit a child passing by on a skateboard. Together with the information gained when following the protocol in Table 27.1, such test results allow an expert statement to be issued that protects potential victims in the future as far as 'reasonably practicable'. In parallel, sensible measures can be put on the dog without compromising its welfare more than is reasonably necessary (Döring et al., 2008). In the above example this could be the leash as a first management tool for certain areas, education for the owner on dog behaviour and risk prevention, and special training for alternative behaviour strategies when the dog again feels anxious, frustrated or distressed.

Any expert has to work as objectively and reliably as possible to find the adequate balance between reduction of risk and compromised welfare. Therefore an expert statement should also include information on training measures, tentative information on where to place the individual dog and whether and when a second assessment should be done.

## 27.7  Conclusion

In conclusion, *prognosis for the future can never be a Yes/No statement*. However, with state-of-the-art knowledge and practical experience it is possible to provide a prognosis of acceptable validity to decide what measures would be required to allow the dog to live a good life while ensuring the risk for third parties is at a very acceptable level for society. It is for this reason it is also essential to show in the expert statement how the conclusion has been reached so that the recommendations can be revised if necessary in light of new information.

## 27.8  References

Böttjer, A. (2003). Untersuchung des Verhaltens von fünf Hunderassen und einem Hundetypus im innerartlichen Kontakt des Wesenstests nach den Richtlinien der Niedersächsischen Gefahrtier-Verordnung vom 05.07.2000. Dissertation. Tierärztliche Hochschule Hannover.

Bradshaw, J. (2011). In defence of dogs: why dogs need our understanding. Allen Lane Penguin Books, London, UK.

Bruns, S. (2003). Fünf Hunderassen und ein Hundetypus im Wesenstest nach der Niedersächsischen Gefahrtier-Verordnung vom 05.07.2000: Faktoren, die beißende von nicht-beißenden Hunden unterscheiden. Dissertation. Tierärztliche Hochschule Hannover.

De Meester, R., Mills, D. S., De Keuster, T., Schöning, B., Muser Leyvraz, A., Da Graca Pereira, G., Gaultier, E., Corridan, C. (2011). ESVCE position paper on risk assessment. Journal of Veterinary Behavior 6, 248–249.

Döring, D., Mittmann, A., Schneider, B. M., Erhard, M. H. (2008). Genereller Leinenzwang für Hunde – ein Tierschutzproblem? Deutsches Tierärzteblatt 12/2008, 1606–1613.

Friedmann, E. (1995). The role of pets in enhancing human well-being: physiological effects. In: The Waltham Book of Human-Animal Interaction: Benefits and responsibilities of pet ownership; Ed. Robinson, I. Pergamon Press; 33–54.

Mittmann, A. (2002). Untersuchung des Verhaltens von 5 Hunderassen und einem Hundetypus im Wesenstest nach den Richtlinien der Niedersächsischen Gefahrtierverordnung vom 05.07.2000. Dissertation, Tierärztliche Hochschule Hannover.

Paroz, G., Gebhardt-Henrich, S. G., Steiger, A. (2008). Reliability and validity of behaviour tests in Hovawart dogs. Applied Animal Behaviour Science 115, 67–81.

Renn, O., Klimke, A. (1998). Risikoevaluierung von Katastrophen. Diskussionspapier (98–304) der Arbeitsgruppe Internationale Politik; Wissenschaftszentrum Berlin für Sozialforschung. URL: http://bibliothek.wz-berlin.de/pdf/1998/p98-304.pdf

Rodricks, J. V. (1994). Risk assessment, the environment and public health. Environmental Health Perspectives 102, 258–264.

Schöning, B. (2006). Evaluation and prediction of agonistic behaviour in the domestic dog. PhD-Thesis, University of Bristol.

Schöning, B. (2014). Gefährliche Hunde? Hundegesetze in Deutschland – Übersicht und Bestandsaufnahme nach 1½ Jahrzehnten. Unser Rassehund 5/2014, 32–38.

WHO (2012). Rapid risk assessment of acute public health events. World Health Organisation, WHO/HSE/GAR/ARO/2012.1.

7

CHAPTER 28

# Case study of Methods for the Rehabilitation of Dogs that have Bitten: Shelter Dogs

## *Susanne David and Katharina Woytalewicz*

## 28.1 Introduction

Rehabilitation means the co-ordinated application of medical, social, pedagogical and technical means influencing the physical and mental condition of an individual, helping the individual to reach the greatest possible improvement in living conditions (WHO Technical Report 668/1981). For example, the rehabilitation of people with disabilities is a process aimed at enabling them to reach and maintain their optimal physical, sensory, intellectual, psychological and social functional levels.

In this chapter rehabilitation is used in the sense of enabling a dog with a biting history to live 'a good life' and in parallel not putting any third party into danger. A 'good life' means that welfare is not unnecessarily compromised and the individual's typical needs are altogether fulfilled.

There is a vast literature on how to deal and work with dogs with problematic aggressive behaviour and it is beyond the scope of this chapter to review these. It should also be noted that each dog is an individual and the use of generic training programmes can be dangerous. Nonetheless, some recommendations such as physically 'dominating the dog', punishing it for aggressive behaviour, etc., are not only ill-advised for efficacy and risk management reasons, but also contra-indicated for achieving the attempted goal: protecting the welfare of the dog and any possible victims (Hiby et al., 2004). Such recommendations will not be discussed further here, but the reader is referred to the further reading at the end of the chapter for details of the principles to be used, following an appropriate risk assessment. This chapter aims to illustrate the process, application and potential of sensible, dog-friendly and scientifically grounded recommendations, means and methods that can help reduce the risk from dogs that have a biting history. It does not seek to cover comprehensively all known methods for working with dogs with an aggressive behaviour problem. Instead it presents some idea about what can be achieved in a public shelter setting, where dogs with a biting history (quite often seized dogs) are housed.

## 28.2  The dog in the shelter environment

Dealing with a biting dog in a shelter has advantages and disadvantages:

*   One advantage is the very structured living conditions in comparison to a privately owned dog, which can allow for more effective training around a daily routine.
*   A disadvantage is the potential lack of 'close social attachment figures'. Although we assign each dog a 'principal care-taker' (and dogs have been shown to form attachment bonds very quickly, see e.g. Horn et al., 2012 and 2013), this is not the same as living close together with an owner.
*   On the other hand, owners can worsen the problem behaviour due to their emotional involvement, and a non-compliant owner will very probably not stick stringently to a training plan.

Dogs that come to our shelter as a result of biting incidents, regardless of whether they have bitten humans or other dogs, usually have a history of aggressive escalation, leading to a final incident. Such dogs usually have learned 'biting' is a successful strategy for conflict resolution. They do not have alternative strategies for 'getting rid of a problem'. Such one-way strategies develop because humans were not able to (or were willing to) see and understand de-escalating behaviours in former conflict situations, or to accept threatening behaviour as a 'desire for distance' and act appropriately to achieve this. Consequently, the dogs have learned that subtle communication elements, that are less harmful, were not helpful for them to solve their individual problem. Thus they learned to not show them any longer and instead went for more overt forms of communication. The vicious circle then develops because humans usually respond even more physically with those dogs, with harsh manipulation or inflicting pain in an attempt to control the dog. For a certain period punishment and harsh manipulation may disguise a problem and feign a solution – until some day the dog can no longer be handled, the number of victims increases and/or wounds become severe.

## 28.3  The process

### 28.3.1  Setting realistic expectations and goals

It is essential to establish realistic expectations for the behaviour modification exercises at the outset. The goal cannot be 'zero aggression' or that the respective dog will never in its life bite again, unless the intervention is euthanasia, since we cannot know the future for sure. The goal for rehabilitation training should be to put the risk the dog poses for others at a level comparable to that of any ordinary dog regarded as 'friendly and non-aggressive' by the general public. The behaviour modification programme must, itself, have its own specific goals that can be measured, so that it can be shown they have been achieved. This needs to relate to the wider goal related to risk management and the resources available for achieving this. The following paragraphs outline our approach for reaching this goal, starting with the wish list for human resources and going through the principal approach used with three individual examples.

## 28.3.2 *Human resource prerequisites*

Human resources for successful rehabilitation training should have the following properties:

- The trainer must be able to see and understand the communication and social behaviour of dogs at large (Chapter 2) and must be able to act accordingly with the goal of de-escalating any conflict arising or reducing distress where necessary.
- The trainer must especially be able to see any warning signals and act accordingly (usually by retreating and not inflicting force upon the dog) to end such critical situations, or redirect the dog's behaviour into a more useful direction.
- The trainer needs the relevant motor skills to handle the dog and needs excellent timing and co-ordination, especially in relation to giving signals and reinforcement.
- The trainer and all others involved must know about useful management measures and be able to implement them; they should create effective training situations without putting others (humans, dogs or other species) at danger.

Looking through this list it becomes clear there are a lot of possible deficits for dogs living with their owners.

## 28.3.3 *Preliminary groundwork*

In the beginning we analyse the dog and the problem (see also Chapter 18). Often information from owners and, if involved, authorities is scarce and biased. Often owners try to trivialise the problem, whereas authorities may see it as more severe than it actually may be. We often have to read between the lines to get the 'real story' and try to get as much information as possible.

The dog gets an initial veterinary health check, is assigned to a principal care taker and is then kept in a single kennel for an initial period, which lasts about one to two weeks. During this time the principal caretaker (PCT) tries to carefully build up a relationship with the dog. In parallel, the PCT tries to learn as much as possible about the dog, its tolerance levels and which stimuli/situations might be critical, e.g. does the dog show an increasing display of distress when the PCT tries to put a leash on, or puts a hand towards the bowl or a toy. The goal of information gaining and training in this first period is that the PCT can handle the dog safely later on and will act as an attachment figure (source of safety and security) in the later training phase.

Social contact and any training in this first phase are built up very slowly and carefully, using positive reinforcement. The dog should build up a trustful relationship and learn that the PCT is a source of safety and security: friendly, reliable, dependable, and predictable. In this period the PCT also sets up a reward system, comprising primary reinforcers (mostly food) with a secondary reinforcer (clicker or words) for future training and, if necessary, trains the dog to wear a muzzle without distress.

## 28.3.4 *The learning goal*

The dog should learn that there are alternative behaviours to biting that can solve a conflict and improve its own situation. Long-term, the subjective benchmarks for interpreting a certain situation/stimulus as 'threatening' will rise as the emotional and motivational reaction of the dog towards these stimuli/situations changes. Which alternative behaviour is the best solution for which individual dog will be decided from the detailed information gained, and the way the dog reacts in training. This approach follows findings in human psychology where it has been shown that by focusing initially on the behaviour (changing reactions to a threatening stimulus) an emotional re-evaluation of formerly threatening stimuli can be brought about (Lowe and Ziemke, 2011; Bekko et al., 2014).

## 28.3.5 Behaviour modification procedures

In short, the dog is trained to show a spontaneous alternative behaviour that it can rely on in conflict situations, such as concentrating on its attachment figure or retreating from the conflict.

In general we work in small increments, rewarding wanted behaviour as much as possible on a regular basis. We use shaping processes and luring (Veeder et al., 2009; Fugazza and Miklosi, 2015) where necessary, in addition to desensitisation (Blackwell et al., 2013; Butler et al., 2011). As a prerequisite for this to be effective, management measures are implemented to reduce the possibility of incidents where the dog might feel it necessary to show aggressive behaviour. Here again lies an advantage in the well-designed shelter compared to the home environment.

To be able to train an alternative strategy quickly and effectively, we look for behaviours the individual dog can show easily and comfortably and which fit its motor abilities. Therefore the approach for each individual dog has to be different. In some dogs we choose to shape alternative behaviour from the beginning, in other dogs we first train a signal to expect the stressful stimulus and orient towards it, and then train the dog to show the alternative behaviour, following training of bite inhibition, and/or improved tolerance levels for frustration and inhibitory control, when necessary.

We start training this alternative behaviour in non-conflict situations, where the dog is relaxed and motivated. Then we carefully look to introduce more and more distractions, changing location, time, presence or absence of other individuals, introducing other trainers or dog walkers, etc. This may lead to the introduction of stressors that formerly elicited aggressive behaviour. When the dog can show the alternative behaviour reliably under 'heavy distractions', we start introducing explicitly the former aggression eliciting situations/stimuli and go through the process of generalisation again. When the dog finally gets adopted, the new owners receive a short analogous training session with the dog.

Ideally, training is done on a daily basis, but as one can see from the case studies, this is not possible in every case. Training may last weeks or even months, as the dog is the one to decide on the speed of training, as well as how and when challenges can be introduced. For some dogs it takes just four weeks to reliably learn an alternative coping strategy and for others it might take four months.

## 28.3.6 Reflections on outcomes

Despite the disadvantages of a shelter situation (presence of certain stressors and distractions, missing attachment figures such as an 'owner', etc.), the results of the last five years, since we implemented this approach on a regular basis, are promising. The dogs are very receptive to any positive social interaction and training with positive reinforcement. Even with just a few training sessions the dogs show a distinct improvement in behaviour; but it is important to have a friendly approach at all times and to reward any desirable behaviour the dog shows in its daily routine. This quickly helps to improve the communication between dog and PCT, improves the learning abilities of the dog in general and leaves it open for effective trial and error training.

In the last five years we have had approximately 300 dogs with a biting history brought to the shelter. When we measure 'success rate' as either 'the dog is adopted for good and is not noticeable or reported with any biting behaviour from adoption to today', or 'the dog is still living in the shelter (in a dog group) without biting behaviour reported', we have a success rate of 87% and 5% respectively (total success rate 92%). The 'unsuccessful 8%' comprise eight dogs that had to be euthanised and sixteen dogs that are still in the training process (e.g. introducing them into group housing).

## 28.4 Case studies

The following case studies provide three examples of the specific training undertaken with dogs with aggressive behaviour problems. They demonstrate the real world context and application of the principles described in the previous section.

### 28.4.1 Case 1 – Aggression towards a family member

P, a Pit Bull Terrier, neutered male, with no health problems; it came to the shelter when eleven months old. It had bitten the owner's brother in the flat of the owner and consequently was seized by the authorities. The circumstances of this incident could not be ascertained.

P was very active and impulsive, and in parallel easily became fearful. Its tolerance level for becoming frustrated was low and it showed poor bite inhibition.

Problematic were the animal's very quick focus and reactions towards quickly moving humans, dogs and objects such as cars: jumping at and running after them with heavy biting.

In the kennels it showed generally high levels of arousal, which further increased when walked on a leash in the shelter grounds and/or seeing any of the aforementioned objects and subjects.

The dog's problem behaviour differed on the basis of the distance between it and the subject. When there was quite a distance, focus and hunting-style behaviour (quick, focused running up to the individual and trying to grip with the teeth) dominated. When the subjects were close, and/or appeared suddenly, and/or had uncommon, potentially 'dangerous' features (e.g. the person staggering), it showed a massive aggressive response and offensive behaviour, which could then only be controlled via leash management. In the first second of such situations, a short glimpse of fear could be seen, but this was only detectable by very experienced people. Videoing of cases in such circumstances can provide an important educational resource. The dog's PCT could manage it after one week of training without any problems and could control it in situations of high arousal via the leash.

After six months of training (one to two times per week, each session lasting roughly sixty minutes, Table 28.1) P became more and more interested in friendly contact with people and showed a wide range of positive social behaviours (sniffing, rubbing against people, deferential display (e.g. submissive behaviour, avoidance behaviour, etc.). Its obedience level had increased and it could be walked well on the leash, although large distractions had a negative effect on its obedience. Moving humans and objects such as cars, etc. were not of much interest. Certain humans, especially when they were close, still elicited fear. P had learned for such situations to move its head away from the fear–eliciting element towards the handler and keep a focus on the PCT. Hunting-style behaviour was still shown towards cats and small wild animals such as squirrels.

P stayed one year in the shelter, before being adopted by a couple (with no children). For two years it has lived now as a family dog in its new home without any problematic behaviour. The new owners were educated in further training methods for P and proceeded intensively with this for some months.

**Table 28.1** behaviour modification goals and methods used in Case 1.

| | |
|---|---|
| Goal | In subjective threatening situations P shall spontaneously and without signal turn, focus towards the handler and hold the focus.<br>In situations where possible huntable objects appear, P shall react the same.<br>In the long run P will stay emotionally stable in the above mentioned encounters |
| General approach | P was taught an 'attention signal' (Step #1 below) to start the shaping and desensitisation process in contact with the trigger of unwanted behaviour.<br>In parallel the PCT did sessions to enhance P's tolerance of frustration, better bite inhibition and impulse control. |
| Step #1 | Signal 'P' (= name of the dog) was presented in a non-distracting environment.<br>The moment P reacted with moving his head towards the PCT, he got rewarded with a treat as primary reinforcer and verbal secondary reinforcer.<br>Sessions comprised 4–5 repetitions; around 10 such sessions per training class were done with essential pauses in between.<br>When P reacted 5/5 successfully over a few sessions, the next step started. |
| Step #2 | Changes in environment and distraction, but not both at one time.<br>It was ensured that P's tolerance levels for stress, frustration and fear were never exceeded. |
| Step #3 | Training especially with the stimuli formerly eliciting unwanted behaviour present (humans, other dogs) in a desensitisation setting. Training should lead to the attention signal not being necessary any longer but that P starts to look spontaneously at the handler, when the stimuli appeared.<br>When the stimulus elicited fear, a second reward was the stimulus moving away. |

## Text box 28.1 Teaching frustration tolerance and impulse control (Susanne David and Barbara Schöning)

Training is aimed at teaching the dog to calmly tolerate an increasingly delayed reward.

A simple method would be to feed the dog three treats and keep the fourth between the fingers, until the dog sits or lies down or moves backwards (free shaping process; the trainer has to decide for the individual dog which behaviour might be appropriate). Most dogs will actively try to lick or grab the treat from the fingers for some time before they 'try something else for problem solution'.

Such training has to be done carefully so as to not overstrain the dog's tolerance level at that time, which could trigger aggressive behaviour.

Some dogs need to be fixed on a leash in the beginning, to maintain a safe distance (Schöning, 2003).

7

**Text box 28.2  Teaching bite inhibition (Susanne David and Barbara Schöning)**

Increasing bite inhibition can be achieved while playing with the dog.

The moment the dog uses its teeth firmly to grab an object or the arm of the person playing (suitably protected), this person stands still and turns slightly away from the dog.

The moment the dog lets loose, the play starts again.

Ultimately the dog learns that grabbing has to be done carefully when it wants the play to continue.

Again, with dogs with an aggression problem this has to be done very carefully and should only start when the dog has bonded to its PCT and the PCT can handle and manipulate the dog without any problems. Safety clothing (e.g. Kevlar sleeves) can be necessary for protection.

**Text box 28.3  Teaching the identity of a safety place (Susanne David and Barbara Schöning)**

The dog should learn there is a certain place (box, bed, etc.) to where it can retreat and, while being there, nothing negative will happen.

The dog is first lured into/on to this place with treats and gets rewarded with the secondary reinforcer as soon as it gets into/on to the place (the primary reinforcer in this case is the treat used for luring). While going there, the dog hears a signal 'bed', etc.

After some repetitions the dog can actively be sent to the place with the signal 'bed' and immediately when there, gets rewarded with primary and secondary reinforcer.

Consequently, the dog is sent from greater distance to the bed and, when it can be sent from several metres away, the reward gets more and more delayed so that the dog will have to stay there for a longer time before it gets the reward. Many dogs will then sit down or even lay down, and those that do not can be helped with a down command.

The goal is that the dog goes there and lays down just using the signal 'bed'. Additionally, the owners reward the dog many times in between should the dog go to this place on its own.

It is important to advise owners to never send the dog there as a form of punishment.

For dogs that should go there on their own in conflict situations, the training has to be done increasingly in the (carefully designed) presence of stressful stimuli, until the stimulus as such becomes a signal for the dog to go to this place.

**Text Box 28.4 Teaching a signal for 'you are going to be touched'**
**(Susanne David and Barbara Schöning)**

Knowing what will happen can have a calming effect and decrease stress as the animal can prepare for what is going to happen. When the dog knows a signal with the information 'a hand is touching you and this will be neither dangerous nor painful', it can be handled much more easily.

Training starts with touching the dog for a short moment on a spot the dog is already happy with, accompanying this action with a signal, e.g. 'hand'.

When the hand is moved away the dog gets rewarded with a primary and secondary reinforcer (the dog has to have stayed relaxed for this moment).

Consequently, and in small increments, the hand slowly moves onwards over the body and subsequently the touches will last longer and the pressure of the hand can be increased.

It is important that the dog always has to stay calm and relaxed during the training process.

## 28.4.2 Case 2 – Aggression towards strangers

S, a Dalmatian–Collie mix, male-neutered, with no health problems; came into the shelter when four years of age. His owner surrendered him because he could no longer care for him due to health conditions. S was a very insecure and fearful dog, showing defensive behaviour (fixing on humans, growling, and attacking with biting) any time someone approached within 3-4m distance, or wanted to touch or manipulate him. When S had the possibility in such confrontations it preferred to move away, but nevertheless it bit two times in its first few days at the shelter.

Communication displays were altogether subtle and discrete, and showed not much variation, in addition he was not very capable of reading communication signals from other dogs. When coming to the shelter, S showed no interest in interaction with dogs and thus no conflict situations arose. It simply moved away, keeping its distance. Interaction was always initiated by the other dog, and never by S.

S stayed two years at the shelter and in this period it learned, besides alternative behaviour strategies for conflict situations, differential and graded communication and especially facial expressions (Table 28.2).

S went then to a couple running a riding stable and into a group of three other dogs. It has been living there for two years at the time of writing and no problems have been reported. S gets on well with humans and other dogs, is friendly and socially open minded, and largely ignores those individuals or moves away from those who comprise something threatening for it. To further reduce incidents, S has a 'safety kennel' which is open at all times, to where it can retreat when something overbearing happens, e.g. a party on the premises.

Training focused on interaction with humans, but this also improved S's behaviour when interacting with dogs.

**Table 28.2** Behaviour modification goals and methods used in Case 2.

| | |
|---|---|
| Goal | In subjectively threatening situations outside the home territory (i.e. outside the stables grounds or house) S shall spontaneously and without signal turn and focus towards the owner and hold the focus. |
| | In threatening situations inside the territory S shall react the same or, when owners are not present, or the situation is subjectively too dangerous, retreat to his safe place. |
| | S shall tolerate any manipulation by the owners and stay relaxed and friendly. |
| | Long-term, S shall gain emotional stability in the above mentioned situations. |
| General approach | Building a trustful relationship between S and PCT was the first big barrier. |
| | S was taught an 'attention signal' to start the shaping and desensitisation process in contact with the trigger for the unwanted behaviour. |
| | In parallel the PCT did sessions to enhance tolerance of frustration, better bite inhibition and impulse control and (in the very beginning) trained S to wear a muzzle. |
| Step #1 | Signal 'S' (= name of the dog) was presented in a non-distracting environment. |
| | The moment S reacted with moving its head towards PCT, it got rewarded (verbal secondary reinforcer and treat). |
| | Sessions comprised 4–5 repetitions; around 10 such sessions per training class were done with any necessary pauses in between. |
| | When S reacted 5/5 successfully over a few sessions, the next step started. |
| | In parallel a signal for 'you are going to be touched' was trained for close interaction with the PCT. |
| Step #2 | Introducing strange people, at different distances and increasingly showing 'unusual behaviours' (jogging, arm lifting, etc.). |
| | It was ensured that S's tolerance levels for stress, frustration and fear were never exceeded. |
| | Introducing strange people below a certain distance was another big hurdle. |
| | The rewarding process was varied: sometimes the PCT gave the complete reward, sometimes PCT only gave the reward signal and then the stranger threw a treat (primary reinforcer) and moved away (functional reward). |
| Step #3 | S is off-leash when the stranger approaches. |
| | Situations and reward system further vary (including a 'keep going' signal) so that the focus on PCT has to be kept for longer period etc., until in the end strangers can approach directly and S can take the treat from their hands. |
| | 'Keep going' signal was developed by reliably presenting the secondary reinforcer every time the dog showed the wanted behaviour, but the primary reinforcer was on average only given about every fifth time in conjunction with the secondary reinforcer. |

### 28.4.3  Case 3 – Aggression towards other dogs and the owner

D, an American Bulldog, male, with no health problems; came into the shelter when nine months of age. The owner had bought it three months previously via a newspaper advertisement and was already the fourth owner.

From the beginning P showed aggressive behaviour towards humans and dogs when walked on the leash. It reacted aggressively towards the owner, e.g. when she wanted to push it from the sofa. As D weighed 40kg, the (small female) owner had problems in walking it safely on leash. She went to a dog trainer who focused on 'training via dominance'. This and the fact that the owner quickly lost her way in stressful situations and had very bad timing, worsened the behaviour quickly. D bit two dogs and severely injured them and the neighbours complaints increased, before D was finally brought into the shelter.

**Table 28.3** Behaviour modification goals and methods used in Case 3.

| | |
|---|---|
| Goal | Other dogs shall elicit pleasure, positive excitement and a friendly approach and interaction. |
| | In subjective threatening situations with other dogs D shall spontaneously and without signal turn to focus towards the handler and hold the focus. |
| | In the long term D will stay emotionally stable in dog–dog encounters. |
| General approach | Classical counter-conditioning was used for baseline training to quickly change D's emotional reaction to other dogs. |
| | When later D was interacting freely with other dogs, free-shaping (rewarding of wanted behaviour) was also implemented. |
| | D was taught an 'attention signal' to be used as a 'security exit', should this be necessary in training. |
| | In parallel the PCT did sessions to enhance tolerance levels to frustration, increase bite inhibition and impulse control. |
| | Management was crucial here and it was important that D did not meet other dogs outside of training as far as possible. |
| Step #1 | Attention signal was trained as already described for the other two cases. Counter-conditioning was done as follows: with D on the leash, he waited in a secure and quiet environment while another dog was presented at a distance which allowed D to still take treats from the PCT's hand. |
| | The stooge dog was presented only for the time the PCT needed to feed D 20 treats one by one. Then the stooge dog moved out of sight. This was repeated several times with pauses in between, and for as long as D reacted to the presence of the stooge dog with positive anticipation and spontaneously looked in the direction of the PCT. |
| | When D reacted 5/5 successfully over a few sessions, the next steps started. |
| Step #2 | The distance between D and the stooge dog was gradually decreased and new locations and dogs (not combined) were successively introduced. |
| Step #3 | When D did not show aggressive behaviour even in very close contact with other dogs on the leash, the same was done gradually for off-leash situations, using a muzzle and long training leashes for the transition (weaned off these later on). |
| | Training started with walking him with a very socially competent bitch, slowly introducing more bitches and then gradually neutered and finally intact male dogs. |

Initially the training was focused on stress-free handling, obedience for controlling D when outside, and desensitisation and alternative coping strategies for interaction with people (Table 28.3). This was soon successful, but interactions with other dogs were still a problem. It still showed spontaneous aggressive behaviour with a quick escalation.

After six months of intensive daily training, D could live without any problems in a group of ten dogs (mixed breeds, mixed sexes). This allowed it to further improve its social competence tremendously and learn a wide variety of communication strategies. Altogether, D stayed three years in the shelter before it was adopted. It has lived with its new family for more than a year and has contact with other dogs on a regular basis.

Not all training against dog–dog aggression problems are this successful. In particular, when the history reveals a lot of traumatic experiences with dog–dog encounters, training can be problematic and long. However, from our experience it can be said that at least some improvement is possible in any case and this usually leads to safe management of the dog in public, allowing the dog a much better life than before.

## 28.5  Conclusion

Dogs displaying aggressive behaviour are not indelibly more dangerous than other dogs, and the labelling of individuals as such is not helpful. These three case studies describe successful approaches to rehabilitating dogs with a biting history. Although set in a shelter/kennel environment, the same principles for an owner working with an aggressive dog should be successful, and protocols similar, however they are more challenging to implement in this context.

## 28.6  References

Bekko, G. M., Franconeri, S. L., Ochsner, K. N., Chiao, J. Y. (2014). Attentional deployment is not necessary for successful emotion regulation via cognitive reappraisal or expressive suppression. Emotion 14, 504–512.

Blackwell, E., Bradshaw, J., Casey, R. (2013). Fear responses to noise in domestic dogs: Prevalence, risk factors and co-occurrence with other fear related behaviour. Appl. Anim. Behav. Sci. 145, 15–25.

Butler, R., Sargisson, R., Elliffe, D. (2011). The efficacy of systematic desensitization for treating separation-related problem behaviour of domestic dogs. Appl. Anim. Behav. Sci. 129, 136–145.

Fugazza, C., Miklosi, A. (2015). Social learning in dog training: The effectiveness of the Do as I do method compared to shaping/clicker training. Appl. Anim. Behav. Sci. 171, 146–151.

Hiby, E. F., Rooney, N. J., Bradshaw, J. W. S. (2004). Dog training methods: their use, Effectiveness and interaction with behaviour and welfare. Animal Welfare, 13 (1): 63–69.

Horn, L., Virányi, Z., Miklósi, A., Huber, L., Range, F. (2012). Domestic dogs (*Canis familiaris*) flexibly adjust their human-directed behavior to the actions of their human partners in a problem situation. *Anim. Cogn.* 15, 57–71.

Horn, L., Huber, L., Range, F. (2013). The importance of the secure base effect for domestic dogs – evidence from a manipulative problem solving task. PLOS ONE 8, e65296.

Lowe, R., Ziemke, T. (2011). The feeling of action tendencies: on the emotional regulation of goal directed behaviour. Frontiers in Psychology 2, article 346.

Schöning, B. (2003). Lernverhalten, Frustration, Bedrohung. In: NMELF – Niedersächsisches Ministerium für den ländlichen Raum, Ernährung, Landwirtschaft und Verbraucherschutz (Hrsg.): Wesenstest für Hunde. 3. Aufl., Hannover, 20–21.

Veeder, C., Bloomsmith, M., McMillan, J., Perlman, J., Martin, A., (2009). Positive reinforcement training to enhance the voluntary movement of group-housed sooty mangabeys (Cercocebus atys atys). J. Am. Assoc. Lab. Anim. 48, 192–195.

## Recommended further reading for behaviour modification protocols

Bowen, J., Heath, S. (2005). Behaviour problems in small animals. Elsevier Saunders, London.

Horwitz, D., Mills, D. (2009). BSAVA Manual of canine and feline behavioural medicine. BSAVA Gloucester, UK.

Landsberg, G., Hunthausen, W., Ackermann, L. (2013). Handbook of behavior problems of the dog and cat. Elsevier Saunders, Toronto.

Overall, K. (2013). Manual of clinical behavioral medicine for cats and dogs. Elsevier Mosby, St Louis.

# Section 8
# Prevention

In section 8 the authors draw on what we know to critically appraise the wider options for dog bite prevention, in particular educational programmes regarding teaching signs that a dog is unhappy and may bite. In contrast, earlier chapters focused on prevention have considered the topic primarily in terms of an immediate practical perspective. In Chapter 29, Melissa Starling and Paul McGreevy provide a deep critique of the current dog bite prevention programmes and approaches. They find that, although such educational initiatives are designed with great intentions, evaluation of the effectiveness of such programmes is rare. They suggest that there needs to be greater recognition that resources may also need to be directed into dog-related legislation and the supply of pet dogs that have a low inclination to bite. Nonetheless, it is well-established that there is no group more vulnerable to dog bites and in need of effective prevention than children. In Chapter 30, Kerstin Meints describes the Blue Dog bite prevention programme for children and shows how evaluations of this intervention, alongside her other research, has contributed to knowledge about how children's developmental psychology underpins why they are frequently bitten and so often on the face. She calls for interdisciplinary collaboration for further data collection into the contexts of dog bite incidents and how education of children and parents may change their behaviour around pet dogs.

Another key to dog bite prevention is often claimed to be the wider societal promotion of 'responsible dog ownership'. In Chapter 31, Heath Keogh presents a case study of multi-agency working in the London Borough of Sutton. Although, as highlighted in Chapter 29, hard evidence of the effectiveness of this initiative in preventing dog bites, like so many others, is lacking, nonetheless, this scheme promoting 'responsible dog ownership' is well regarded and serves as a model on which we can potentially build proper evaluation tools. It may also provide a framework for other locations where the value of cross-agency collaboration surrounding reporting and managing dog-related issues is recognised.

In summary, despite many programmes and educational initiatives being designed to prevent dog bites, there is often a lack of evidence that they are truly effective in changing both dog and human behaviour. Nonetheless, we are now in a much stronger position to identify those with the most promising characteristics and prioritise these for assessment.

# CHAPTER 29

# Prevention of Dog Bites – Resources and their Value

## *Melissa Starling and Paul McGreevy*

## 29.1 Introduction

Dogs are social predators, semi-feral scavengers, living alongside humans, as both companions and family members. It does not, therefore, seem surprising that people are bitten regularly by dogs. Indeed, it is more surprising that serious dog bites are, comparatively speaking, so rare. For example, some breeds bite so rarely in a way that causes concern that they do not feature in dog bite statistics. Nonetheless, dogs have the capacity to do serious harm and even to kill humans. In some countries, where dogs are the main vector for human rabies infection, bites alone represent a significant threat to life. It is estimated that the annual frequency of dog bites to children is around twenty-two per 1,000 children, both in the USA (Kahn et al., 2004) and Belgium (Keuster et al., 2006). The cost of medical care for dog bite victims is a concern for governments, and there may also be significant psychological costs. One study reported more than half of children bitten by dogs showed signs of post-traumatic stress disorder (Keuster et al., 2006). Considering the potential for dog bites to be costly to humans and to governments, it is worth investing resources into their prevention. Parties most commonly willing to make this investment include local, state and federal governments, but also some health organisations, hospitals and dog advocacy groups.

There are several tactics employed to prevent dog bites to humans, many based on scientific research into who gets bitten, where, by which dogs, and why, which is covered elsewhere in this volume. Therefore this chapter will focus on education programmes to prevent dog bites and how successful they are, and finishes with possible future directions for dog bite prevention.

## 29.2 Dog bite prevention

Dog bites are widely held to be preventable (Dixon et al., 2012), although this is yet to be shown clearly and has been challenged elsewhere in this volume (see Chapter 4). Nonetheless, there are many education programmes and policies that aim at prevention. These can be divided into two broad strategies: education and legislation. This chapter will deal only with educational resources.

## 29.3 Education programmes

Education initiatives to reduce the prevalence of dog bites are typically aimed at groups most at risk. These are generally children, but also adults in jobs where risk of dog bites is high, such as the postal service. There are numerous dog bite prevention programmes run by local governments, private companies, and interest groups, and it is impossible to address them all here. Table 1 captures details on prevention programmes readily accessible to the English speaker and where details of the programme are available. This table was generated through internet searches using the terms: 'dog bite prevention', 'dog bite programme', 'dog safety' and 'dog education'. The key points of the programmes have been streamlined to reveal similarities and differences between them. Advice on dog bite prevention is also available on the websites of dog trainers, humane societies, animal shelters, local governments, hospitals and kennel clubs, with many of the same points as those outlined in Table 29.1.

**Table 29.1** A list of readily accessible dog bite prevention programmes, where they are in use, and their key features.

| Programme | Country | Key points |
|---|---|---|
| For Kids' Sake Canine Threat Assessment Guide (C-TAG) | USA (Texas) Australia (QLD) | Positive interactions between dogs and children. For those in animal-management industries. Identifying high-risk dogs before bites, with 'risk score' based on a scoring procedure that includes containment, aggressive behaviour, purpose of breed, and presence of stressors, among other factors. |
| Minnesota Veterinary Medical Association (MVMA) | USA | How to approach pet dogs safely. Safe and unsafe behaviour around dogs. Dog body language. Stand like a tree, or lie like a log, if a strange dog approaches. |
| Dog Buddies | Canada (Ottawa) Ottawa Humane Society/Ottawa Public Health | Know – ask before petting. Slow – move slowly around dogs. Freeze – be still and look away if a dog is scary. |
| Dogs 'n' Kids | Australia (Royal Children's Hospital) UK | Dog body language. Teaching children safe interactions with dogs. Identifying high-risk situations, such as dogs eating, sleeping, children playing. |
| American Veterinary Medical Association (AVMA) | USA, also adapted for children in several languages and distributed in World Animal Protection programmes | Emphasises parental supervision. Children not to approach strange dogs. Identifying high-risk situations. Stay still if approached by a dog. |
| Prevent-A-Bite | Australia | Ask owners before touching a dog. How to pat a dog safely. How to behave when approached by a strange dog. Identifying high-risk situations. |

| | | |
|---|---|---|
| Doggone Safe | Canada, USA, regional coordinators also in Australia, France, India, Italy, Ireland, Liberia, New Zealand, Spain, South Africa, UK | 'Be a tree', stand still, keep hands close to body and eyes down.<br>If a dog knocks you down, protect back of neck with arms and keep feet together.<br>Dog body language.<br>Also programme for adults working around dogs, which covers dog body language and risk assessment. |
| Blue Dog | Belgium, also in use in other countries. Interactive software | Dog body language.<br>Choosing a dog for the family.<br>Responsible dog ownership. |
| Prevent A Bite | Germany, Switzerland | Children are taught how to approach or behave around dogs in different contexts, then practise alone, then practise with a person in a dog suit and finally with real dogs. |
| Keeping our children safe around dogs (booklet) | New Zealand, University of Waikato | Be a statue or a stone (still, limbs close to body).<br>Adult supervision.<br>Teach children dog body language.<br>Appropriate and inappropriate behaviour around dogs.<br>Responsible dog ownership. |
| Delta Dogsafe™ | Australia | Dog body language.<br>How to safely approach a dog.<br>Uses life-sized dog toy. |
| Blue Cross for Pets – Be Safe With Dogs | UK | Dog body language.<br>How to safely approach a dog.<br>House rules.<br>How to behave when a dog threatens you. |
| The Dogs Trust – Learn With Dogs<br>Be Dog Smart | UK | Adult supervision.<br>Reasons dogs may bite.<br>Training the family dog.<br>Safe games children can play with dogs.<br>Behaviour children should not be allowed to engage in around dogs.<br>How to behave when a dog threatens you. |
| University of Tennessee College of Veterinary Medicine – Dog Bite Prevention in Children | USA | Emphasises that not all dogs are friendly.<br>How to behave when a dog threatens you.<br>How to safely approach a dog. |
| The Kennel Club – Safe and Sound | UK | Safe and unsafe behaviour around dogs.<br>Identifying high-risk situations.<br>How to behave if a dog approaches or knocks you down. |
| BARK – Be Aware, Responsible, and Kind | USA – The National Association for Humane and Environmental Education (NAHEE) | Teaches children dog body language.<br>Appropriate behaviour around dogs. |

## 29.4  Are education programmes effective?

Common advice from education programmes includes how and when to approach dogs, how to recognise dog body language that may signal fear, anxiety, uneasiness, conflict, or aggression, and how to keep safe when approached by a strange dog, as well as parental supervision at all times. The advice makes sense intuitively, but the efficacy of these programmes and recommendations is questionable, and surprisingly few studies have attempted to address this. The 'Blue Dog' programme is one that has been examined scientifically (see Chapter 30). It was developed in Belgium to teach children under seven years and their parents to recognise situations where dog bites may be triggered in the household (Meints and de Keuster, 2009). Children of the target age can transfer visualised lessons to real life, and it has been concluded that improved knowledge from the framework of the Blue Dog programme will translate to safer behaviour around dogs in the home (Meints and de Keuster, 2009). There is a precedent for this assumption, as a similar programme aimed at bicycle safety has reported significant increases in bicycle safety as measured by computer tests and correct helmet adjustment (McLaughlin and Glang, 2010). However, family dogs are not just objects – they are active, animate, social members of the family that may seek interactions.

The temptations that dogs can present to children may be more complex than is applicable to a simple safety assessment of images of unfamiliar dogs on a screen. It is difficult to test long-term effects of a programme on everyday behaviour around dogs, but a value assessment of any dog bite prevention programme should consider long-term efficacy. The researchers studying the Blue Dog programme concluded accurately that it can serve as a useful learning and awareness tool, but wondered whether it changed the way children behaved towards dogs or if it prevented dog bites. A second study found that children did retain improved basic knowledge of safe behaviour around dogs from the Blue Dog programme, but that this did not translate to adopting safer behaviour around dogs or being able to recall the lessons and apply them to a novel situation (Schwebel et al., 2012). Indeed, children who participated in the Blue Dog programme actually showed, for reasons unknown, a trend for more risky behaviour around a live dog (Schwebel et al., 2012).

An Australian study on a dog bite prevention programme called 'Prevent-A-Bite' aimed at increasing precautionary behaviour in children around dogs. It found that children of primary school age did show an increase in precautionary behaviour around dogs after participating in the programme (Chapman et al., 2000). It is not known if this increased precautionary behaviour persists in the long term (Chapman et al., 2000), or if it generalises unfamiliar dogs to those the children know and live with.

A second Australian study examined the efficacy of the Delta Dogsafe programme by measuring children's responses to photos of dogs when asked would they pat the dog before and after children and their parents participated in the programme (Wilson et al., 2002). It found a moderate increase in knowledge if children participated in the programme, and effects were augmented if parents were also given complementary material (Wilson et al., 2002). A similar study of the BARK programme in the USA had similar findings, with children showing improved knowledge about dogs and how to behave around them (Spiegel, 2000), but neither study investigated whether that knowledge transferred to changes in behaviour around dogs in everyday life.

Taken together, these studies show that education programmes can improve general knowledge of dog body language and appropriate behaviour around dogs in children of primary school age. However, whether that translates to changed behaviour in everyday life is unclear, with only one study showing this and doing so only in the short-term (Chapman et al., 2000). Presumably these programmes have not been carried out in a broad enough area over an extended period to allow an examination of dog bite statistics and whether any reduction in dog bites in children can be detected in areas where these programmes are commonplace. Education initiatives aimed at children may lack effectiveness if they do not successfully change the behaviour of parents. It is assumed that supervision would reduce bite risk, as children may trigger up to 86% of bite incidents at home (Meints and de Keuster, 2009 – no data cited), and it has been reported that most dog bites in children occur in the absence of adult supervision (Kahn et al., 2004). However, a study of the effect of the Blue Dog programme on parental supervision practices found that it made no difference at all to the extent to which parents supervised children around dogs (Morrongiello et al., 2013). An Australian study found that 70% of parents with at least one dog allowed their children to play unsupervised with the family dog at times (Wilson et al., 2002), and one of the studies on the Blue Dog programme showed that half of parents read 'most of' the guide sent home for parents to read, while 36% read 'a little bit' and 7% did not read any (Schwebel et al., 2012). This may reflect parents' belief that their children already know the material (Schwebel et al., 2012), or that their children would not deliberately hurt or tease a dog (Wilson et al., 2002), or may simply reflect the priorities of a busy parent.

As well as the presence or absence of adult supervision of children around dogs, the quality of supervision must also be considered. In some studies, it has been reported that when a child is bitten by a dog, an adult is present more often than not (Reisner et al., n.d.; Cassell and Ashby, 2009), but adults are not necessarily good at assessing critical risks in this context (Mathews and Lattal, 1994; Vilar et al., 1998), and may believe the family dog would never bite a child (Wilson et al., 2002). It is also likely that people have repeated positive experiences with companion dogs that may shape the belief that particular dogs are safe (Schwebel et al., 2012), which may make changing attitudes and behaviour difficult. Parents are also known to encourage children to approach dogs they know almost nothing about, and model that behaviour themselves if their child shows caution, rather than reinforcing them for their cautious behaviour (Morrongiello et al., 2013). For adult supervision to be effective in preventing dog bites in children, the following conditions would need to be met:

1. The supervising adult must have his or her full attention on the interactions between child and dog. This means he or she must not be watching television, preparing meals, tidying the room, or supervising another child. Clearly, dangerous situations can escalate quickly with only subtle warning signs.
2. The supervising adult is sufficiently good at interpreting dog body language to identify high-risk situations before they escalate to a bite. There is no research that assesses this to date.
3. The supervising adult must be in a position to intervene if it becomes necessary before escalation to a bite. This may mean being within arm's reach of child and/or dog and unencumbered with younger children, laptops, other pets, etc.

## 29.5  What might work?

As outlined in Chapter 4, interventions to prevent dog bites may need to take a broader perspective. Some thoughts are outlined below.

## 29.5.1 Legislation

It is possible that legislation aimed more broadly at responsible dog ownership could help to reduce dog bites. Regardless of their breed, dogs are not required to attend any training classes even though such classes may potentially reduce dog aggression towards humans (Grey, 2002). It is believed that a lack of socialisation in early life may lead to an increased risk of behavioural problems such as aggression, as evidenced by Duffy et al.'s findings (2008) that dogs obtained from commercial businesses rather than breeders or friends are more likely to exhibit nearly all kinds of behavioural problems, including aggression. It has also been found that attending puppy socialisation classes is associated with a decreased risk of aggressive behaviour towards visitors to the home (Casey et al., 2014), which is consistent with other findings that a lack of experience with urban environments in early life is associated with increased aggression towards people (Appleby et al., 2002). In addition, it is believed there is a genetic component to dog temperament, and selecting breeding stock for temperaments compatible with modern living with humans may be a worthwhile goal for breeders to embark on, provided that better temperament-testing tools are developed (King et al., 2012).

In recent times, the 'Calgary model' has received considerable attention from stakeholders interested in correctly identifying potentially dangerous dogs and reducing the clash between dogs and humans. The city of Calgary, in Canada, has experienced a steady decline in dog bite incidents since the 1980s – a trend that appears unusual. Calgary's focus on education for compliance ultimately led to Responsible Pet Ownership bylaws being enacted in 2006. These bylaws mandated the licensing of dogs and cats by three months of age, and legislated for penalties to dog owners who allowed their dog to become a threat or nuisance, transported their dog unrestrained in trucks, allowed their dog in prohibited areas, failed to keep their dog from obstructing pathways, failed to clean up animal waste, and failed to keep their dog on a leash except in designated off-leash areas (City of Calgary, 2006).

The city also launched a responsible pet ownership education programme that addressed the bylaws and also encouraged people to gonadectomise their pets, provide training and socialisation, and procure dogs from ethical sources such as rescue organisations or breeders (City of Calgary Animal & Bylaw Services, 2013). The city also provides brochures on preventing and reporting dog bites. The city currently enjoys 90% compliance in dog licensing and 50% compliance in cat licensing, resulting in the majority of impounded animals being collected by their owners (Outreach, 2007). Although the decline in dog bites over the past thirty years in Calgary suggests that the general approach is effective, it is difficult to pinpoint the mechanisms that have had the most critical influence. Research into owners' compliance with dog-related laws, the broader community's perception of responsible pet ownership and the effect of these factors on dog bites in the community may begin to address the problem more holistically. Other community-based initiatives such as that described by Keogh (Chapter 31) in this text, are emerging and appear to be having a positive impact but good research into these perceived effects is essential.

## 29.5.2 Education programmes

In addition to problems with the efficacy of education programmes, there may be a problem with the dissemination of educational material. For example, an online survey by the Morris Animal Foundation found that only 21% of veterinarians and 5% of physicians acquired their knowledge of dog bite prevention from medical or veterinary school, and only 14% of veterinarians and 4% of physicians followed a formal protocol when it came to educating dog owners on bite prevention (MAF, 2010).

The focus of education programmes may need to be broadened. Currently, education programmes are focused on children and how they should behave around dogs to avoid being bitten. Education for adults is generally focused on supporting children with supervision and enforcing house rules. Perhaps education programmes aimed at teaching adults how to interpret dog body language and provide effective supervision, as well as reinforcing cautious behaviour rather than encouraging children to approach dogs, would be beneficial.

Further, as outlined in Chapter 4, an ongoing problem may be that adults do not have accurate perceptions and beliefs regarding risk of dog bites (Westgarth and Watkins, 2015). In particular this may be an issue regarding the risks of dogs to children, because the adults are accumulating positive or neutral experiences themselves with dogs or simply cannot comprehend that their dog would do that to their child. Quantifying risks associated with different dog signals and human behaviour around dogs so that parents can be shown a concrete figure may help them adjust their risk perception regarding dogs and children.

Education programmes and legislative measures should be assessed properly for efficacy, but such assessments remain elusive due to the inconsistent quality of dog bite data. It may be beneficial to improve that quality by examining what should be reported and how, and settling on a standardised method of reporting.

### 29.5.3 The dogs, not the owners

Given persistent questions about the effectiveness of human education programmes, perhaps a shift of focus towards the dogs may prove more fruitful. Encouraging owners to take dogs to socialisation and training classes as early as possible may help set dogs up for long-term success in a human world. At the same time such classes should equip owners with better skills for training their dog and interpreting body language for correct risk assessment. A study in Rome found that, in a sample of about twenty serious dog aggression cases, most of the dogs involved were unruly and poorly controlled or trained by their owners, 37% of them were removed from their parents before eight weeks old, and 37% of them slept on couches or people's beds (Maragliano et al., 2007). Another study similarly found that sleeping on an owner's bed in the first two months of ownership was associated with a greater incidence of biting (Guy et al., 2001), and it has also since been reported that dogs removed from their litters at less than eight weeks of age are more likely to show behavioural problems (Pierantoni et al., 2011). These findings are moderately consistent in the literature but contrary results have also been reported (Westgarth et al., 2012), (also see Chapter 10 for a critique and summary of the dog bite risk factor literature). In summary, there may be measures dog owners can be encouraged to take that will reduce the likelihood of dogs biting when they are older. A randomised control trial for each intervention would be needed to confirm this.

It may also prove beneficial to better understand the dogs that do not show aggression towards humans. Are these dogs particularly tolerant or amicable? Have they benefited from care, housing, or training practices that are associated with a reduced risk of biting? As others have identified (see Chapter 10), aggression appears to have a heritable component but there is a need to better define this construct rather than consider it a simple phenotypic feature of an animal (see Chapter 1). With better definition and understand of the biological basis of aggressive behaviour is it possible to devise a temperament test to aid breeders in selectively breeding for low-risk dogs?

## 29.6 Conclusion

Dog bite prevention is considered an important issue for many governments, yet there has been very little research into which preventative measures are effective and, if they are effective, why. Indeed, while there might be an outcry against ineffective breed-specific legislation, it seems many other less discriminatory measures may be equally ineffective, even if well meaning. Dissemination of educational material appears incomplete, and ability and willingness of supervising adults to comply with advice is poorly understood. Furthermore, the factors influencing bite risk have not been fully elucidated, and the circumstances surrounding dog bite incidents are largely just best guesses from witnesses. Many of the problems with dog bite data are perennial and difficult to address but, if this issue is to be understood properly, data collection should be standardised and of high quality.

## 29.7 References

Appleby, D. L., Bradshaw, J. W. S., Casey, R. A. (2002). Relationship between aggressive and avoidance behaviour by dogs and their experience in the first six months of life. *The Veterinary Record*, 150(14), pp.434–438.

Casey, R. A. et al. (2014). Applied Animal Behaviour Science. *Applied Animal Behaviour Science*, 152, pp.52–63.

Cassell, E., Ashby, K. (2009). Unintentional dog bite injury in Victoria: 2005–7. Hazard.

Chapman, S. et al. (2000). Preventing dog bites in children: randomized controlled trial of an educational intervention. *The Western Journal of Medicine*, 173(4), pp.233–234.

City of Calgary Animal & Bylaw Services (2013). Responsible dog ownership. Available at: http://www.calgary.ca/CSPS/ABS/Documents/Animal-Services/Responsible-Pet-Ownership-Bylaw/responsible_dog_ownership.pdf.

Dixon, C. A. et al. (2012). Dog bite prevention: A new screening tool. *The Journal of Pediatrics*, 160(2), pp.3 37–341.

Duffy, D. L., Hsu, Y., Serpell, J. A. (2008). Breed differences in canine aggression. *Applied Animal Behaviour Science*, 114(3-4), pp.441–460.

Grey, K. (2002). Breed-Specific Legislation Revisited: Canine Racism or the Answer to Florida's Dog Control Problems. Nova L Rev.

Guy, N. C. et al. (2001). Risk factors for dog bites to owners in a general veterinary caseload. *Applied Animal …*, 74(1), pp.29–42.

Kahn, A. et al. (2004). Prevalence of dog bites in children: a telephone survey. *European Journal of Pediatrics*, 163(7), pp.424–424.

de Keuster T., Lamoureux, J., Kahn, A. (2006). Epidemiology of dog bites: A Belgian experience of canine behaviour and public health concerns. *The Veterinary Journal*, 172(3), pp.482–487.

King, T., Marston, L. C., Bennett, P. C. (2012). Breeding dogs for beauty and behaviour: Why scientists need to do more to develop valid and reliable behaviour assessments for dogs kept as companions. *Applied Animal Behaviour Science*, 137(1–2), pp.1–12.

MAF (2010). Online Survey Helps Improve Bite Prevention Programs. Available at: www.morrisan-imalfoundation.org/blog/category/dog/survey-improves-bite-prevention.html#.VQehdRDLfzE [Accessed 17 March 2015].

Maragliano, L. et al. (2007). Biting dogs in Rome (Italy). *International Journal of Pest Management*, 53(4), pp.329–334.

Mathews, J. R., Lattal, K. A. (1994). A behavioral analysis of dog bites to children. *Journal of Developmental Behavioral Pediatrics*, 15(1), pp.44–52.

McLaughlin, K.A., Glang, A. (2010). The effectiveness of a bicycle safety program for improving safety-related knowledge and behavior in young elementary students. *Journal of Pediatric Psychology*, 35(4), pp.343–353.

Meints, K., de Keuster, T. (2009). Brief Report: Don't Kiss a Sleeping Dog: The First Assessment of 'The Blue Dog' Bite Prevention Program. *Journal of Pediatric Psychology*, 34(10), pp.1084–1090.

Morrongiello, B. A. et al. (2013). Examining parents' behaviors and supervision of their children in the presence of an unfamiliar dog: Does The Blue Dog intervention improve parent practices? *Accident Analysis and Prevention*, 54, pp.108–113.

Outreach, A. N. (2007). City of Calgary: Dog Licensing Program. pp.1–7.

Pierantoni, L., Albertini, M., Pirrone, F. (2011). Prevalence of owner-reported behaviours in dogs separated from the litter at two different ages. *Veterinary Record*, 169(18), pp.468–468.

Reisner, I. R. et al., Behavioural characteristics associated with dog bites to children presenting to an urban trauma centre. *Injury prevention*, 17(5), pp.348–353.

Schwebel, D. C. et al. (2012). The Blue Dog: Evaluation of an Interactive Software Program to Teach Young Children How to Interact Safely With Dogs. *Journal of Pediatric Psychology*, 37(3), pp.272–281.

Spiegel, I. B. (2000). A pilot study to evaluate an elementary school-based dog bite prevention program. *Anthrozoos*, 13(3), pp.164–173.

Vilar, R. G. et al. (1998). Parent and pediatrician knowledge, attitudes, and practices regarding pet-associated hazards. Archives of pediatrics adolescent medicine, 152(10), pp.1035–1037.

Westgarth, C., Watkins, F. (2015). A qualitative investigation of the perceptions of female dog-bite victims and implications for the prevention of dog bites. *Journal of Veterinary Behavior: Clinical Applications and Research*, 10(6), pp.479–488.

Westgarth, C., Reevell, K., Barclay, R. (2012). Association between prospective owner viewing of the parents of a puppy and later referral for behavioural problems. *Veterinary Record*, 170(20), pp.517–517.

Wilson, F., Dwyer, F., Bennett, P. C. (2002). Prevention of dog bites: Evaluation of a brief educational intervention program for preschool children. *Journal of Community Psychology*, 31(1), pp.75–86.

# CHAPTER 30

# Children and Dogs – Risks and Effective Dog Bite Prevention

## Kerstin Meints

## 30.1 Introduction

This chapter focuses on child–dog interactions and misinterpretations of situations and behaviours. It also focuses on how we can teach children and their parents about safe behaviour with dogs.

First, we will briefly describe benefits and risks of human–dog interactions. Second, we will offer a new explanation as to why children under the age of eight may get bitten in the face more often than older children. We will then focus on typical situations in the home with the pet dog and introduce the Blue Dog Bite prevention tool, its purpose and how it works. We will explain how it was first assessed for its efficacy as well as reflect on others' assessments of the tool. We will also show that the Blue Dog tool changes children's and parents' behaviour in real life, having assessed the programme for its effectiveness and longitudinal learning success.

Next, we will move from creating awareness of typical risk situations in the home to awareness of a dog's distress signalling. We will describe how humans misinterpret still images of dogs' facial expressions with the majority of four-, five-, six- and even seven-year-old children misinterpreting dogs' facial expressions, often misunderstanding dogs' aggressive expression as 'happy'. Finally, we will demonstrate using videos clips how children and adults show a considerable lack of knowledge and misunderstanding of dogs' facial expressions and body language. We also show how we can improve knowledge in this area by teaching children and their parents to understand dog signalling correctly. Given the results of these studies, we can educate children and parents and other relevant parties and stakeholders, as well as inform dog bite prevention programmes to help prevent dog bite incidents and therefore contribute to children's safety and dogs' welfare alike.

## 30.2 Benefits of dog–child interaction

Numerous studies have claimed benefits of human–dog interaction for human health (Raina et al., 1999; Bufford et al., 2008; Cutt et al., 2008; Yabroff et al., 2008), in pet therapy (Wilson, 1991) and in relation to children's development (e.g. Kidd and Kidd, 1987; Poresky and Hendrix, 1990; Triebenbacher, 1998; Melson et al., 1992). Dogs function as social facilitators (Raina et al., 1999) and are seen as a friend and social partner (Filiatre et al., 1986) as well as family members, (see also Wells, 2007; McCardle et al., 2011a; McCardle et al., 2011b; Fine, 2010; Johnson, Beck and McCune, 2011, for overviews and case studies). In children, cognitive improvements were found when a dog was present during problem-solving tasks (Gee et al., 2010a), instructions were followed better (Gee et al., 2010b) and children were more attentive and calm in classroom situations (Kotrschal and Ortbauer, 2003). In hospitals, physiological measures revealed that animal-assisted therapy leads to less anxiety and less distress in children (Vagnoli et al., 2015). Studies have demonstrated that toy animals do not have such effects (e.g. Nielson and Delude, 1989; Beetz et al., 2012). Effective benefits have been associated with dogs, both familiar and unknown (Friedmann and Son, 2009). Children with ASD and children with behaviour problems seem to relax in the presence of a dog (e.g. Beetz et al., 2012) and for children with autism spectrum disorder (ASD) animals may serve as catalysts (Burrows et al., 2008; O'Haire, 2012). It is commonly believed that children with pets have more self-esteem and children show more empathy after being around a pet. It has been suggested that children with behaviour problems and from deprived backgrounds may be taught empathy through education, exposure and direct experience with animals (see Beetz et al. for an overview). Pets are seen as family members and are often a child's best friend with the ability to help children overcome anxiety and isolation (Melson, 2001).

As far as numbers are concerned, in the UK about 24–30% of households have a dog (Murray et al., 2010; PFMA, 2015). In the US today around 40% of households own a dog (AVMA, 2015; APPA, 2015) and, strikingly, a child in the US is more likely to grow up with a pet than with a father (Melson, 2001).

## 30.3 Risks of dog–child interaction

However, while clear benefits exist, there are also risks to consider, primarily dog bites. Accurate statistics are difficult to collect and interpret (See Chapter 3). It has been suggested that each year, 1.5% of the general population suffers a dog bite that requires medical attention (Gisle et al., 2001; Gilchrist et al., 2008). In the UK, recent Hospital Episode Statistics show steep increases in hospital admissions from 991 dog bite and strike injuries in 1989 to 6,740 in 2014 (HSCIS, 2014). Approximately 210,000 people a year are attacked by dogs in England alone (Department for Environment, 2012). The prevalence of dog bites in children is twice that of other age groups (Horisberger et al., 2004; Kahn et al., 2004). A recent study of patients with dog bites admitted to a maxillofacial department in a district general hospital in the UK over a twenty-one-month period showed that 43% of these patients were children under the age of ten (Mannion et al., 2015). Young children suffer more often from bites to the neck and head areas (Kahn et al., 2003; Schalamon et al., 2006; Dwyer,

Douglas, van As, 2007; Morgan, 2007; Reisner et al., 2011; HSCIS, 2014) and 55% of children who were bitten severely suffer from post-traumatic stress disorder (Peters et al., 2004).

The UK National Health Service (NHS) data from April 2014 confirm that children under nine are bitten most often, suffer most bites to the face/head and dog bite rates are three times as high in most deprived areas compared to least deprived areas (HSCIS, 2014, see also Dwyer et al., 2007).

Costs to the NHS are estimated around £10 million (Anon, 2013) and effective prevention has recently and repeatedly been demanded by the medical and veterinary professions (e.g. Mannion and Mills, 2013; Mannion and Shepherd, 2014; Mannion et al., 2015).

In contrast to hospital emergency data, interview data from children and adolescents show an even more disconcerting picture. Research showed that 20% of dog-owning parents admitted that their child had been bitten (Wilson, Dwyer and Bennett, 2003; see also Lakestani, Donaldson, Verga and Waran, 2006). However, when interviewed themselves, almost 50% of five to twelve year old children report to have been bitten (e.g. Spiegel, 2000; see also Beck and Jones, 1985; Sacks, 1989) with interviewees stating that they were mostly bitten by familiar dogs.

It is important to dispel the myths that:

* Most bites occur in the street
* Most bites occur by unfamiliar dogs
* The main problem is caused by 'dangerous breeds'
* Bites to the face occur because children are small.

In reality, the majority of bites to younger children occur with familiar dogs (72–75%) and in the home environment (Overall and Love, 2001; Bernardo, Gardner, Rosenfield, Cohen and Pitetti, 2002; Kahn et al., 2003, Schalamon et al., 2006; Dwyer et al., 2007; Reisner et al., 2011). It is often reported that in the vast majority of cases (e.g. 86% of cases, see Kahn et al., 2003) an interaction from the child towards the dog appears to trigger the bite (Kahn et al., 2003, for more data see Reisner et al., 2007; Reisner et al., 2011). All dog breeds have the potential to bite, including mixed breeds and the most commonly owned breeds, large or small (see Cornelissen and Hopster, 2010, for overview and discussion, also Horisberger et al., 2004; Schalamon et al., 2006). Further, most bites occur while there is no active parental supervision (Kahn et al., 2003; Reisner et al., 2007).

## 30.4 Understanding bites to the face and head

There is no evidence supporting a relationship between a dog's breed or size and facial injuries in children – instead, the child's age is known to be a significant factor related to bites to the face and head area (Bernardo et al., 2002; Kahn et al., 2003; Schalamon 2006, Hon et al., 2007). It is still unclear why young children get bitten mainly in the face and neck area (Dwyer et al., 2007). One study indicates that, in young children, bites to the face are associated with the dog *lying down* (Reisner et al., 2011) and the child's interaction prior to biting is reported to be *positive/benign* from the viewpoint of the child (Reisner et al., 2011). Interestingly, other research has shown that 67% of three- to four-year-olds' interactions with a dog involves touching (Millot et al., 1986). Photographic analysis demonstrated that 97% of photos show people in physical contact with dogs, generally with their heads close together (Katcher and Beck, 1985). There is currently no detailed analysis of other media, for example, YouTube clips that at times display unsafe interactions of children and dogs. However, recently, a 'Put the camera down' campaign was launched by *DogSEE.org* to create awareness of this and to encourage responsible parenting in order to avoid bite incidents (www.youtube.com/watch?v=_z0yPs9sdS8&feature=player_detailpage).

We conducted a specific investigation as to why young children get bitten in the face. As children's behaviour triggers bite injuries in the majority of cases, and as we had observed previously that children lean in very closely on objects they are interested in, almost touching the object of interest with their noses, we studied if and how children close in on items they are interested in (Meints, Syrnyk, and de Keuster, 2010).[1] We selected a range of objects, novel static and self-propelling objects as well as familiar static and moving toy animals. We varied children's physical distance to an object and also studied the role of smell of an object on children's facial proximity (or leaning in) behaviour. We tested children from two to six years, twenty-four children per age group, with about half of them female. We were able to demonstrate that children showed significant intrusive facial proximity behaviours, especially with moving items and novel items. Children at two and three years showed significantly more intrusive leaning-in behaviours than four-, five- and six-year-old children. In addition, in a related pilot study, we also gathered first evidence that children show clear leaning in behaviour with small animals (creepy crawlies and snails).

It is important that parents and carers of younger children are aware of this intrusive inspection behaviour; this often happens very quickly, and as animals may trigger this behaviour even more easily, it is a possibility that children get bitten in the face because they prefer close facial proximity to objects and animals they are interested in. By leaning in very closely towards a dog, they can put themselves at risk for a bite injury. This may not be the only cause for facial bites to younger children, but in combination with other interactions initiated by children, their close facial proximity behaviour could well be a major contributing factor. Raising awareness of this behaviour by young children will hopefully lead to better and closer supervision of small children in contact with dogs, and in turn can contribute to a reduction in bite injuries, especially to children's faces. Further research, ideally with parents and medical professionals, could enhance our knowledge by gathering much improved information detail on the circumstances of facial bites – unfortunately, we currently lack this kind of information on a larger scale.

## 30.5 Teaching children about typical household situations with familiar dogs

The Blue Dog bite prevention tool was created with the aim to provide the first empirically evaluated dog bite prevention tool for children under the age of seven (Meints and

---

1   The project was funded by the Waltham Centre for Pet Nutrition, a division of Mars, Incorporated, and by the Blue Dog Trust.

de Keuster, 2009).[2] It is vital that prevention tools are assessed (see Zeedyk and Wallace, 2003) as without assessment of their effectiveness we simply do not know if an educational tool works or not. So far only very few programmes have been assessed to measure their effectiveness; Chapman et al. (2000) and Spiegel (2000) have evaluated programmes focused on public safety with unfamiliar dogs and targeting children over seven years of age, while Wilson et al. (2003) looked at a programme targeted towards younger children, testing them with photographs of unfamiliar dogs.

The Blue Dog is the only programme that is directed at helping children under seven years of age to understand how to behave safely with the family dog in a home setting. It teaches them about safety with familiar dogs and has been evaluated for its learning success. It consists of a DVD with a 'test yourself' module and a 'Blue Dog stories' module. The accompanying parent booklet contains explanations on the fifteen assessed typical household situations in which children were found to get bitten most according to hospital data (Kahn et al., 2003).

It was tested empirically whether children's knowledge and assessment of a potential risk situation in the home improved. In addition, we also assessed if their behaviour with respect to their own dog changed as a result of using the test yourself module and the Blue Dog stories. This assessment occurred in two steps.

First, the test yourself module was used to assess children's knowledge improvement before and after a training session integrated into the module. The module combined training via presentations of cartoons depicting child–dog interactions and assessment of outcomes via questions about the scenarios, which probed children's knowledge before and after training. Ninety-six children were tested. Children were aged three to six years, with half of them receiving verbal feedback and half receiving additional parental support. Children were retested after two weeks. Children showed significant improvement in knowledge about safe behaviour with familiar dogs and they retained this knowledge over time. Older children performed consistently better than younger children. Verbal feedback had no influence on learning, but parental support was especially useful for younger children (Meints and de Keuster, 2009). There were no effects for participants' gender or dog ownership status. Thus, the Blue Dog programme successfully improves children's knowledge about safe behaviour with dogs. These findings have been replicated by ourselves and by others (e.g. Schwebel, Morrongiello, Davi, Stewart and Bell, 2012; Morrongiello et al., 2013).

We were also interested to find out if the educational Blue Dog stories on the DVD increased children's knowledge about safe behaviour with familiar dogs. As knowledge gain does not automatically translate into changed behaviour in practice, we were further interested to see if children who have a dog at home use the acquired knowledge and change their behaviour in real life with their own dog (Meints, Lakestani and de Keusteri, 2010; Meints, Lakestani and de Keuster, 2014).

Baseline measures of children's knowledge were taken for the different scenarios in the Blue Dog programme, similar to Meints and De Keuster (2009). In the following training

---

2   The research was funded by the Federation of European Companion Animal Veterinary Associations (FECAVA) and Groep Geneeskunde Gezelschapsdieren.

phase children were allowed to watch the Blue Dog stories. Then, in the testing phase, the stories' effectiveness was assessed via presentation of a set of novel child–dog interaction vignettes. Testing occurred longitudinally (before/after story exposure, retest after eight weeks, six months, one year) with thirty-six children aged three to five years in two groups; one group had the DVD at home and the other group only took the parent booklet home. Again, children showed successful learning and significantly increased knowledge, with older children achieving higher scores. Younger children with the DVD at home showed higher improvements than the group who only received the parent booklet to take home, suggesting that for younger children it is useful to be able to play repeatedly with the DVD. In addition, we found high compliance in reading the parent booklet: 95% of parents had read the booklet and about 70% of parents found the booklet useful to teach their children safe behaviour with dogs. Of the parents, 86% found the parent booklet easy to understand and 95% found the messages and behaviour advice clear. Some 71% of parents found the DVD for children useful.

Most importantly, we found that almost half of parents (48%) stated that after the intervention their children behaved more safely with dogs in general, and 38% of parents said their children behaved more safely around their own dog. Further, about 30% of parents said they themselves changed their behaviour with their own dog and about 30% now supervise their children more closely (Meints, Lakestani and de Keuster, 2014).

Thus, we have clear evidence that the Blue Dog programme helps to educate children to behave more safely with dogs and thus it is plausible to hypothesise that it can aid in dog bite prevention. The research validated the effectiveness of both modules on the DVD and evidenced that children not only learn successfully about safer behaviour with familiar dogs in typical home situations, but parents also observed a change in real-life behaviour in their children – with retention lasting up to one year.

In their recent joint papers, Schwebel et al. (2012) and Morrongiello et al. (2013) also claim to have tested Blue Dog's effectiveness in real-life conditions. A novel feature of their approach was to assess children with their parents in an unfamiliar location (a university psychology lab) with an unfamiliar dog and an unfamiliar person associated with the dog. They instructed the child to 'do whatever they wanted' (Morrongiello et al., 2013) or to 'play with any of the items in the room, including the dog' and showed the child how to play with the dog (Schwebel et al., 2012: 275). The experimenter then told the children the dog needed to rest and left the room, but with the explicit instruction to the child to 'do whatever *they* (the children) preferred' (see Schwebel et al., 2012 for full instructions; see Morrongiello et al. for very similar instructions). In this set-up and instructed as described, it is not surprising that children chose to interact with the dog. It is also not surprising that adults did not stop them: a clear authority figure allowed the children explicitly to do as they preferred. As the authors state themselves 'it is likely that parents assumed the dog was safe because of the context' (Morrongiello et al., 2013). To test Blue Dog's effectiveness, it would have been appropriate if these researchers had tested their participants with their own dogs in their own homes and on a wider range of fifteen Blue Dog scenarios.

However, as parental judgements (48%) suggest that Blue Dog does transfer to situations with unknown dogs (see above), it would be useful if further and appropriately operationalised empirical testing were to be carried out with the Blue Dog scenarios to investigate Blue Dog's transferability to unknown dogs.

## 30.6 Teaching children about dogs' distress signalling

While raising awareness and teaching children about safe behaviour with their family dog in the home environment is very useful indeed and helps to reduce risk situations, we also need to address a related problem: children's – and dog owners' – ability to interpret dogs' body language. When trying to enable safe interaction between children and dogs, it is vital that children are able to interpret the animal's signalling correctly to avoid injury and distress. However, it has been shown that children and adults often do not understand dogs' body signalling (Reisner and Shofer, 2008; Kerswell, Bennett, Butler and Hemsworth, 2009; Mariti, Gazzano, Moore, Baragli, Chelli and Sigheri, 2012; Bloom and Friedman, 2013). Interpretations in adults can vary with experience, but dog ownership does not predict correct interpretations (e.g. Tami and Gallagher, 2009; Wan, Bolger and Champagne, 2012).

Furthermore, there is a general lack of knowledge regarding dog behaviour and safety practices for child–dog interactions (Reisner and Shofer, 2008; Dixon et al., 2012). Children often confuse a fearful or angry dog with a friendly one (Meints, Racca and Hickey, 2010; Meints, Racca and Hickey, submitted; Racca, Guo, Meints, Mills, 2012). When four-, five-, six- and seven-year old children and adults were tested on photographs of neutral, aggressive and friendly human and dog facial expressions, adults made fewer than 1% mistakes, but the majority of four-, five-, six- and even seven-year-olds make many more errors. For example, looking only at the angry dog faces, 40% of four-year old children misinterpret these and 78% of these misinterpret aggressive dog faces as 'happy'. In contrast, children were very able to read human faces, often exceeding 90% correct responses. These results indicate a severe lack in interpretation abilities in children of facial expressions of dogs which could contribute to the high incidence of dog bites, especially in younger children. Further, children often commented how happy they thought these (angry-looking) dogs were and how they would approach and 'cuddle and kiss' them. Given these results and this worrying misinterpretation, children and parents *need* to be advised in order to prevent injuries and dog bite prevention programmes and puppy classes should be among the first to integrate this message to help prevent further incidents.

One could argue that photographs are static and that more realistic video stimuli would be more effective, thus, we have also tested children's and parents' assessments of dogs' body language and facial expressions using videos of real-life dogs. We carried out two studies that pioneer this new research on human perception and categorisation of dogs' signalling – one cross-sectional study using videos with and without sound and one longitudinal study.

In the first study we tested twenty-two four-year-olds and twenty-four five-year-olds by showing them videos of dogs according to the distress signals on Shepherd's 'ladder of aggression' (Shepherd, 2002). These consist of distress behaviours ranging through various steps, from 'low' (e.g. nose-licking, eye-blinking, turning head away) via 'medium' (e.g. crouching, tail tucked under) to 'high' distress (e.g. staring, growling, showing teeth, biting). However, these steps are not to be understood as a simple linear progression; their relationship to each other differ from individual to individual and depending on the situation the dog is experiencing. Often more than one signal is displayed, and also, the dog can move directly from the 'lowest' to the 'highest' step on the ladder, depending on what it has learned (e.g. signalling being ignored), how it feels and depending on the dog's perception of the situation, i.e. if the signalling results in more comfort from the dog's perspective.

We investigated children's evaluations by using a child–appropriate five-point scale with faces that ranged from happy (1) via neutral to unhappy/angry (5). As recent studies by Flom et al. (2009) and Pongrácz et al. (2011) suggest that additional acoustic input may enhance children's recognition and correct interpretation of dog signalling, we also tested if audible distress signalling (i.e. growling, snarling) influences children's judgement of the displayed dog's expression. Results show that children only distinguished high distress dog behaviours from low and medium distress displays (as defined by Meints et al., 2014), however, they did not discriminate between medium and low distress. Children interpreted videos of friendly dogs more correctly. While scores for the high distress group are significantly higher than for the other groups, overall, these scores are still lower (average of 3.2) than expected, possibly due to 81% of children scoring some of the dog videos in this group as 'very happy'. Children often chose 'very happy' when dogs exposed their teeth in the video (Meints et al., 2014; Meints et al., in prep.).

We then specifically compared children on a subset of the high distress displays (i.e. growling and snarling, dogs with exposed teeth) by showing them video stimuli with or without sound to investigate if audible growling or snarling increased children's correct answers. While there were no age group differences, there was a significant increase in scores when stimuli were shown with sound, raising their mean scores from 3.2 to 3.8 (out of 5). However, scores still did not reach the expected higher scores for angry (4) or very angry (5) (Meints and Just, 2014; Meints and Just in prep.).

In sum, this research confirms that children routinely commit errors interpreting dogs' facial expressions: even when videos instead of still images are used, children still misinterpret highly distressed displays as 'happy' and relaxed. While sounds increase children's awareness, overall this awareness does not fully reflect the displayed risk of the situation. This highlights the urgent need to teach children to recognise and interpret dogs' distress signalling appropriately to avoid future injury. In further research and in interventions teaching children dogs' distress signalling it is advisable to use training stimuli with sound as this seems to enhance correct recognition of dog signalling for the higher risk signals.

In a further study we integrated this finding and investigated longitudinally how three-, four- and five-year old children interpret dogs' signalling (Meints, Brelsford, Just and De Keuster, 2014).[3] We again used Shepherd's (2002) 'ladder of aggression' as our basis to create categories of low, medium and high distress dog signalling and created videos for sixteen different situations, plus an additional four 'happy' dog videos. Videos had been assessed independently by three experienced dog behaviour experts and were then grouped into four categories (high distress, medium distress, low distress and 'happy'). We first ran

8

3   This research project was co-funded by the *Eunice Kennedy Shriver* National Institute of Child Health and Human Development (NICHD) and the Waltham Centre for Pet Nutrition, a division of Mars, Incorporated. The project described is supported by Grant Number 1R03HD071161-01 from the *Eunice Kennedy Shriver* National Institute of Child Health & Human Development and Mars-Waltham.

a baseline test to gauge participants' knowledge before the training intervention and then tested them again straight after the training. We tested again after six months and after one year without any more interspersed training sessions. Thirty-three parents also took part in separate sessions and underwent the same procedure – 52% of these had been bitten at some point in their life, which fits the interview data described above.

The results show that knowledge in all participants improved significantly after training. The older the participants, the more correct the interpretation of the dog's distress signalling and facial expression. However, the 'lower' distress signals (e.g. nose licking, eye blinking, yawning, turning head away) were less likely to be recognised. Importantly, children displayed the same kind of misinterpretation error with videos as with photographs. Before training, four-year-olds made 53% errors in the highest of categories (staring, snarling, growling, snapping, biting) and of these, 65% were interpreted as happy. In five-year-olds we saw 36% errors and 52% of these as 'happy', and even in parents we saw 17% errors for highly distressed dogs, of which 13% were categorised as 'happy'.

These misinterpretations were reduced after training to 34% in the youngest children (result after 1 year), to 24% in the four-year-old group, to 19% in the five-year-old group and to no mistakes in the adult group. Thus, compared to the static photo stimuli there were even more misinterpretations. There were no effects of gender or dog ownership, nor parental education or socio-economic status (Meints, Brelsford, Just and De Keuster, 2014).

In sum, successful teaching of dogs' distress signalling within a given context may be a promising way forward for dog bite prevention. Children from three years onwards profit from appropriate intervention, showing significant improvements in knowledge immediately afterwards but also over a protracted time period. Increased awareness and knowledge can lead to perceived safer behaviour with dogs, potential risk reduction and potentially less bite incidents while dogs will profit as families' awareness of dogs' distress signalling is raised, hopefully resulting in more appropriate management. Future research on dog body language should also address differences in anatomy (hair, skin folds, short noses) and strategies of individual dogs that may change within a context.

## 30.7 Conclusion

When trying to enable safer interaction between children and dogs, it is vital that children and their parents are able to recognise situations in the household that can increase the risk for a dog bite. It is equally important for children and their parents to learn to interpret their dog's signalling correctly to avoid injury and distress to both parties. It is also vital that parents are aware of both – potential risk situations and dogs' body language – in order to act responsible and safeguard and educate their children and to guarantee the welfare of the family dog.

The striking lack of knowledge on dogs' behaviour and signalling (Reisner and Shofer, 2008; Bloom and Friedman, 2013) and the lack of knowledge in safety practices and safe behaviour in child–dog interactions (Reisner and Shofer, 2008; Dixon et al., 2012) mixed with common misconceptions on treatment and education of dogs (and children), does not make this task easy to fulfil.

Our research has for the first time highlighted in detail where the knowledge gaps are and how we can address them. We have summarised promising results and are hopeful to keep developing our pioneering programme of research and interventions to contribute to reducing future dog bite incidents, using a variety of empirically assessed prevention tools and messages.

Despite all prevention efforts it needs to be clear that we will not be able to prevent all dog bite incidents just by rolling out prevention programmes. While it is important that we raise awareness and educate all concerned via as many channels as possible, it is vital that parents are vigilant and supervise and educate their children, and give their dog the respect and welfare it needs. More scientifically sound research on effective prevention strategies for all ages is required. Further, gathering of accurate dog bite incident figures together with systematically recorded contexts of bite injuries will also increase knowledge regarding the extent of the public health problem and most suitable prevention strategies.

In order to tackle this complex issue, we need all concerned, from researchers to policy makers, dog breeders, puppy class tutors, dog trainers and veterinarians, as well as dog owners, families and medical practitioners to be involved in a joint, multi-disciplinary and evidence-based approach to human–dog interaction, giving education and prevention a central role so we can enjoy the benefits of the human–animal bond and reduce its risk.

## 30.8 References

AVMA. (2015). US Pet Ownership Statistics. Retrieved on 27 April 2015 from https://www.avma. org/KB/Resources/Statistics/Pages/Market-research-statistics-US-pet-ownership.aspx

APPA. (2015). 2015–2016 APPA National Pet Owners Survey Statistics: Pet Ownership & Annual Expenses retrieved on 27 May 2015 from www.americanpetproducts.org/press_industrytrends.asp

Beck, A. M., Jones, B. A. (1985). Unreported dog bites in children. *Public Health Report*, 100, 315–321.

Beetz, A., Kotrschal, K., Turner, D. C., Hediger, K., Uvnäs-Moberg, K., Julius, H. (2003). The Effect of a Real Dog, Toy Dog and Friendly Person on Insecurely Attached Children During a Stressful Task: An Exploratory Study. *Anthrozoos*, 24, 349–368.

Beetz, A., Uvnäs-Moberg, K., Julius, H., Kotrschal, K. (2012). Psychosocial and Psychophysiological Effects of Human-Animal Interactions: The Possible Role of Oxytocin. Frontiers in Psychology, 3, 234.

Bernardo, L. M., Gardner, M. J., Rosenfield, R. L., Cohen, B., Pitetti, R. (2002). A Comparison of Dog Bite Injuries in Younger and Older Children Treated in a Pediatric Emergency Department. *Pediatric Emergency Care*, 18, 247–249.

Bloom, T., Friedman, H. (2013). Classifying dogs' (*Canis familiaris*) facial expressions from photo-graphs. *Behavioural Processes*, 96, 1–10.

Bufford, J. D., Reardon, C. L., Li, Z., Roberg, K. A., DaSilva, D., Eggleston, P. A., Liu, A. H., Milton, D., Alwis, U., Gangnon, R., Lemanske, R. F. Jr., Gern, J. E. (2008). Effects of dog ownership in early childhood on immune development and atopic diseases. *Clin Exp Allergy.*, 38, 1635–43.

Burrows, K. E., Adams, C. L., Spiers, J. (2008). Sentinels of safety: Service dogs ensure safety and enhance freedom and well-being for families with autistic children. *Qualitative Health Research*, 18, 1642–1649.

Chapman, S., Cornwall, J., Righetti, J., Sung, L. (2000). Preventing Dog Bites in Children: Randomized Controlled Trial of an Educational Intervention. *British Medical Journal*, 320, 1512–1513.

Cornelissen, J. M. R., Hopster, H. (2010). Dog bites in The Netherlands: A study of victims, injuries, circumstances and aggressors to support evaluation of breed specific legislation. *The Veterinary Journal,* 186, 292–298.

Cutt, H. E., Knuiman, M. W., Giles-Corti, B. (2008). Does getting a dog increase recreational walking? *International Journal of Behavioral Nutrition and Physical Activity*, 5, 17.

Dixon, C. A., Mahabee-Gittens, E. M., Hart, K. W., Lindsell, C. J. (2012). Dog bite prevention: an assessment of child knowledge. *J Pediatrics,* 160, 337–341.e2.

DogSEE.org. (2015). Put the camera down campaign. Available at https://www.youtube.com/watch?v=z0yPs9sdS8&feature=playerdetailpage. (accessed 25 April 2015).

Dwyer, J. P., Douglas, T. S., van As, A. B. (2007). Dog bite injury in children – a review of data from a South African pediatric unit. *South African medical Journal*, 97, 597–600.

Filiatre, J. C., Millot, J. L., Montagner, H. (1986).New data on communication behaviour between the young child and his pet dog. *Behav. Process.* 12, 33–44.

Fine, A.H. (2010). Handbook of Animal-Assisted Therapy. London: Academic Press.

Flom, R., Whipple, H., Hyde, D. (2009). Infants' intermodal perception of canine (Canis familiaris) facial expressions and vocalizations. *Developmental Psychology*, 45, 1143–1151.

Friedmann, E., Son, H. (2009) The human–animal bond: How humans benefit. *Vet. Clin. North Am. Small Anim Practice,* 39, 293–326.

Gee, N. R., Church, M. T., Altobelli, C. L. (2010a). Preschoolers make fewer errors on an object categorization task in the presence of a dog. *Anthrozoös, 23,* 223–230.

Gee, N. R., Crist, E. N., Carr, D. N. (2010b). Preschool children require fewer instructional prompts to perform a memory task in the presence of a dog. *Anthrozoös, 23,* 178–184.

Gilchrist, J., Sacks, J. J., White, D. D., Kresnow, M.-J. (2008). Dog bites: still a problem? *Injury Prevention*, 14, 296–30.

Gisle, L., Buziarsist, J., Van der Heyden, J., Demarest, S., Miermans, P. J., Sartor, F., Van Oyen, H., Tafforeau J. (2002). Health Enquiry by Interview, Institute of Public Health, IPH/EPI Report N° 2002–22.

Hon, K. E., Fu, C. A., Chor, C., Tang, P. H., Leung, T., Man, C. Y., Ng, P. (2007). Issues associated with dog bite injuries in children and adolescents assessed at the emergency department. *Pediatr. Emerg. Care*, 23, 445–449.

Horisberger, U., Stärk, K. D. C., Rüfenacht, J., Pillonel, C., Steiger, A. (2004). The epidemiology of dog bite injuries in Switzerland – characteristics of victims, biting dogs and circumstances. *Anthrozoös*, 17, 320–339.

HSCIS (2014). Health and Social Care Information centre: admissions caused by dogs and other mammals. Retrieved April 27 2015, from www.hscic.gov.uk/catalogue/PUB14030/prov-mont-hes-admi-outp-ae-April%202013%20to%20January%202014-toi-rep.pdf

Johnson, R. A., Beck, A. M., McCune, S. (2011). *The Health benefits of Dog Walking for Pets & People.* Purdue: Purdue University Press.

Kahn, A., Bauche, P., Lamoureux, J., Dog Bites Research Team. (2003). Child victims of dog bites treated in emergency departments. *European Journal of Pediatrics*, 162, 254–258.

Kahn, A., Robert, E., Piette, D., De Keuster, T., Lamoureux, J., Leveque, A. (2004). Prevalence of dog bites in children. A telephone survey. *European Journal of Pediatrics*, 163, 424.

Katcher, A. H., Beck, A. M. (1985). Safety and Intimacy: Physiological and Behavioral Responses to Interaction with Companion Animals. *Proc of the International Symposium on the Human–Pet*

*Relationship,* on the occasion of the 80th birthday of Konrad Lorenz, Vienna, 1983. Austrian Academy of Sciences, Vienna, Austria, pp.122–128.

Kerswell, K. J., Bennett, P. J., Butler, K. L., Hemsworth, P. H. (2009). Self-reported comprehension ratings of dog behaviour by puppy owners. *Anthrozoös,* 22, 183–193.

Kidd, A. H., Kidd, R. M. (1987). Reactions of infants and toddlers to live and toy animals. *Psychological Reports,* 61, 455–464.

Kotrschal, K., Ortbauer, B. (2003). Behavioral effects of the presence of a dog in a classroom. *Anthrozoos: A Multidisciplinary Journal of The Interactions of People & Animals,* 16, 147–159.

Lakestani, N. N., Donaldson, M., Verga, M., Waran, N. (2006). Keeping children safe: how reliable are children at interpreting dog behavior? *Proceedings of the 40th International Congress of the International Society for Applied Ethology,* 233. ISAE Committee: Cranfield University Press.

Mannion C. J., Mills, D. S. (2013). Injuries sustained by dog bites. *British Journal for Oral Maxillofacial Surgery,* 51, 368–9.

Mannion C. J., Shepherd, K. (2014). One Health approach to dog bite prevention. *Veterinary Records,* 174, 151–2.

Mannion, C., Graham, A., Shepherd, K., Greenberg, D. (2015). Dog bites and maxillofacial surgery: what can we do? *British Journal of Oral and Maxillofacial Surgery,* 56, 479–484.

Mariti, C., Gazzano, A., Moore, J. L., Baragli, P., Chelli, L., Sigheri, C. (2012). Perception of dogs' stress by their owners. *J Vet behaviour,* 7, 213–219.

McCardle, P., McCune, S., Griffin, J. A., Eposito, L., Freund, L.S. (2011a). *Animals in our lives.* Baltimore: Brookes.

McCardle, P., McCune, S., Griffin, J. A., Maholmes, V. (2011b). *How Animals Affect Us.* Washington: APA.

Meints, K., de Keuster, T. (2009). Don't Kiss a Sleeping Dog: The First Assessment of 'The Blue Dog' Bite Prevention Program. *Journal of Pediatric Psychology,* 34(10), 1084–1090.

Meints K., Racca, A., Hickey, N. (2010). How to prevent dog bite injuries? Children misinterpret dog facial expressions. *Injury Prevention,* 16, suppl 1, A68.

Meints, K., Syrnyk, C., De Keuster, T. (2010). 'Why do children get bitten in the face?' *Injury Prevention,* 16, suppl 1, A172.

Meints, K., De Keuster, T., Lakestani, N. (2010). 'Children and dogs: How the "Blue Dog" help to prevent dog bite injuries'. *Proceedings of the Canine Science Forum,* 25–28 July, Vienna Austria, p.140.

Meints, K., Brelsford, V., Just, J., de Keuster, T. (2014). How children and parents (mis)interpret dogs' body language: a longitudinal study. *Poster presentation at the International Conference for Anthrozoology (ISAZ) in Vienna, July 2014.*

Meints, K., Racca, A., Hickey, N. (in prep) 'How to prevent dog bite injuries? Children misinterpret dogs' facial expressions'.

Meints, K., Lakestani, N., De Keuster, T. (2014). 'Does the Blue Dog change behaviour?' The First Longitudinal Assessment of the Blue Dog Bite Prevention Programme. *Poster presentation at the International Conference for Anthrozoology (ISAZ) in Vienna, Austria, July 2014.*

Meints, K., Just, J. (2014). Growl or no growl? Differences in children's interpretation of dogs' distress signalling. *Poster presentation at the International Conference for Anthrozoology (ISAZ) in Vienna, July 2014.*

Melson, G. F. (2001). *Why the wild things are: Animals in the lives of children.* Cambridge, MA: Harvard University Press.

8

Melson, G. F., Peet, S., Sparks, C. (1992). Children's attachment to their pets: Links to socio-emotional development. *Children's Environments Quarterly*, 8, 55–65.

Millot, J. L., Filiatre, J. C., Eckerlin, A., Gagnon, A. C., Montagner, H. (1986). Olfactory cues in the relations between children and their pet dogs. *Applied Animal Behaviour Science*, 19: 189–195.

Morgan, M., Palmer, J. (2007). Clinical review: Dog bites. BMJ, 334, 413–417.

Morrongiello, B. A., Schwebel, D. C., Stewart, J., Bell, M., Davis, A. L., Corbett, M. R. (2013). Examining parents' behaviors and supervision of their children in the presence of an unfamiliar dog: Does The Blue Dog intervention improve parent practices? *Accid. Anal. Prevent.*54, 108–113.

Murray, J. K., Browne, W. J., Roberts, M. A., Whitmarsh, A., Gruffydd-Jones, T. J. (2010). Number and ownership profiles of cats and dogs in the UK. *Veterinary Record*, 166, 163–168.

Nielson, J. A., Delude, L.A. (1989). Behavior of young children in the presence of different kinds of animals. *Anthrozoos*, 3, 119–129.

O'Haire, M. E. (2012). Animal-assisted intervention for autism spectrum disorder: A systematic literature review. *J Autism Dev Disord.* 43: 1006–1022.

Overall, K. L., Love, M. (2001). Dog bites to humans—demography, epidemiology, injury, and risk. *J Am Vet Med Assoc.*, 218, 1923–1934.

Peters, V., Scottiaux, M., Appelboom, J., Kahn, A. (2004). Post-traumatic stress disorder following dog bites in children. *Journal of Pediatrics*, 144, 121–122.

PFMA (2015). Retrieved from: www.pfma.org.uk/pet-population-2015 on 27 April 2015.

Pongrácz, P., Molnár, C., Dóka, A., Miklósi, A. (2011). Do children understand man's best friend? Classification of dog barks by pre-adolescents and adults. *Applied Animal Behaviour Science*, 135, 95–102.

Poresky, R. H., Hendrix, C. (1990). Differential effects of pet presence and pet-bonding on young children. *Psychological Reports*, 67, 51–4.

Pongracz, P., Csaba, M., Doka, A., Miklosi, A. (2011). Do children understand man's best friend? Classification of dog barks by pre-adolescents and adults. *Applied Animal Behaviour Science*, 135, 95–102.

Raina, P., Waltner-Toews, D., Bonnett, B., Woodward, C., Abernathy, T. (1999). Influence of companion animals on the physical and psychological health of older people: an analysis of a one-year longitudinal study. *J Am Geriatr Society*, 47, 323–9.

Racca, A., Guo, K., Meints, K., Mills, K. (2012). Reading faces: differential lateral gaze bias in processing canine and human facial expressions in dogs and 4-year-old children. *PLOS ONE*, 7(4): e36076.

Reisner, I., Shofer, F., Nance, M. (2007). Behavioral assessment of child-directed canine aggression. *Injury Prevention*, 13, 348–351.

Reisner, I. R., Shofer, F. S. (2008). Effects of gender and parental status on knowledge and attitudes of dog owners regarding dog aggression toward children. *Journal of the American Veterinary Medical Association*, 233, 1412–1419.

Reisner, I. R., Nance, M. L., Zeller, J. S., Houseknecht, E. M., Kassam-Adams, N., Weibe, D. J. (2011) Behavioral characteristics associated with dog bites to children presenting to an urban trauma center. *Injury Prevention*, 17: 348–53.

Sacks, J. J., Sattin, R. W., Bonzo, S. E. (1989). Dog bite-related fatalities from 1979 through 1988. *Journal of the American Medical Association*, 262: 1489–1492.

Schalamon, J., Ainoedhofer, H., Singer, G., Petnehazy, T., Mayr, J., Kiss, K., Höllwarth, M. E., 2006. Analysis of dog bites in children who are younger than 17 years. *Pediatrics*, 117, e374–e379.

Schwebel, D. C., Morrongiello, B.A., Davis, A.L., Stewart, J., Bell, M. (2012). The Blue Dog: Evaluation of an interactive software program to teach young children how to interact safely With dogs. *J. Pediat. Psychology*, 37, 272–281.

Shepherd, K. (2002). Development of behaviour, social behaviour and communication in dogs. In: *BSAVA Manual of canine and feline behavioural medicine*. Ed. D. Horwitz, D. Mills, S. Heath, British Small Animal Veterinary Association, pp.8–20, ISBN 0-905214-59-5.

Spiegel, I. B. (2000). A pilot study to evaluate an elementary school-based dog bite. Prevention program. *Anthrozoös*, 13, 164–173.

Tami, G., Gallagher, A. (2009). Description of the behaviour of domestic dog (Canis familiaris) by experienced and inexperienced people. *Applied Animal Behaviour Science,* 120, 159–169.

Triebenbacher, S. (1998). Pets as transitional objects: Their role in children 's emotional development. *Psychology Reports* 82, 191–200.

Vagnoli, L., Caprilli, S., Vernucci, C., Zagni, S., Mugnai, F., Messeri A. (2015). Can Presence of a Dog Reduce Pain and Distress in Children during Venipuncture? *Pain Management Nursing*, 16, 89–95.

Wan, M., Bolger, N., Champagne, F.A. (2012). Human Perception of Fear in Dogs Varies According to Experience with Dogs. PLoS ONE 7, e51775.

Wells, D. L. (2007). *Domestic dogs and human health: An overview. British Journal of Health Psychology,* 12, 145–56.

Wilson, F., Dwyer, F., Bennet, P. (2003). Prevention of dog bites: evaluation of a brief educational intervention program for preschool children. *Journal of Community Psychology*, 31, 75–86.

Yabroff, K. R., Troiano, R. P., Berriganet, D. (2008), Walking the Dog: Is Pet Ownership Associated With Physical Activity in California? *Journal of Physical Activity and Health*, 5: 216–228.

Zeedyk, M. S., Wallace, L. (2003). Tackling Children's road safety through edutainment: an evaluation of effectiveness. *Health Education Research*, 18, 493–505.

8

# CHAPTER 31

# Case study – Multi-Agency Collaboration for the Prevention of Dog Bites: The LEAD Initiative

## Police Constable Heath Keogh, Community Intelligence Officer and LEAD Initiative Dog

*SPOC (Single Point of Contact) Sutton Police Station*

*'A dog's behaviour or actions are only a reflection on its owner's inability and irresponsibility to take an interest in their dog's behaviour, actions and well-being.'*

Heath Keogh, 2016

## 31.1 Introduction

**L**ocal **E**nvironmental **A**wareness on **D**ogs (LEAD) is a UK-based initiative led by the Metropolitan Police. It was founded in the London borough of Sutton, a low crime and park-rich borough in south-west London, bordering Surrey.

LEAD seeks to encourage 'responsible ownership' of all breeds of dog, regardless of the owners' social background. The programme encompasses engagement, intervention, prevention and, where needed, enforcement.

- It offers advice to the public on dog issues including fouling, noise nuisance, dog-on-dog/pet attacks and offences under the Dangerous Dogs Act 1991.
- It works to improve dog safety and dog welfare in the borough.
- It also aims to tackle criminal, anti-social and irresponsible behaviour by individuals with dogs in a way that protects and reassures the public to improve residents' safety and their perception of safety.

The LEAD initiative requires the co-operation of a number of organisations to be fully effective, and so successful partnership working is an essential prerequisite. In January 2005, the Metropolitan Police and its then commissioner, Sir John Stevens, and Sutton Council took the bold and pioneering step to bring *together under a single line management* their community safety services to make Sutton borough safer. This new venture was called the Safer Sutton Partnership Service (SSPS) – a joint team of police officers and council community safety staff based at Sutton police station. In January 2015, the SSPS held a tenth anniversary exhibition to highlight its overall achievements, which included a 35% fall in overall crime over the period, a 40% fall in calls about anti-social behaviour, a fall in the fear of crime across all major crime types, and £750,000 cashable, year-on-year, savings to local residents (see http://content.met. police.uk/News/10-years-of-making-the-borough-safer/1400029153911/1257246745756).

It was against this background that the LEAD initiative concerning dogs was launched and flourished, albeit in response to a specific incident two days before Christmas in December 2010 that made national press headlines.

## 31.2 The triggers to action

LEAD was launched in 2011 following the tragic death of a woman, in her fifties inside a property in Wallington, part of the borough of Sutton, on Thursday, 23 December 2010. The victim was attacked by a large Molosser/Mastiff-type dog. It was not a prohibited breed as set out under s.1 of the UK Dangerous Dogs Act 1991, nor a recognised breed as set out by the UK Kennel Club breed standards.

- Within twenty-four hours of this event, members of the community were interviewed on national television media and by national/local newspapers.
- Many of those interviewed mentioned that they had brought the behaviour of the dogs at the address to the attention of the local policing team and the local authority/government departments.
- They told journalists that they had raised issues about noise nuisance, dog fouling and the dogs being allowed to jump into other residents' gardens.
- The Metropolitan Police's Territorial Policing Headquarters (TPHQ) voiced its concerns about what had happened and instructed the senior management at Sutton to carry out a review to include how police engaged with dog owners.
- The author of this case study was requested to undertake this work and proceeded to search police databases for any records concerning the dog at the address in Wallington. He found that no record had been kept on police systems of any contact that had been raised between members of the local community and police. This may have been because the issues raised were too low level to be recorded in this way.

In general, my research found that low level anti-social behaviour concerning dogs was not being recorded unless there had been a concern that the dog may be a prohibited breed or that an offence under the Dangerous Dogs Act 1991 had been committed. The research continued and contact was made with the local authority departments and all registered social landlords to ascertain:

- How they recorded dog-related incidents
- Who they shared this information with
- How many dogs were within their properties.

The results found the following:

- Registered social landlords could not provide figures in relation to dogs within their properties. Only that 'Tenants must seek permission' or that 'Dogs/pets are not permitted'.
- There was also a problem with the recording of low level incidents and the sharing of information from partners to police and police to partner organisations.

Although the dog attack in Wallington proved to be a catalyst for action, there had been a high level of concern expressed by Sutton residents in surveys over recent years about nuisance dogs, such as dog-on-dog attacks and dog fouling in the borough. It was clear that there was a need for a structured and co-ordinated, borough-wide approach to encourage 'responsible dog ownership'. It needed to be relevant to all dog owners – those in private and rented accommodation – and open to all types and breeds of dog.

However, addressing the impact of dog ownership – whether responsible or irresponsible – in local communities was never going to be solely a police matter. Key to success was going to be the involvement of partner organisations, which had a vested interest in also promoting responsible dog ownership. These organisations include:

- Sutton Council
- Sutton Housing Partnership – the biggest landlord in Sutton
- Registered social landlords including Roundshaw Homes
- The RSPCA and the local Riverside Animal (rescue) Centre.

## 31.3  Managing LEAD

My work is within the borough's Anti-Social Behaviour Unit, a collaborative unit funded by the Metropolitan Police, Sutton Council and Sutton Housing Partnership. It deals with all reports of anti-social behaviour, which includes physical and verbal abuse targeting individuals or groups, and incidents involving nuisance, noise and damage resulting in victims suffering harassment, alarm or distress. This unit actively encourages reporting of anti-social behaviour and responds to incidents, issues and concerns promptly. The unit gathers intelligence and evidence and responds in a way that is commensurate with the level of the seriousness and urgency of each report. Victims and witnesses are given regular updates on how incidents are being dealt with and progressed. As a result of the work of the unit, the number of calls about anti-social behaviour is falling in the borough and so too are the number of repeat victims.

Thus this was an ideal home for the LEAD initiative regarding issues with dogs.

## 31.4  LEAD objectives

LEAD's objectives are as follows:

- To proactively and positively promote responsible dog ownership, defined such as establishing daily routine, good animal care, identification by chipping, teaching children to respect animals, health, well-being and welfare, and pet insurance.

- To promote safety and welfare of all types and breeds of dogs through public engagement activities, such as dog roadshows and police talks to groups.
- To work in partnership with other organisations including Sutton Council, Sutton Housing Partnership, registered social landlords, the Riverside Animal Centre, Dogs Trust and others.
- To support local residents with education, training and responsibility towards their dogs, including providing updates on dog legislation, such as the need for all dogs to be microchipped by April 2016.
- To encourage owners in social housing to register their dogs with their landlord.
- To reduce criminal and anti-social behaviour by individuals with dogs by intervention and legislation in a way that offers protection and reassurance to residents.
- To deal actively with other irresponsible actions by individuals with dogs such as the misuse and mistreatment of dogs.
- To deal with prohibited types/breeds using enforcement when necessary.
- To publicise LEAD community and enforcement activities and LEAD performance through regular communications, press activity and promotional materials.

## 31.5 How LEAD works

A pillar of how LEAD works is keeping records of all dog-related incidents and sharing that information with key partners. Records are kept of all dog-related incidents regardless of dog breed. These records are shared with partner agencies, such as the local authority, registered social landlords and national animal charities. This generates an audit trail of engagement, which helps manage risk.

There are two key strands to the LEAD initiative. One is the proactive engagement with dog owners in local communities and the other is early intervention and enforcement.

### 31.5.1 Proactive engagement

The vast majority of dog owners appear to be responsible and respond positively to initiatives to help them become more knowledgeable about their pet's care, well-being and safety. This is especially appreciated when this advice service is delivered to their local community in a roadshow backed by police and local authority with specialists on hand including the RSPCA, Dogs Trust or Riverside Animal Centre. These roadshows seek to encourage dog owners to be better owners and to network the message to other dog owners about what is being done to promote responsible ownership in the borough.

LEAD engagement activities include:

- Engaging with dog owners during regular police patrols.
- Arranging dog roadshows in local parks and open spaces to offer dog advice and free or discounted dog microchipping.
- Encouraging owners (if a social housing resident) to register their dog with their landlord.
- Publicising activities to promote responsible dog ownership and distributing advice and support materials.

## 31.5.2 Early intervention and enforcement

It is felt by the author that there is a tiny minority of dog owners whose dogs become involved in criminal, anti-social and irresponsible behaviour – and it is important for public reassurance that such incidents are dealt with promptly and robustly. Police will intervene early, initiate control measures and ultimately prosecute offenders when a dog:

- Has committed an offence;
  - Where someone has reasonable apprehension that they would be injured or attacked by a dog;
  - Is a prohibited type/breed in the UK (see Chapter 13); or
- Has been linked with anti-social behaviour.

Officers take steps to protect the community wherever legislation permits. For example, court proceedings could result in a control order, which may require the owner/keeper to meet certain conditions, such as the dog being muzzled in public places or only walked by an adult aged eighteen or over. Failure to meet any conditions set could result in the dog being destroyed. In addition, there is an education requirement around enforcement messages, because owners/keepers are often unaware of the law on dogs. For example, it is not widely known that in the UK residents only have to be in reasonable apprehension/fear of being attacked by a dog for a crime to have been committed.

LEAD enforcement activities include:

- In all cases where a dog owner or keeper comes to the attention of police or the local authority, contact being made with that person, regardless of whether a criminal offence has been committed (see two-stage letter process below).
- Any contact being documented and shared with partner organisations. Such records provide an important source of evidence should enforcement prove necessary and if matters were to progress to prosecution and court proceedings. Courts would expect detailed records to be presented to them by the authorities when considering a case.
  - Information captured should include:
    - Details of the owner
    - The person in charge of the dog at the time
    - Details of the housing provider (where appropriate)
    - A full account of the incident
    - Details of the dog including its name, breed/type, colour, age, gender
    - Whether it has been neutered/spayed and microchipped.

## 31.5.3 Two-stage letter process

LEAD has created a two-stage letter process following reports of criminal, anti-social or irresponsible behaviour:

- 1st 'Coming to Notice' letter

  A letter is posted to an owner/keeper from police to acknowledge that an incident has come to police attention. The letter will include details of where, when, why, who, the time and the nature of the incident, such as a dog being allowed to behave in such a way that it will have a detrimental effect on the local community such as a dog on pet attack, fighting with other animals or dog fouling.

These details, when appropriate, will be shared with relevant partners, such as Sutton Council's Environmental Health Team, Sutton Housing Partnership and a registered social landlord. Other documents enclosed with this first letter include:

- LEAD leaflet and brief background to the initiative
- The Kennel Club Safe and Sound Scheme and Good Citizen Dog Scheme information; www.thekennelclub.org.uk/training/good-citizen-dog-training-scheme
- RSPCA leaflet on dealing with care, training and welfare, and behaviour around unfamiliar dogs, www.rspca.org.uk/adviceandwelfare
- Battersea Dogs and Cats Home Breed Fact Sheet, www.battersea.org.uk/apex/webbreeds?pageId=031-dogbreeds&type=dog
- Sutton Council bye-laws. https://www.sutton.gov.uk

- 2nd 'Coming to Notice' letter

Should the dog's behaviour come to police notice again, a second letter will be hand-delivered by the local Safer Neighbourhoods police team – information that again will be shared with relevant partner organisations.

At the same time as the second letter is sent, an Acceptable Behaviour Contract will be sought. This is a voluntary agreement between the police and the individual. If this is declined, the police Anti-Social Behaviour Unit will monitor the dog's behaviour for at least six months. The letter will state that police may pursue one of the following court orders if anti-social behaviour persists:

- Anti-Social Behaviour Order (ASBO) or Criminal Behaviour Order (CBO)
- Contingency Destruction Order (CDO) on conviction (under the Dangerous Dogs Act 1991)
- Dog Control Order (DCO) (under Section 2 of the Dogs Act 1871)
- Community Protection Notice (CPN)

## Additional actions during this letter process

It is important to note that an ASBO, CDO, DCO or CPN can be sought at any time during this letter process depending on the seriousness of the incident. In the most serious of cases, police have powers to seize the dog and summons owners to court. In addition, if the dog owner resides in social housing, the landlord, who would have been notified of this correspondence, will send a letter or visit the dog owner/keeper within seven working days to remind him or her of, or enforce, the tenancy agreement. Continued anti-social behaviour could result in permission to have a dog being withdrawn (assuming permission has been sought already and granted) or even the property being repossessed and the tenant evicted. Landlords are required to keep police informed of any actions taken.

## 31.6  Evidence of effectiveness

Since January 2011 (to June 2016), actions taken by police in Sutton include:

- 297 letters to dog owners (283, CTN1 and 14, CTN2). Therefore 95% required no further action. Only four have proceeded to commit an offence under the Dangerous Dogs Act; if the assumption is made that without intervention all of these would have gone on to commit an offence (of which proportion in reality we do not know), this suggests a success rate of more than 98% through early intervention
- Thirteen Acceptable Behaviour Contracts (ABCs)
- Forty-seven Dog Control Orders/Contingent Destruction Orders
- One injunction (working with a local registered social landlord)
- Four disqualifications (convictions under the AWA 2006 and DDA 1991)
- Sixteen LEAD roadshow days (Riverside Animal Centre, Dogs Trust and registered social landlords)
- More than 635 dogs microchipped.

We were contacted by a family whose family pet dog attacked two children. The family reacted by arranging for the dog to be moved to the home of another relative. Police continued to work with the family and the matter was resolved with a Section 2 Control Order under the 1871 Dogs Act. This meant no family member received a criminal record and meant that the dog was able to stay within the family circle, although restrictions were put in place regarding its behaviour, particularly relating to children under the age of eighteen.

We believe that the programme is effective, however, no data are available at this time to confirm an actual reduction in dog bites as a result of our efforts. However, an increase in intelligence reports over the last twelve months suggests better identification of dog issues, improved referrals to police, and improved police recording of incidents. Clearly the programme provides a useful framework for addressing the wider social and behavioural issues associated with dog bites, and data will need to be gathered over an extended time to show real world impact.

## 31.7  LEAD recognition and accomplishments

LEAD has been recognised as being a model of best practice for engaging with responsible and irresponsible dog owners in other UK areas beyond Sutton and London. In addition, LEAD has been endorsed by: the UK Kennel Club; Battersea Dogs and Cats Home; and the Department for Environment, Food and Rural Affairs (Defra). In addition, LEAD has been used as a case study by Defra for its new 'Dealing with Irresponsible Dog Ownership Practitioner's Manual', which accompanies the Anti-Social Behaviour Crime and Police Act (October 2014). https://www.gov.uk/government/policies/protecting-animal-welfare/activity. LEAD was nominated as a finalist in the Kennel Club National Good Citizen Dog Scheme Awards 2013.

## 31.8  Strengths and weaknesses

Strengths:

* Based within a joint organisation rather than single
* Recording information of all dog incidents (regardless of whether they are deemed criminal) and sharing that information with partner organisations to manage risk and create an audit trail and evidence for court
* Proactive education to encourage responsible dog ownership of all breeds of dog
* Proactive enforcement to encourage owners to realise there will be consequences to irresponsible ownership and to reassure residents that the authorities are taking action to keep the borough safe
* Non-breed-specific initiative
* Encompassing all dog owners regardless of social background
* Identifying key stakeholders
* Improving reporting pathways from local agencies
* Building up trust and rapport through integrated working
* Establishing joint outcomes with registered social landlords.

Weaknesses:

* Information not being recorded and shared by police officers and other partner organisations
* Failing to take action when action is necessary
* Malicious reporting by partner organisations or members of the public.

## 31.9  Summary/recommendations

The LEAD dog initiative in Sutton has highlighted an important need to record all dog-related incidents. All relevant organisations need to sign up to share that information and to work together to co-ordinate appropriate engagement and intervention at the earliest opportunity. Local agencies need to establish appropriate mechanisms for assessing risk and develop an understanding of how to escalate cases into multi-agency risk management and intervention as required.

Sutton's LEAD initiative has been shared among many UK police forces and local authorities that have felt the need to learn from LEAD to help them address the issue of dog-related incidents in their areas. This is part of a general move to increasingly work to deliver greater customer or resident focus to the services they provide.

In a relatively short time, LEAD has become an important strategy in Sutton to address dog-related incidents as part of wider initiatives and operations to combat anti-social behaviour and criminal activity. It is also a key part of addressing residents' concerns around nuisance dogs and to continue to make Sutton a low crime borough and one of the safest boroughs in London. The Annual Community Safety Survey (SENSOR) has highlighted responsible dog ownership as a top-ranking concern over the last five years.

## 31.10  Further reading

www.slough.gov.uk/moderngov/documents/s35388/5a%20-%20Dog%20Initiative%20
   Booklet%20A5.pdf

# Section 9
# Concluding Comments

In our final concluding comments section, Rachel Orritt and Todd Hogue, in Chapter 32, draw on their combined expertise in forensic psychology and animal behaviour to reflect on an alternative way forward for assessing risk. This is based on methods used in other potentially high-risk situations for the public where there is a lack of clear scientific evidence but growing professional expertise. Forensic risk assessment using structured professional judgment allows the synthesis of scientific data with expert opinion in an organised way to allow best use of these resources. It may not be perfect but it provides a clearly traceable basis for both action and accountability.

In the final piece we briefly reflect on the messages presented throughout the text, the lessons we should learn and specific priorities for moving forward in a more cohesive and evidence based way.

# CHAPTER 32

# Reconciling Opinion and Evidence on Dog Bites – A Suggested Way Forward Using Forensic Risk Assessment

*Rachel Orritt and Todd E. Hogue*

## 32.1 Introduction

As highlighted at many points throughout this text, the study of human-directed aggressive behaviour (HDAB), and the strategies employed to address it, are hampered by the way it is perceived and rationalised by the public, the media and to some extent policy makers. Dog bites in particular invoke a certain degree of dread because of their perceived unpredictability (Hogue et al., 2015, unpublished results). Many dog bite prevention strategies have been conceived and employed, and their development accelerated by the consistently high level of media and public interest. Unfortunately most of these strategies have not been the product of good quality evidence, instead being purposed for the perceived rather than actual reduction of risk. In this chapter, we draw on the experience of forensic psychology for managing the risk associated with repeat violent behaviour to propose an alternative strategy for the understanding and reduction of HDAB risk, through evidence-based risk prediction and structured professional judgement.

## 32.2 Current approaches to addressing human-directed aggressive behaviour

### 32.2.1 Current strategies

In an attempt to address HDAB and dog biting incidents, a variety of different strategies are currently in use. They can be found at all levels, from behavioural rehabilitation programmes followed by the individual dog–carer partnership (Chapters 25, 26 and 28), educational programmes about canine behaviour (Chapters 29, 30 and 31), temperament tests to screen dogs (Chapters 9 and 27) and legislation to implement national policy (Chapter 13).

At a national level, jurisdictions are often motivated to be seen to be confronting the issue, particularly if there is a heavy media or public focus on particularly severe dog bites. Unfortunately the reactive legislation that results is not always based upon scientific evidence, but seeks to appease the public by targeting a minority of dogs and owners (Chapter 5, 6 and 7). For example, rather than taking note of any potential evidence for breed-specific risk (Cornelissen and Hopster, 2010; Schalke et al., 2008, see also Chapter 10), the response in the UK and EU and some US states has been to maintain and 'strengthen' their own breed-specific legislation (National Canine Research Council, 2013). This may involve increasing the application of the current law or simply increasing the maximum associated fines and/or jail sentences.

On an individual assessor level, the European Society for Veterinary Clinical Ethology (ESVCE) has produced a brief framework for veterinary behaviourists to follow when assessing a dog for aggressive behaviour (Corridan et al., 2011). These guidelines represent one of the only points of professional reference for an assessor tasked with a HDAB risk assessment. However, they provide more of a general code of good practice rather than specific instructions as to the formulation and implementation of a useful risk assessment. Widespread use of these guidelines would, at the very least, ensure some degree of consistency between assessors. However, the extent of uptake of these guidelines is unknown, and there has been no testing whether the clinical assessment of HDAB is accurate and/or consistent between assessors.

Temperament tests (also known as provocation tests or test batteries) and clinical assessments are often employed to assess working or companion dogs (Taylor and Mills, 2006). The assumption is that the behaviours shown during the test translate to response to similar stimuli outside of the test. However, as reviewed in Chapter 9, there are many issues associated with these types of test, not least their predictive validity (Barnard et al., 2012). With the notable exception of the Socially Acceptable Behaviour (SAB) test (Planta and De Meester, 2007), few have demonstrable predictive power and then only for limited situations.

An alternative approach is to target the potential victims of dog bites. Behaviour education initiatives, such as the Blue Dog project (Chapter 30; Meints et al., 2010) are usually targeted towards children. These initiatives aim to educate the public as to the behaviour of dogs in order to promote safe human–dog interactions. While these educational programmes are popular with academics and the public, it is unreasonable to expect educational strategies to provide the ultimate solution to this public health issue (see Chapters 29 and 4). Instead, they should be seen as a component of a rigorous suite of methods, used appropriately and consistently, to prevent, predict and manage HDAB.

## 32.2.2 Roadblocks for prevention

Unfortunately, an evidence-based approach that is purposeful, widely accepted and adopted at national level is rarely achieved. The reasons for this are numerous, but two of the most prominent obstructions to progress are summarised below.

1.  Firstly, the relationship between the news media, the public and policy makers promotes punitive legislation in place of effective preventative strategies (Orritt and Harper, 2015). In this view the news media is the main driving force, encouraging the perception that severe and fatal dog bites are a common occurrence and can be attributed to the presence of 'dangerous dogs' and irresponsible owners. This perception is encouraged through various mechanisms, including an overrepresentation of fatal dog bite stories, and oversimplification of those stories to conform to 'good versus evil' frameworks (see

Chapters 5, 7 and 11). To facilitate this framework, the media present the characters in the story in binary terms – a dog is either dangerous or not, an owner responsible or irresponsible. This media depiction calls the public to action to demand immediate development or 'strengthening' of laws relating to the control of dogs. Following legislative change, any further reports of dog biting incidents by the news media result in public judgement of the law as ineffective. This is then reflected back to the public by the news media, which restarts the cycle.

2.  The problem with the resulting punitive legislation is not just its lack of intentioned effect, but the fact that, from a political perspective, the problem has been addressed. Politically, measures are in place to protect the public by 'rid[ding] the country of the menace of these fighting dogs' (Dorey, 2005, p.38). Secondly, whether or not any measure really does protect the public is, in actuality, almost completely unknown to both politicians and scientists alike. This is because to know whether a reduction has been achieved requires baseline knowledge of the frequency of injurious dog bite occurrences and the systematic evaluation of the effect of any change in strategy. Approximating baseline rates for dog bites is extremely problematic (See Chapter 3). Depending on the severity, injuries from some bites will go untreated or be treated at home, while more severe bites and bites to children or other vulnerable parties will be overrepresented in hospital data. Kahn et al. (2004) estimated that half of all dog bites go unreported. Those bitten by their own dog might even be motivated to lie about the cause of their injury to protect their dog or themselves (see Chapter 23). Without an accurate base rate for dog bite incidences, representative of the demographics of victims, the effectiveness of new measures cannot be assessed accurately. This renders approximation of dog bite incidence across the population of primary importance.

## 32.3  A new direction in dog bite prevention

### 32.3.1  A psychological approach to predicting risk

Techniques and approaches first developed for humans are often adapted to great success for use in non-human animals, and the relationship between the two health disciplines is proving ever more fruitful, driven by 'One Health' principles (One Health, n.d.). Historically, the discipline of psychology has benefited from the study of animal behaviour, including development of key theories and frameworks such as behaviorism (Skinner, 1974) and classical conditioning (Pavlov, 1927). However, the transfer of knowledge between the newer areas of psychology, such as forensic psychology, and applied animal behaviour, has perhaps been less widely embraced as a paradigmatic level.

Historically, the forensic psychology approach to violent offending resembled the veterinary and behaviourist approach to HDAB in dogs (Monahan and Skeem, 2014). Typically the clinician would apply a 'clinical' approach, meaning that he or she would appraise the history of the individual being assessed and use personal clinical experience to form a prognosis for future behaviour, which would inform management and treatment of the individual. Monahan (1981) reported that this system resulted in risk predictions that were less accurate than chance, followed by concerns that the criteria for clinical assessments were inconsistent and largely opinion based (Pfohl, 1978). Following these criticisms, the

9

field of forensic psychology refocused on identifying factors linked to the prediction of violent offending, leading to the first usable risk assessments (Conroy and Murrie, 2007). Researchers then started to develop predictively valid risk assessments as tools to inform the management and treatment of future violence risk, in place of oversimplified measures of 'dangerousness' (Singh et al., 2011). Currently there are a wide variety of risk assessments available to the forensic psychologist for use in the clinical setting (Douglas et al., 1999; Otto and Douglas, 2010) and the potential to apply these to HDAB is a current focus of the authors' research.

## 32.3.2 Forensic risk assessment

Forensic risk assessments can be constructed by identifying the relevant risk factors following appraisal of the literature pertaining to a specific group (e.g. adolescents or adults, men or women) and behaviour (e.g. violence, sexual offences, etc.). It is important to note here that risk factors do not have to be direct causes of the behaviour of concern, only associated with it. Therefore a group of factors that simply have a statistical relationship to behaviour of concern can still be used. A trained professional (the assessor) appraises each risk factor in turn when considering an individual's predisposition for the behaviour of interest, and the resulting information is amalgamated into an overall prediction of risk. Risk factors do not just serve to inform the prediction, but also highlight areas that could be addressed in the future management of the individual's behaviour.

Risk factors can be subdivided into categories based upon their nature and use in the risk assessment itself.

- *Static risk factors*, broadly speaking, are those that cannot realistically be changed. Demographic factors such as gender, social class and ethnicity are examples of static risk factors, as are historical factors such as previous behaviour and childhood experiences.
- *Dynamic factors* are those that at least have the potential to change. In the case of *stable dynamic factors*, this change might not be immediately or quickly achievable with change happening over time. One's attitudes, for example, can be particularly resistant to sudden change, but cannot be considered static. *Acute dynamic factors* are those that can be changed over a short period of time, for example drug use/intoxication or acute changes in mood (e.g., fear or anger).

The split between static and dynamic factors is particularly important when it comes to risk management. Stable risk factors provide the base rate of risk related to the individual, whereas the appraisal of dynamic risk factors can be used to formulate management strategies that are evidence-based and specific to the individual. The inclusion of dynamic factors also means that the same risk assessment process can be used to assess an individual's risk multiple times; meaning that changes in risk level can be monitored over time. The composition of risk factors in an assessment and the type of inferences that one can justifiably make from them differs dependent on the type of risk assessment used.

Forensic risk assessments are broadly categorised into two main types: actuarial risk assessments and structured professional judgement assessments:

- *Actuarial risk assessments* make predictions of future risk on the basis of existing evidence from individuals with similar risk levels/factors. Examples of actuarial assessments include the VRAG (Quinsey, Harris, Rice and Cormier, 1998) to predict violent and the Static-99 (Boer, Hart, Kropp and Webster, 1997) to predict sexual offending.
- *Structured professional judgement* (SPJ) systems on the other hand guide experienced clinicians to make a professional judgement structured by the current knowledge of risk prediction in that area. Examples of this would include the HCR-20 (Webster, Douglas, Eaves and Hart, 1997) for violence risk and the SVR-20 (Hanson and Thornton, 1999) for sexual offending risk.

These are summarised in Table 32.1.

**Table 32.1** Risk assessment types (table content is informed by Skeem and Monahan (2011)).

| Risk Assessment Type | Strengths | Limitations |
| --- | --- | --- |
| Structured Professional Judgement (SPJ) | Factors unique to the case and not included in the assessment can be considered. | The degree of certainty for a single individual risk prediction cannot be known. |
| Actuarial | Weighting of individual factors is left up to the assessors judgement. Prediction can be made with an identified level of accuracy about groups of individuals. | Cannot be used to monitor risk over time. Cannot be used to inform risk management strategies. |

The way in which risk factors are scored and amalgamated is entirely dependent upon the type of risk assessment being used (Monahan and Skeem, 2014).

Skeem and Monahan (2011) suggest that there is little difference between the two types in terms of predictive efficiency. However, there may be advantages to using one type of risk assessment over the other in certain situations.

It is anticipated that an SPJ-type risk assessment for use in predicting and managing HDAB in dogs would be the most appropriate type of tool. Due to the variety of owner–dog–environment groupings, this type of assessment can be flexible enough to allow the clinician to appraise unique factors that may not be identified in the risk assessment itself. The inclusion of both static and dynamic factors allows the assessment to be used to assess the risk associated with an individual animal in its current situation, as well as it to be responsive to changes such as medical and/or behavioural therapy, or other risk management practices. As such, an SPJ method allows for a more tailored approach to risk assessment and the greater inclusion of individual differences in the risk formulation.

## 32.4 Applying forensic risk assessment to the domestic dog

### 32.4.1 Defining behaviour

A critical problem in the area has been the failure to define clearly and accurately what constitutes human-directed aggressive behaviour (HDAB) in the dog (Chapter 1). Definitions and descriptions of varying terms (e.g. bites, aggression, injury) are not always provided, which has limited the extent to which it is possible to develop a clear evidence base in the HDAB area (Chapter 10, Newman, 2012, unpublished results).

Clear case definitions of HDAB are critical for the following reasons, they:

- Provide clarity for participants completing questionnaires
- Contribute to testable hypotheses and repeatable experiments, including comparison of survey findings between studies
- Facilitate scientific communication to the public and other interested parties
- Limit miscommunication in academic discussion
- Avoid ratifying sensationalised terms used by the media.

A clear and consistent definition of the behaviour of concern is a required first step for risk assessment development, as it drives the risk assessment question. In the case of a forensic risk assessment for dogs, that question could be, 'Will this dog be involved in an injurious bite to a human in the next twelve months?' This question can only be answered if the term 'injurious bite' is defined, so that the behaviour is measurable and we can evaluate the effectiveness of the prediction. In qualitative investigations into perceptions of aggressive behaviour in dogs (Orritt et al., 2015; Westgarth et al., 2015) researchers have found that participants have a wide variation in interpretation of aggression and severity of bites, often selecting words such as 'nip', 'maul', 'savage', 'rip', etc. to clarify the severity and intentionality of the behaviour. For this reason it is appropriate to provide a definition for 'bite' prior to collecting data from participants about dog behaviour, rather than assume that a consistent definition is held between participants. For example:

> **'Dog bite, Bite or Bit:** *in reference to injury caused by a dog's teeth to a human of any severity level, from bruises and scratches to puncture wounds and lacerations. This is inclusive of all circumstances and motivations. For example, accidental bites, warning bites, predatory bites, play bites and intentional bites would all be included as types of dog bite.' (Orritt et al., 2015, unpublished results)*

Notably this definition does not exclude bites that occur in the context of play, as in the instance from which this definition was taken the intention was to amass information on all types of injurious dog bite. Where contextual distinction is important, a different functional definition may be more appropriate, such as those indicated by questions to participants in a study by Messam et al. (2008).

## 32.4.2  A closer look at behaviour

In the prediction of violent offending, risk assessments are now able to be much more specific in the behaviour they predict. For example, specific and different assessments exist for predicting sexual offending and domestic violence, which are both subsets of general violent offending. This is achievable because of the existing level of knowledge and the relative maturity of each field of interest.

For a comprehensive risk assessment of human injury to be applied to dogs, the full range of human-directed aggressive behaviour would have to be covered. This should include everything from non-injurious through to serious injurious bites or even death. All instances should be accounted for by the assessment as possible precursors to and predictors of future HDAB. However, many forms of HDAB are difficult to quantify (e.g. attempted bite, 'nips', etc.), particularly when the owner conveys the information after the event. For validating a risk assessment it may be more useful to use a specific and measurable outcome, such as injurious bites, particularly in the initial development stages.

## 32.4.3 Evidence required

In order to identify risk factors for a predictive tool, sufficient evidence must be gathered so that the presence of each individual risk factor used in the assessment is well supported. The existing evidence for risk factors that are linked to different forms of HDAB is lacking in many key areas (Chapter 10 and Newman, 2012, unpublished results). For example, not all studies compare cases with a control sample of dogs that are not showing problematic HDAB in order to infer differences in risk; further even if this is attempted it is often not a truly appropriate control population. Additionally, the samples in many studies are unrepresentative of the wider population, particularly where samples are derived from veterinary presentations, hospital data or extreme groups (such as dog bite deaths). This has been discussed in detail in Chapter 10 and will not be repeated here.

In addition to lack of rigour, the investigation of HDAB risk factors is biased towards dog-specific factors, such as dog signalment (eg. breed, neuter status), and neglects to investigate the full range of dog and non-dog factors that could influence the presentation of HDAB. In order to provide a holistic picture, research should also investigate 'non-dog' risk factors, such as environmental and contextual factors as well as owner or family factors.

Finally, although behaviour science is often dismissive of data acquired through owner self-report, it is important to note that, in a risk assessment scenario, the majority of information will come directly from the owner. Therefore, what the owner considers to be a 'problem' in terms of HDAB is critically important. Studies should take steps to increase the reliability of owner self-report of dog behaviour in a number of ways, starting with the provision of clear definitions of the behaviours being studied. These definitions should be used in questionnaire studies, and open-ended questions should be included to gather richer information. Questionnaire design should be based on initial qualitative enquiries for clarity. For example, if an owner is asked to provide information regarding the severity of his or her dog's most injurious bite, it would be inappropriate to word answers using bite classifications from the Lackmann scale (Lackmann et al., 1992, Chapter 21), or from Dunbar's dog bite scale (Association of Pet Dog Trainers, n.d.), see also chapter 16. Bite classification descriptions from these scales are likely to be misunderstood and incorrectly interpreted by participants on account of the medical jargon used. Instead, a selection of jargon-free items based upon qualitative investigation of terminology clearly understood and interpreted by all using is more appropriate, to ensure that the participant then classifies the bite as accurately as possible.

## 32.4.4 Factors required

It is necessary to consider what it is that we are specifically trying to predict. Risk of harm, which in this case would be the severity of the bite should it occur (encapsulating the extent

9

**Table 32.2** Example Risk Factors (for illustrative purposes only).

| Example Risk Factor | Risk Factor Type | Considerations |
|---|---|---|
| Breed | Static | • Size relative to potential targets<br>• Exercise requirements |
| Fear | Stable dynamic | • Presence of fear/anxiety<br>• Fear related to humans (e.g. Stranger-directed)<br>• Typical response to fearful stimuli |
| Family Members | Static | • Presence of vulnerable humans in home (children/elderly/disabled)<br>• Consistency of treatment between family members |
| Training | Acute/Stable dynamic | • Punitive methods<br>• Reliability of recall |
| Home Security | Acute dynamic | • Security of garden parameter<br>• Security of house |

of the bite, length of recovery, potential scarring of the victim and psychological harm) is entirely different from risk of incidence (the probability that an injurious bite occurs, regardless of severity). Both types of risk are important and necessary, but different factors may inform one or the other, rather than both. For example, a dog with the jaw anatomy (Chapter 12), neck musculature and size conducive to an extensive bite injury may be associated with a high risk of severity of outcome, but may be no more likely to bite than a dog whose anatomy is less conducive to an extensive bite injury.

The published evidence available is currently insufficient to support the ultimate inclusion or exclusion of certain risk factors in a risk assessment format. However, we have attempted to explain how certain factors that could be linked to HDAB might be used (see Table 32.2) in light of the fact that risk factors do not have to be causal to the behaviour of interest to be included in a risk assessment. Please note that the examples given in the table do not represent a definitive list of risk factors for HDAB.

Dynamic factors might be used to manage the level of risk associated with an animal in a certain situation. For example, 'House and garden security', an example of an acute dynamic factor, could be targeted as part of a risk management strategy. If a dog–owner pairing were initially given a high score for this factor (indicating that the dog could leave the property at will) improvement in this area would have obvious risk management benefits. On the other hand 'Training methods used' could be an example of a stable dynamic factor; for example if the owner believes that a dog should be verbally or physically punished as part of training, or he/she may be reluctant to modify their practices. The static factor 'dog breed' cannot be changed as part of a risk management strategy, but can inform the level of risk associated with a dog in a certain situation. It is up to the assessor to work through the considerations of each factor. Rather than just giving a score, each dynamic factor should be considered in the development of management and prevention strategies.

## 32.4.5 The end product

The final risk assessment could be used in a variety of different contexts where assessment of the HDAB risk associated with a specific dog, in a certain situation, was required (see

**Table 32.3** Possible uses of SPJ tool.

| User Group | Problem Presentation | Use of the SPJ tool |
|---|---|---|
| Veterinarian | A dog presents at a veterinary surgery after a display of HDAB. | The veterinary surgeon needs to quickly and accurately assess the immediate risk in order to discern the appropriate course of action in the limited time frame of a veterinary consult. |
| Rescue Shelter Staff | A rescue centre or shelter is considering rehoming a dog with uncertain history to a family. | The rescue centre staff need to select the most appropriate family and environment for the dog, therefore minimising the risk over a longer period of time. |
| Animal Behaviourist | A behaviourist wants to construct a risk management protocol for a dog that is frightened of strangers. | The behaviourist needs to identify the areas that will offer the most scope for positive change, and may need to repeat the assessment at a later date to see if the strategies used have affected actual risk. |
| Expert Witness | An expert witness is required to assess the risk of a dog that has previously bitten, should it be returned to live with its owner. | The expert witness needs to predict with a high level of accuracy the likelihood of a repeated bite incident. |

Table 32.3). Therefore, flexibility of use is one of the most important features of a structured professional judgement (SPJ) risk assessment relating to dogs.

The risk assessment, in all of these scenarios, maintains its flexibility of use by structuring, rather than dictating, the assessor's judgement. To ensure that this structure is a significant improvement on current practice, a range of tests are required to confirm validity and reliability over time.

Predictive validity is the most obvious validation test that would be required after the development of a risk assessment prototype. It is essential to approximate the degree of accuracy to which judgements can be made using the assessment, and the time frame over which these judgements retain their accuracy. Further to this, inter-rater reliability tests, in which different assessors score the same case, would be required to check that assessment outcomes are consistent between assessors, who may vary in terms of attitudes, experience and education. Providing training and a manual to assist scoring of items maximises inter-rater reliability, by highlighting the ways in which individual items affect risk.

In the same way that the validity of the assessment must be discerned, so too must the efficacy of complementary training, including manual information. This would need to be investigated both in the immediate sense, to discern improvement to predictive validity and inter-rater reliability, and in the long term, to assess if trained individuals use the risk assessment consistently over time.

Only when the validity of the risk assessment tool and its associated training has been confirmed should it be used on a wider scale, to inform risk prediction and risk management of dogs.

## 32.5 Conclusion

A forensic risk assessment tool for the prediction and management of HDAB in dogs has the potential to reduce dog bite incidence and other consequences of this behaviour. This can be achieved if the development of the risk assessment is:

1. Based on appraisal of high quality evidence
2. Clearly defines the terms and parameters of the behaviours of interest
3. Includes both static and dynamic factors that cover a broad range of dog, owner and environment variables
4. Is subject to rigorous testing before its common use.

Crucially, the risk assessment should be used to address behaviour resulting in all bite severities, rather than selectively focusing on severe or fatal bites. Ultimately, the development of a forensically informed risk assessment represents a conceptual change away from the reliance on unstructured expert opinion and towards accurate and consistent predictions resulting from the structured judgement of trained professionals, working from the same protocols.

## 32.6 References

Association of Pet Dog Trainers (n.d.) Dr. Ian Dunbar's Dog Bite Scale. Available at: www.dogtalk. com/BiteAssessmentScalesDunbarDTMRoss.pdf (Accessed 12 September 2015).

Barnard, S., Siracusa, C., Reisner, I. Valsecchi, P., Serpell, J. A. (2012). Validity of model devices used to assess canine temperament in behavioral tests. *Applied Animal Behaviour Science* 138, 79–87.

Boer, D. P., Hart, S. D., Kropp, P. R., Webster, C. D. (1997). Manual for the Sexual Violence Risk-20. Professional guidelines for assessing risk of sexual violence. Burnaby, B. C.: Simon Fraser University, Mental Health, Law, and Policy Institute.

Casey, R. A., Loftus, B., Bolster, C., Richards, G. J., Blackwell, E. J. (2014). Human directed aggression in domestic dogs (Canis familiaris): Occurrence in different contexts and risk factors. *Applied Animal Behaviour Science* 152, 52–63.

Conroy, M. A., Murrie, D. C. (2007). Historical overview of risk assessment. In Forensic assessment of violence risk: A guide for risk assessment and risk management. John Wiley & Sons, Hoboken, New Jersey, pp.6–8.

Cornelissen, J. M. R., Hopster, H. (2010). Dog bites in The Netherlands: A study of victims, injuries, circumstances and aggressors to support evaluation of breed specific legislation. *Veterinary Journal* 186, 292–298.

Corridan, C., Gaultier, E., Pereira, G. D. G., De Keuster, T., De Meester, R., Mills, D., Leyvraz, A. M., Shoening, B. (2011). ESVCE position statement on risk assessment European Society of Veterinary Clinical Ethology.

Dorey, P. (2005). *Policy Making in Britain: An Introduction*, 1st edn. London: Sage, London, UK.

Douglas, K. S., Cox, D. N., Webster, C. D. (1999). Violence risk assessment: Science and practice. *Legal and Criminal Psychology* 4, 149–184.

Hanson, R. K., Thornton, D. (1999). Static-99: Improving actuarial risk assessments for sex offenders (User Report 99–02).Ottawa, ON: Department of the Solicitor General of Canada.

Kahn, A. Robert, E., Piette, D., De Keuster, T., Lamoureux, J., Leveque, A. (2004) Prevalence of dog bites in children: a telephone survey. *European Journal of Pediatrics* 163, 424.

Lackmann, G. M. Draf, W., Isselstein, G., Tollner, U. (1992). Surgical treatment of facial dog bite injuries in children. *Journal of Cranio-Maxillo-Facial Surgery* 20, 81–86.

Meints, K., De Keuster, T., Butcher, R. (2010). How to prevent dog bite injuries? The Blue Dog. In *IP Safety*. pp.171–172.

Messam, L. L. M., Kass, P. H., Chomel, B. B., Hart, L. A. (2008). The human–canine environment: a risk factor for non-play bites? *The Veterinary Journal* 177, 205–215.

Monahan, J. (1981). The clinical prediction of violent behaviour. Aggressive behavior 8, 85–86.

Monahan, J. and Skeem, J. L. (2014). The evolution of violence risk assessment. *CNS Spectrums* 19, 419–424.

National Canine Research Council (2013). Breed-Specific Legislation (BSL) FAQs. Available at: http://nationalcanineresearchcouncil.com/dog-legislation/breed-specific-legislation-bsl-faq/ (Accessed 12 September 2015).

Newman, J. (2012). Human-directed dog aggression; A systematic review. MPhil thesis. University of Liverpool, Liverpool, UK.

One Health (n.d.). Mission Statement. Available at: www.onehealthinitiative.com/mission.php (Accessed 12 September 2015).

Orritt, R., Gross, H., Hogue, T. E. (2015). His bark is worse than his bite: Perceptions and rationalization of canine aggressive behaviour. *Human-Animal Interaction Bulletin* (in press).

Orritt, R., Harper, C. (2015). Similarities Between the Representation of 'Aggressive Dogs' and 'Sex Offenders' in the British News Media. In: Blanco, C., Deering, B. (eds.) *Who's Talking Now? Multispecies relations from human and animals' points of view*. Inter-disciplinary Press, Oxford, UK, pp.245–248.

Otto, R. K., Douglas, K. S. (2010). Historical-clinical-risk management-20 (hcr-20) violence risk assessment scheme: Rationale, application, and empirical overview. In: Roesch, R., Hart, S. (eds.) *Handbook of Violence Risk Assessment*. Routledge, New York City, New York, pp.153–155.

Pavlov, I. (1927). *Conditioned Reflexes*. Oxford: Oxford University Press, Oxford, UK.

Pfohl, S. (1978). *Predicting Dangerousness*, Lexington Books, New York City, New York.

Planta, J. U. D., De Meester, R. H. W. M. (2007). Validity of the Socially Acceptable Behavior (SAB) test as a measure of aggression in dogs towards non-familiar humans. *Vlaams Diergeneeskundig Tijdschrift* 76, 359–368.

Quinsey, V. L., Harris, G. T., Rice, M. E., Cormier, C. A. (1998). Violent offenders: Appraising and managing risk. Washington, DC: American Psychological Association.

Schalke, E., Ott, S. A., Von Gaertner, A. M., Hackbarth, H., Mittmann, A. (2008) Is breed-specific legislation justified? Study of the results of the temperament test of Lower Saxony. *Journal of Veterinary Behavior: Clinical Applications and Research* 3, 97–103.

Singh, J. P., Grann, M., Fazel, S. (2011). A comparative study of violence risk assessment tools: a systematic review and metaregression analysis of 68 studies involving 25,980 participants. *Clinical Psychology Review* 31, 499–513.

Skeem, J. L., Monahan, J. (2011). Current Directions in Violence Risk Assessment. Current Directions in Psychological Science 20, 38–42.

Skinner, B. F. (1974). About Behaviourism. Random House Inc., New York City, New York.

Taylor, K. D., Mills, D. S. (2006.) The development and assessment of temperament tests for adult companion dogs. Journal of Veterinary Behavior: Clinical Applications and Research 1, 94–108.

Webster, C. D., Douglas, K. S., Eaves, D., Hart, S. D. (1997). HCR-20: Assessing risk for violence (version 2). Burnaby, BC: Simon Fraser University, Mental Health, Law, and Policy Institute.

# Dog Bites – a Multidisciplinary Perspective

*Carri Westgarth and Daniel Mills*

It should be clear from the chapters of this book that the subject of dog bites is an important area of academic study for many different disciplines, and that we need these different disciplines to work with each other to improve our knowledge base and generate solutions on how to best prevent and manage dog bites. In this sense, the issue of dog bites is not just a multidisciplinary challenge (i.e. one requiring different disciplines to examine the problem) but also a transdisciplinary one (i.e. one that extends across traditional boundaries). Contrary to the views often presented by individual experts, we still do not know how to prevent dog bites. There are large gaps in our understanding of the contexts in which bites occur, factors that increase or decrease the risk, and truly effective things we can do to prevent them. However, that does not mean that solutions are simply a matter of opinion or personal preference. Clearly some beliefs are better evidenced than others and some carry more risk if they are wrong. Both of these need to be considered before making practical recommendations. We must also make sure we do not confuse a lack of evidence of importance of a particular factor with evidence of a lack of importance of a particular factor. Science does not deal with absolutes and knowledge reflects our best understanding at a given time. In the face of scientific uncertainty, pragmatic answers do not necessarily lie in the areas that are best researched, but in those that are well grounded theoretically and carry least risk for the potential benefit they bring. At the same time we must not be complacent and be satisfied with the status quo. We hope this book, by highlighting the many deficiencies in our understanding, will inspire rather than demoralise. Inspire people to come together to better address these challenges, helping in any way they can to further this important subject.

The problems arising from what we do not know begin with our understanding of, and agreement on, what a dog bite actually is. Without agreement on a case definition, we cannot design studies to test risk factors or prevention methods. For example, if a dog is playing and 'accidentally' bruises or punctures skin, is this a dog bite? It may require medical treatment, but the cause of the bite would require vastly different prevention methods than a bite in a different context such as fear. Dog bites are a heterogeneous phenomenon, and so cannot be understood as a single entity or statistical outcome. We need to ask ourselves,

9

what exactly are we seeking to manage and prevent? We must avoid oversimplification or overgeneralisation, rather we must be specific and define what we mean in any given context.

Despite the ubiquity of quoted statistics, it is also pertinent to note that we do not know how common dog bites are. Even with a case definition, we have little comprehension of the scale of the problem beyond what is recorded in hospital admission data (or possibly emergency room attendance) and we know this to be a poor metric with population bias. Many bites do not contribute to these statistics, but they still have the potential to impact on both individual and societal well-being. However, to what extent and in what way we do not know. Indeed, it might even be that exposure to a mild risk in one context is protective of a more serious bite in another. Without relevant data, we simply do not know. We also need to investigate the proportion of bites that occur in different contexts. Although many epidemiological studies have been performed to analyse for risk factors for dog bites, these studies are usually not robust enough to tell us much. Even where studies are robust and comparable, their findings may contradict due to unrecognised confounders. This is not actually surprising considering the multitude of different situations and possible 'reasons' as to why a dog bite event may present. Rather than thinking that dog bites have simple 'causes', we must recognise that they arise from the interplay between complex series of events relating to the history of both the dog and victim, together with the immediate preceding circumstances. No single aspect is the 'cause' that needs to be addressed to change the outcome. To believe this is to overlook the risk as we have seen from single issue initiatives, e.g. breed-specific legislation that assumes certain types of dog are the main problem). Thus, when we have contradictory results we should not dismiss them but rather seek to understand them better and the apparent contradiction. This is no easy task.

It seems that current prevention initiatives focus largely on educational interventions aimed at increasing people's knowledge of dog signalling and appropriate responses to this. There is a widespread belief that the key to bite prevention is helping people to understand the signs that a dog is unhappy and may bite. However, it is clear that this deficit is not simply due to lack of information or knowledge, and addressing this problem is not simply a matter of providing information. Even 'experts' in dog behaviour get bitten. The message needs to be communicated effectively, i.e. in a way that allows the learner to assimilate the information in a meaningful way that brings about not just increased knowledge but also behaviour change. Unfortunately this issue is further confounded by our lack of knowledge of dog communication, which is largely based on expert belief and anecdote rather than rigorous scientific observation. We require further experimental observational core research into dog communication. If we are to design educational initiatives based on understanding dog emotion and behaviour, we first need a comprehensive understanding of what dogs are really telling us. In addition, even if we accept that people often lack some of the skills required for interpreting dog behaviour, we do not know that this is why bites happen. The human inclination to blame the victim for behaving in a way to cause their own demise is deep rooted and may be misleading. In essence, when it comes to prevention we need to be able to not only identify what needs to be learnt or put in place, but also how to deliver any messages and the most effective intervention point. These are all important gaps in our knowledge.

As the chapters contained within this book demonstrate, there is much myth and popularist construction of the scale, nature and solution to the problem circulating within modern day society. The conviction with which these beliefs are held must not be confused with the evidence that supports them. Stigmatised 'banned' breeds, and blame directed at the 'otherness' of 'irresponsible' owners is ingrained into legislation widely deemed ineffective by many, and even scientifically unsound. However, there is clear evidence that the propensity for a dog to bite does have an inherited component. This does not mean that it transcends environmental effects to allow simple stereotypes. Nonetheless, there are simple measures that can be undertaken to help to reduce the risk from the pet dog, who is so often the source of a bite. This begins with choosing the right dog as a pet in the first place. Unfortunately, many owners select a puppy based on inappropriate criteria and without meeting the mother or appreciating her temperament, let alone that of the sire.

If we are to learn from the problems of the past, we need to agree on the systematic process for investigation and collection of data relating to at least all fatal and serious dog bites requiring medical treatment. Gold standard protocols to shape this investigation are outlined clearly within this book, and we hope their publication here will serve to improve the quality of evidence and data in future. The primary piece of evidence required in such situations is the dog itself and its behaviour, however it is extremely rare for a dog to be detained for investigative purposes. Too often they are euthanised at the scene or shortly after, precluding the gathering of potentially important data from which we can learn and inform future prevention strategies. A cultural shift is required towards retention of dogs until a thorough behavioural examination has been made; it can then be euthanised afterwards if necessary. This would require funding to cover kennelling care, although it need only be temporary. A register of willing and suitably qualified animal behaviour experts able to undertake the necessary evaluations is also required. Our own experience indicates that many meeting this requirement would volunteer their services at minimal cost in order to further our knowledge of this most important topic. Although dog behavioural experts are integral to any investigation surrounding the risk of dog bites, this book emphasises that a multidisciplinary team is required to thoroughly investigate, understand and manage the issues pertaining to dog bites. Human perceptions, beliefs and behaviours regarding dogs and the issue of risk perception are key areas that have only just begun to receive specific investigation by social science and public health experts. In addition, as outlined in this book, experts in animal law, forensics and medical treatment also have much to offer the field. Key to the furtherance of knowledge on dog bite prevention is collaboration between these diverse disciplinary fields.

It is also clear that there is a need for research of a higher standard in terms of contribution of evidence. In particular, where suitable, there now needs to be a move towards well-designed randomised controlled trials and cohort studies of both risk factors and the efficacy of potential prevention strategies. To achieve this requires greater investment regarding resources (both time and cost). Pooling of resources towards larger, comprehensive projects is one way to achieve this. Project leadership by epidemiologists and public health experts will also facilitate the best value study design to provide robust evidence.

The dog bite issue has often been conceived as a 'dog-related problem' rather than 'another injury prevention scenario'. Prevention strategies will benefit greatly from input from injury prevention and public health experts, applying proven methods and techniques lent from other effective preventative strategies. It is also paramount that any well-meaning prevention initiatives, whether educational or legislative, are thoroughly tested for efficacy. It is only then that they can be hailed as a success and applied more widely. However well-intended, there is considerable duplication of efforts regarding educational programmes. This means duplication of resources spent designing, promoting and delivering them, along with the potential for mixed messages being given to the public. Collaborative working between stakeholders should be fostered to streamline this.

Clearly there is much still to do, but through the creation of this text we hope we have offered a point of reference not just to the problems but also the solutions to this issue. By bringing together experts from such diverse fields, we hope that all can gain a deeper appreciation of the nature of the challenges we face and the most professional way to operate, whatever our specialism or interest.

# INDEX